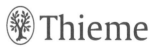

Synopsis of Hip Surgery

Shane J. Nho, MD, MS
Associate Professor
Head, Section of Young Adult Hip Surgery
Co-Director, Division of Sports Medicine
Department of Orthopedic Surgery
Rush Medical College of Rush University
Rush University Medical Center
Chicago, Illinois, USA

Joshua D. Harris, MD
Associate Professor
Houston Methodist Institute of Academic Medicine
Houston Methodist Department of Orthopedics & Sports Medicine Outpatient Center;
Adjunct Assistant Professor
Texas A&M University
Houston, Texas;
Associate Professor
Weill Cornell Medical College
New York City, New York, USA

Brett R. Levine, MD, MS
Associate Professor
Department of Orthopedic Surgery
Rush University Medical Center
Chicago, Illinois;
Service Line Director
Elmhurst Memorial Hospital
Elmhurst, Illinois, USA

236 illustrations

Thieme
New York • Stuttgart • Delhi • Rio de Janeiro

Library of Congress Cataloging-in-Publication Data is available with the publisher.

Important note: Medicine is an ever-changing science undergoing continual development. Research and clinical experience are continually expanding our knowledge, in particular our knowledge of proper treatment and drug therapy. Insofar as this book mentions any dosage or application, readers may rest assured that the authors, editors, and publishers have made every effort to ensure that such references are in accordance with **the state of knowledge at the time of production of the book.**

Nevertheless, this does not involve, imply, or express any guarantee or responsibility on the part of the publishers in respect to any dosage instructions and forms of applications stated in the book. **Every user is requested to examine carefully** the manufacturers' leaflets accompanying each drug and to check, if necessary in consultation with a physician or specialist, whether the dosage schedules mentioned therein or the contraindications stated by the manufacturers differ from the statements made in the present book. Such examination is particularly important with drugs that are either rarely used or have been newly released on the market. Every dosage schedule or every form of application used is entirely at the user's own risk and responsibility. The authors and publishers request every user to report to the publishers any discrepancies or inaccuracies noticed. If errors in this work are found after publication, errata will be posted at www.thieme.com on the product description page.

Some of the product names, patents, and registered designs referred to in this book are in fact registered trademarks or proprietary names even though specific reference to this fact is not always made in the text. Therefore, the appearance of a name without designation as proprietary is not to be construed as a representation by the publisher that it is in the public domain.

Thieme Publishers New York
333 Seventh Avenue, New York, NY 10001, USA
+1-800-782-3488, customerservice@thieme.com

Georg Thieme Verlag KG
Rüdigerstrasse 14, 70469 Stuttgart, Germany
+49 [0]711 8931 421, customerservice@thieme.de

Thieme Publishers Delhi
A-12, Second Floor, Sector-2, Noida-201301
Uttar Pradesh, India
+91 120 45 566 00, customerservice@thieme.in

Thieme Publishers Rio
Thieme Publicações Ltda.
Edifício Rodolpho de Paoli, 25° andar
Av. Nilo Peçanha, 50 – Sala 2508
Rio de Janeiro 20020-906 Brasil
+55 21 3172 2297

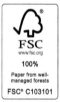

FSC
www.fsc.org
100%
Paper from well-managed forests
FSC® C103101

Cover design: Thieme Publishing Group
Typesetting by Thomson Digital, India
Printed in the United States of America by King Printing Co., Inc.
ISBN 978-1-62623-524-3

Also available as an e-book:
eISBN 978-1-62623-525-0

To my family, for their endless support and sacrifice. Thank you, Sloane, Connor, and Charlie, for your love and encouragement!

Shane J. Nho, MD, MS

I would like to dedicate this book to Lisa, whose grit, passion, beauty, intelligence, and wit have inspired me for years. I would also like to thank Cinnamon and Totoro and their never-ending loyalty, joy, and love. Finally, I must acknowledge my father and mother, whose absolute dedication, leadership, and devotion have made me everything I am today.

Joshua D. Harris, MD

I would like to dedicate this book to my wife, Kari, for sticking with me through all of the years of studying, training, and working. Without her love and support, I would not be in the position that I am in today. In addition, I want to thank my kids, Kylie and AJ, for keeping me honest and up to date with the current times. I would also like to acknowledge my mentors at all levels (undergraduate through fellowship), as without their "tough love" approach to teaching I would not have this opportunity to contribute to my profession. Lastly, I would like to dedicate this book to my late father, Nathan, who inspired me to be the person I am today.

Brett R. Levine, MD, MS

Contents

Section II

Preface

The evaluation and management of patients with hip pain has undergone enormous growth in recent times. Our understanding of both arthritic and nonarthritic conditions has led to meaningful improvements for the care of individuals with both acute traumatic and chronic ailments. International collaborations have developed multiple agreements and guidelines that help clinicians assimilate patient symptoms and physical examination findings with imaging. Short- and midterm outcomes of both surgical and nonsurgical treatment of nonarthritic hip conditions continue to expand the evidence base for hip preservation. Advanced imaging techniques and longer follow-up will determine if our treatments stand the test of time and truly preserve the joint with high-quality prospective registries and randomized trials. Long-term published outcomes of hip arthroplasty confirm high degrees of success and satisfaction, with considerable benefits bestowed upon the patient and society.

Reinhold Ganz and his team have contributed immensely to the field of hip preservation surgery, both open and arthroscopic techniques. Their efforts paved the way for understanding the effects of morphological abnormalities on hip degeneration. Their seminal work on femoroacetabular impingement and dysplasia predominates the literature and forms the basis for current and future research in hip preservation. Open procedures, including surgical dislocation and periacetabular osteotomy, have demonstrated consistent high reliability for excellent, durable subjective and objective outcomes. Arthroscopic and endoscopic procedures have revolutionized the surgical treatment of nearly all hip conditions. These minimally invasive approaches have shown outcomes as good, and in some cases better, as open approaches in the management of intra-articular chondrolabral and osseous pathology and extra-articular peritrochanteric and deep gluteal space problems.

Hip arthroplasty outcomes continue to demonstrate the highest levels of success within all of orthopedic surgery and musculoskeletal medicine. Improved understanding of surgical techniques and enormous progress in technology have truly refined the art and science of the procedure to the highest level. As our active population has generated a group of very young individuals with advanced hip disease undergoing arthroplasty, patients are returning to active, healthy lifestyles and continuing to be contributing members to society. Improved evidence on managing revision arthroplasty has led to durable, excellent outcomes even in these challenging multifactorial clinical scenarios.

It is with utmost excitement and optimism that we, the editors of *Synopsis of Hip Surgery*, present this text. Our students, residents, fellows, surgeons, physicians, researchers, therapists and, most importantly, our patients, will find this book to be a terrific resource for quick acquisition of knowledge on everything related to the hip. We are truly indebted to the authors of all the chapters in this book, whose efforts made this vast work possible.

Shane J. Nho, MD, MS
Joshua D. Harris, MD
Brett R. Levine, MD, MS

Acknowledgments

I want to acknowledge several individuals who helped me with not only this text but in my development as a clinician–scientist hip surgeon. First, I must recognize Lisa, my better half, an incredible surgeon herself, for her love, humor, patience, encouragement, support, guidance, and teaching. Cinnamon and Totoro, our pups, embody love, laughter, and joy. Every day with them is a blessing. My parents, Jeff and Glenola, are the basis of my passion, work ethic, respect, and integrity in my professional and personal life. Finally, all my mentors, the exemplary role models, whom I have looked up to throughout my training and practice: Nina Wilson, Tom Williams, Dave Flanigan, Bernie Bach, Brian Cole, and especially my co-editor, Shane J. Nho. In and out of the classroom, clinic, laboratory, and operating room, the value of their insight and instruction, critique and commentary, and advice and mentorship is immeasurable.

Joshua D. Harris, MD

Contributors

Hassan Alosh, MD
Orthopedic Surgeon
Hip and Knee Arthroplasty
Centers for Advanced Orthopedics
Washington, DC, USA

Edward C. Beck, MD, MPH
Physician Scientist
Department of Orthopedic Surgery
Wake Forest Baptist Health
Winston-Salem, North Carolina, USA

Joshua Alan Bell, MD
Orthopedic Surgeon
Division of Adult Reconstruction
Department of Orthopedic Surgery
OrthoAtlanta
Atlanta, Georgia, USA

Ian Clapp, MS
Research Fellow
Section of Young Adult Hip Surgery
Division of Sports Medicine
Department of Orthopedic Surgery
Rush University Medical Center
Chicago, Illinois, USA

Matthew Colman, MD
Assistant Professor
Division of Orthopedic Oncology and Spine,
   Back, and Neck
Department of Orthopedic Surgery
Rush University Medical Center
Chicago, Illinois, USA

Brian M. Culp, MD
Orthopedic Surgeon
Department of Orthopedic Surgery
Princeton Orthopedic Associates
Princeton, New Jersey, USA

Gift Echefu, MD
Resident
Section of Young Adult Hip Surgery
Division of Sports Medicine
Department of Orthopedic Surgery
Rush University Medical Center
Chicago, Illinois, USA

Yale A. Fillingham, MD
Assistant Professor
Division of Adult Reconstruction
Department of Orthopedic Surgery
Dartmouth Hitchcock Medical Center
Lebanon, New Hampshire, USA

Michael A. Flierl, MD, FAAOS
Michigan Orthopedic Surgeons
Assistant Professor
Department of Orthopedic Surgery
Oakland University/William Beaumont
Royal Oak, Michigan, USA

Joshua D. Harris, MD
Associate Professor
Houston Methodist Institute of Academic
   Medicine
Houston Methodist Department of
   Orthopedics & Sports Medicine
Outpatient Center
Adjunct Assistant Professor
Texas A&M University
Houston, Texas;
Associate Professor
Weill Cornell Medical College
New York City, New York, USA

Robert A. Jack II, MD
Orthopedic Surgery Resident
Department of Orthopedic Surgery
Houston Methodist Orthopedics and Sports
   Medicine
Houston, Texas, USA

Kyleen Jan, BS
Medical Student
Section of Young Adult Hip Surgery
Division of Sports Medicine
Department of Orthopedic Surgery
Rush University Medical Center
Chicago, Illinois, USA

Jahanzeb Kalkaus, MD
Resident
Department of Surgery
University of Louisville Hospital
Louisville, Kentucky, USA

David J. Kaufman, MD
Orthopedic Surgeon
Division of Adult Reconstruction
Department of Orthopedic Surgery
Northwestern Lakeforest Hospital
Northwestern Feinberg School of Medicine
Chicago, Illinois, USA

Matthew Knedel, MD
Orthopedic Surgeon
Saint Agnes Care Orthopedic Institute
Fresno, California, USA

Robert C. Kollmorgen, DO
Assistant Professor
Fresno Department of Orthopedic Surgery
Hip Preservation
University of California, San Francisco
Fresno, California, USA

Kyle Kunze, MD
Orthopedic Surgery Resident
Department of Orthopedic Surgery
Hospital for Special Surgery
New York City, New York, USA

Brett R. Levine, MD, MS
Associate Professor
Rush University Medical Center
Chicago, Illinois;
Service Line Director
Elmhurst Memorial Hospital
Elmhurst, Illinois, USA

Brian D. Lewis, MD
Assistant Professor
Hip Preservation Surgery
Duke Orthopedic Surgery
Durham, North Carolina, USA

Carlos J. Meheux, MD
Orthopedic Surgeon
Kelsey-Seybold Clinic
Houston, Texas, USA

Kamran Movassaghi, MD, MS
Resident
Department of Orthopedic Surgery
University of California San Francisco
Fresno, USA

William H. Neal, MD
Orthopedic Surgery Resident
Department of Orthopedic Surgery
NYU Langone Health
New York city, New York, USA

Shane J. Nho, MD, MS
Associate Professor
Head, Section of Young Adult Hip Surgery
Co-Director, Division of Sports Medicine
Department of Orthopedic Surgery
Rush Medical College of Rush University
Rush University Medical Center
Chicago, Illinois, USA

Alexander Newhouse, BS
Research Assistant
Section of Young Adult Hip Surgery
Division of Sports Medicine
Department of Orthopedic Surgery
Rush University Medical Center
Chicago, Illinois, USA

Luis F. Pulido-Sierra, MD
Assistant Professor
University of Florida
Gainesville, Florida, USA

Roshan P. Shah, MD, JD
Assistant Professor
Division of Adult Reconstruction
Department of Orthopedic Surgery
Columbia University
New York City, New York, USA

Robert Axel Sershon, MD
Orthopedic Surgeon
Hip and Knee Arthroplasty
Anderson Orthopedic Research Institute
Alexandria, Virginia, USA

Matthew W. Tetreault, MD
Attending Surgeon
Orthopedic Surgery
Albany Medical Center
Capital Region Orthopedics
Albany, New York City, New York, USA

Brian R. Waterman, MD
Associate Professor
Sports Medicine
Department of Orthopedic Surgery;
Fellowship Director
Orthopedic Sports Medicine and Shoulder
  Surgery;
Team Physician
Wake Forest University Athletics
Wake Forest University School of Medicine
Winston-Salem, North Carolina, USA

Section I

1 Anatomy of the Hip and Surgical Approaches

Brian R. Waterman, Edward C. Beck, Gift Echefu, Ian Clapp, William H. Neal, Shane J. Nho

Basic Anatomy of the Hip and Pelvis

Femur

I. The femur bone is a near-cylindrical long bone with high cortical bone density, separated from each other by the breadth of the pelvis. The anterior femoral bow is angled medially for relative valgus alignment. There is a gender difference in pelvic breadth, with it being wider in females.

II. It is divided into the body and two extremities, upper and lower (**Fig. 1.1**).

    A. The upper extremity consists of the head, neck, and greater and lesser trochanter:

        1. The head:

            a. It is globular, convex, and hemispheric. It is superiorly, medially, and slightly anterior directed.

            b. It has a smooth, articular surface covered in hyaline cartilage normally.

            c. The fovea capitis is a small, concave, depression within the medial side of the head, directed superior to posteroinferiorly. It is deficient in articular cartilage and provides attachment for the ligamentum teres: the acetabular branch of the obturator artery runs within and disruption results in avascular necrosis of the head.

        2. Neck:

            a. The neck is relatively flat and pyramidal. It connects the head to the shaft of the femur.

            b. It is flattened anterior to posterior, constricted in the middle, and broadens from medial to lateral.

            c. The anterior surface is perforated by numerous vascular foramina. Along the junction of the anterior surface with the head is a shallow groove. It is prominent in the elderly and provides attachment to orbicular fibers of the hip joint capsule.

            d. The inferior border, long and narrow, curves slightly posteriorly and ends at the lesser trochanter.

            e. The angle of inclination is formed by intersection of a line drawn along the shaft of the femur and a line drawn down the neck of the femur. It is widest in infancy and decreases with age. The normal angle is between 120 degrees and 125 degrees. It shows height and gender variability: less in shorter individuals and right angle in females than in males. Angle greater than 125 degrees results in coxa valga, and decreased angle results in coxa vara.

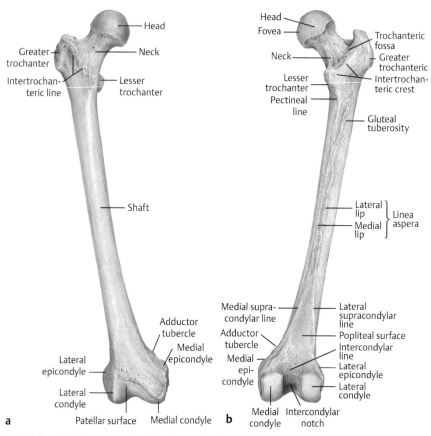

Fig. 1.1 The right femur: anterior (**a**) and posterior (**b**) views. (Source: Schuenke M, Schulte E, Schumacher U. Thieme Atlas of Anatomy. General Anatomy and Musculoskeletal System. 2nd edition, ©2014, Thieme Publishers, New York. Illustrations by Voll M and Wesker K.)

3. The trochanter is divided into lesser and greater trochanters; they are connected by the intertrochanteric line.

    a. The lesser trochanter is a conical eminence. From its apex, three borders extend: medial, lateral, and inferior. The inferior border is continuous with the middle division of the linea aspera. The apex provides attachment to the psoas major muscle.

    b. The greater trochanter is a large, irregular, quadrilateral eminence. It is located at the junction of the neck with the upper part of the body. It has two surfaces (medial and lateral surfaces) and four borders (superior, inferior, anterior, and posterior borders).

B. Lower extremity:

    1. The distal end of the femur is cuboid and has a greater transverse diameter than the anteroposterior diameter. It is prominent on both sides as the medial and lateral condyles, separated by the intercondylar fossa.

    2. Inferior to the lateral condyle is an oblique groove that provides attachment to the popliteus muscles.

C. Body:

    1. The body of the femur is cylindrical, broader superiorly, flattens, and narrows downward. It is convex anteriorly and concave posteriorly. The prominent longitudinal ridge, linea aspera, lies posteriorly.

    2. It has three borders (posterior, lateral, and medial) and three surfaces, separated by the borders.

    3. The linea aspera is a crest on the posterior aspect of the femur. It is composed of the medial and lateral lips, and an intermediate line. The lateral ridge extends upward from the lateral lip to the base of the greater trochanter, forming the gluteal tuberosity and providing attachment to the gluteus maximus. The intermediate ridge extends upward as the pectineal line toward the base of the lesser trochanter, providing attachment to the pectineus muscle.

    4. The lateral border runs from the greater trochanter to the anterior extremity of the lateral condyle. The medial border runs from the intertrochanteric line to the anterior extremity of the medial condyle.

    5. The anterior surface is situated between the lateral and medial borders. it is smooth, convex, broader superiorly and inferiorly with a narrow center. It provides attachment for the vastus intermedius.

    6. The lateral surface is the portion between the lateral border and the linea aspera. The superior three-fourths provide attachment for the vastus intermedius.

    7. The medial surface includes the area between the medial border and the linea aspera; it provides attachment for the vastus medialis.

Pelvis and Acetabulum

Fig. 1.2 shows a three-dimensional reconstruction of the hip.

I. The pelvis is formed by the bones of the ilium, ischium, and pubis. It is a large and flat bone.

II. Ossification is from three primary centers for the ilium, ischium, and pubis.

III. The primary centers fuse by age 13 to 14 at a **Y**-shaped triradiate cartilage at the center of the acetabulum.[1]

IV. The right and left hemipelvis articulate with each other anteriorly at the pubic symphysis and posteriorly at the sacral ala to form the sacroiliac joint.

V. The pelvis offers the primary connection between the axial skeleton and the bones of the lower limb, forming a bridge for structures passing from the axial skeleton to the lower limb.

VI. Bones of the hip offer stability and attachment for soft tissues.

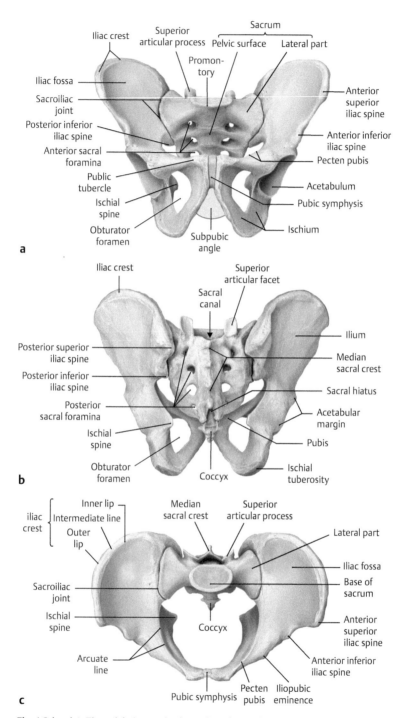

Fig. 1.2 (a–c) 1. The pelvis (example shown here is male). (Source: Schuenke M, Schulte E, Schumacher U. Thieme Atlas of Anatomy. General Anatomy and Musculoskeletal system. 2nd edition, ©2014, Thieme Publishers, New York. Illustrations by Voll M and Wesker K.)

Ilium

I. The ilium is the widest and the largest of the three parts of the hemipelvis.

II. It is divided into the ala and the body, which are separated by the arcuate line anteriorly and the acetabular margin externally.

III. Ala:

    A. The ilium expands superiorly to form the ala:

        1. The concave inner surface of the ala forms the iliac fossa, giving attachment to the iliacus.

        2. The convex external surface forms the gluteal fossa from which originates the gluteal muscles.

    B. The superior margin thickens to form the iliac crest. The crest projects forward and backward, forming the anterior and posterior iliac spines.

        1. The superior margin provides an inferior attachment for the abdominal wall muscles.

        2. The anterior and posterior iliac spines further subdivide into the superior and inferior spines.

        3. The anterosuperior iliac spine (ASIS) is an important landmark; it provides attachment for the inguinal ligament and the sartorius muscle.

        4. The anteroinferior iliac spine (AIIS) projects outward from the wing of the ilium. The superior portion of the AIIS provides attachment to the direct head of the rectus femoris. Avulsion fracture may occur at this site of attachment. The inferior portion provides attachment to the iliofemoral ligament of the hip joint, slightly superior to the acetabular rim. In some individuals, the AIIS may project distally to impinge on the femoral neck during motion. Subspine impingement may limit hip motion and cause labral injuries.[2]

IV. Body:

    A. The body of the ilium forms a part of the acetabulum and provides attachment to the obturator internus.

Ischium

I. It is inferior to the ileum and posterior to the pubis. The superior portion forms one-third of the acetabulum.

II. Parts: superior, inferior rami, and the body:

    A. Superior ramus:

        1. It extends inferiorly and posteriorly from the body.

        2. Its three surfaces are the posterior, inner, and external surfaces.

        3. It extends anteriorly to form the posteroinferior margin of the obturator foramen.

        4. It expands posteriorly to form the ischial tuberosity.

B. Inferior ramus:
   1. It is flat and thin and ascends from the superior ramus to join the pubis anteriorly.
   2. It has two surfaces, inner and external, and two borders, medial and lateral.
C. Body of the ischium:
   1. It contributes to the formation of the acetabulum.
   2. It has two surfaces, external and inner surfaces, and two borders, posterior and anterior.

Pubis

I. The anterior aspect of the hip and pelvis comprises three parts: the body and the inferior and superior pubic rami.
   A. The body forms a part of the acetabulum; it projects anteromedially toward midline to connect with the opposite body of the pubis at the pubic symphysis.
   B. The superior and inferior rami form a part of the obturator foramen.

Acetabulum

I.   It is formed by the fusion of the three hip bones marked by the triradiate cartilage.
II. The acetabular rim surrounds the fossa and is limited inferiorly by the acetabular notch.
III. The fossa provides attachment for the ligamentum teres.
IV. The acetabular notch is converted into a foramen by the transverse acetabular ligament.
V.   The acetabular labrum is attached to the rim. The labrum deepens the acetabular surface for articulation with the femoral head.
VI. The standard clock-face reference provides reliable surgical landmark of the intra-articular hip structures.[3] Irrespective of laterality, the 3 o'clock position always marks the anterior aspect, the 9 o'clock position the posterior aspect, the 12 o'clock position the superior aspect, and the 6 o'clock position the inferior aspect (**Fig. 1.3**).

Joints

I. Hip joint:
   A. Osseous structures: The ball-and-socket synovial joint is formed by the head of the femur and the acetabulum.
      1. The articular surfaces are lined by the hyaline cartilage.
      2. The acetabulum is deepened by the acetabular labrum and articulates with the head of the femur.

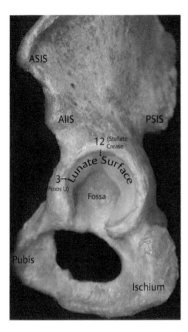

ASIS

AIIS   PSIS

12 (Stellate Crease)

Lunate Surface

3— (Psoas U)

Fossa

Pubis

Ischium

Fig. 1.3 Clock face of the acetabulum.

3. The hip joint connects the trunk and pelvis to the bones of the lower extremity.

B. Capsule: It is attached to the acetabulum superiorly and the neck of the femur inferiorly, and blends anteriorly with the iliofemoral ligament.[4] It is composed of two sets of fibers: circular fibers (that invest the femoral neck) and longitudinal fibers.

C. Ligaments:

1. The hip joint ligament is divided into the intracapsular and extracapsular ligaments (**Fig. 1.4**).

2. The extracapsular ligaments are divided into the "**Y**"-shaped iliofemoral (anterior), ischiofemoral (posterior), and pubofemoral (inferior) ligaments.

3. The ligamentum teres forms the intracapsular ligament.

D. Angles:

1. Lateral center-edge angle:

a. The angle between a vertical line and a line from the center of the femoral head to the most lateral bony part of the acetabulum.[5]

b. Normal: 25 to 40 degrees; less than 20 degrees indicate developmental dysplasia of the hip (DDH).[6]

c. It is used in femoroacetabular impingement syndrome (FAIS) diagnosis.

d. It evaluates the acetabular lateral coverage.

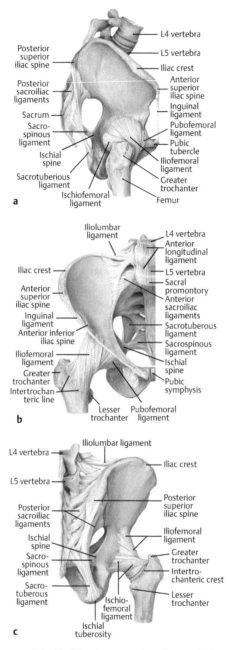

Fig. 1.4 (a–c) The ligaments of the hip joint. (Source: Schuenke M, Schulte E, Schumacher U. Thieme Atlas of Anatomy. General Anatomy and Musculoskeletal System. 2nd edition, ©2014, Thieme Publishers, New York. Illustrations by Voll M and Wesker K.)

2. Anterior center-edge angle:

   a. On false profile, the angle formed by intersection of a vertical line through the center of the femoral head and a line extending through the center of the femoral head to the anterior sourcil.[7]

   b. It is obtained from the false profile view (allows assessment to the degree of femoral head anterior coverage), measures anterior dysplasia.

   c. Normal: 25 to 40 degrees; less than 20 degrees indicates DDH.[8]

   d. It evaluates the acetabular anterior coverage.

3. Transverse (acetabular) angle: It is the angle between a line drawn from the superior to the inferior acetabular rim and the horizontal plane.

4. Femoral version:

   a. Each limb is measured individually.

   b. On axial computed tomography (CT), find the slice that best reveals the femoral neck and the condylar alignments.

   c. Measure the condyle-horizontal angle (CH) and the neck horizontal angle (NH) (**Fig. 1.5**).

   d. Calculate the angle of the neck relative to the condyles (NC = NH − CH).

   e. In internal rotation, the CH is added to the NH. In external rotation, the CH is subtracted from the NH angle.

5. Tonnis angle: on anteroposterior (AP) plain radiograph. The angle is formed between a horizontal line and a line extending from the medial to lateral edges of the sourcil. Normal: less than 10 degrees.[6,9]

6. Acetabular version:

   a. On axial CT, each limb is measured individually. Find the slice that best reveals the deepest floor of the acetabulum.

   b. The angle is measured between a line drawn tangent to the anterior and posterior walls of the acetabulum and a true sagittal line.

7. Acetabular angle (of Sharp):

   a. It measures the acetabular inclination on the AP plain radiograph.

   b. The angle is formed between a horizontal line and a line from the tear-drop to lateral acetabulum. Normal: 33 to 38 degrees.[6]

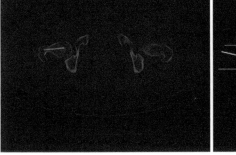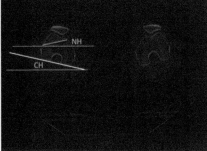

Fig. 1.5 Analysis of the femoral version. Abbreviations: CH, condyle-horizontal angle; NH, neck-horizontal angle.

8. Femoral neck angle: It is the widest in infancy and reduces to average of 125 degrees in the adult. It varies among individuals and gender.
    a. Coxa vara: reduced angle (<120 degrees).
    b. Coxa valga: increased angle (>135 degrees).
E. Movements: Varying ranges of motion—flexion, extension, abduction, adduction, medial, and lateral rotations and circumduction.
F. Blood supply: Medial and lateral circumflex arteries; branches off the deep artery of the thigh. Sometimes it may directly branch off the femoral artery. The foveal artery lies within the ligamentum teres, branches off the posterior division of the obturator artery, and supplies the femoral head. Disruption of blood supply from the foveal artery may lead to avascular necrosis.

II. Sacroiliac joint:
A. It is formed by the sacrum (triangular bone formed from fused lower vertebrae) and the ilium on either side of the posterior midline.
B. Movement about the joint is planar. Reinforced by joint capsule and numerous ligaments: anterior, posterior, and interosseous sacroiliac ligaments, and sacrotuberous and sacrospinous ligaments.[10]
C. It connects the axial skeleton to the pelvis and transmits upper body weight to the lower extremities.

III. Sacrococcygeal symphysis:
A. It is formed between the coccyx and the sacrum. The interosseous ligament connecting both structures is analogous to the intervertebral disk.[11]
B. It is reinforced by the anterior, posterior and lateral sacrococcygeal ligaments.
C. Movements are limited to flexion and extension.[11]

IV. Pubic symphysis:
A. It is an amphiarthrodial joint formed in the midline by the left and right pubic bones. Between the articulation is the fibrocartilaginous disk that is strengthened by the superior and inferior pubic ligaments.[12]
B. It allows limited movement.

Musculature

The hip is surrounded by six groups of muscles: flexors, extensors, adductors, abductors, internal rotators, and external rotators (**Table 1.1**).

Surgical Anatomy

Surface Anatomy (Fig. 1.6)

I. Skin:
A. Anteriorly, the skin of the abdomen and the thigh on each side is clearly demarcated by a line, marking the site for the inguinal ligament. The skin of the anterior and medial thigh is thin, smooth, and elastic.

Table 1.1 Groups of muscles, function and neurovascular supply

Group of muscles	Muscle	Function	Blood supply	Innervation
Flexors	Adductor brevis	Adducts the thigh at the hip, internally rotates the thigh, weak hip flexor	Profunda femoris, medial circumflex, and obturator arteries	Obturator nerve
	Adductor longus	Adducts and flexes the thigh, helps internally rotate the thigh	Profunda femoris, medial circumflex arteries	Obturator nerve (anterior division)
	Adductor magnus	Adductor part: adducts, flexes, and internally rotates the thigh	Femoral, profunda femoris, and obturator arteries	Adductor part: obturator nerve
		Hamstring part: extends thigh		Hamstring part: sciatic nerve (tibial division
	Iliacus (iliopsoas)	Flexes the thigh and stabilizes the hip joint	Iliac branches of iliolumbar artery	Femoral nerve
	Pectineus	Adducts and flexes the thigh	Medial circumflex artery, obturator artery	Femoral nerve and occasionally anterior division of obturator nerve
	Psoas major (iliopsoas)	Flexes thigh	Lumbar branches of the iliolumbar artery	Ventral rami of the first lumbar nerve
	Rectus femoris	Flexes the thigh	Profunda femoris and lateral circumflex arteries	Femoral nerve
	Sartorius	Abducts, externally rotates, and flexes the thigh	Femoral artery	Femoral nerve
	Tensor fasciae latae	Abducts, internally rotates, and flexes the thigh	Ascending branch of lateral circumflex femoral artery	Superior gluteal nerve
Extensors	Adductor magnus	Adductor part: adducts, flexes and internally rotates the thigh	Femoral, profunda femoris, and obturator arteries	Adductor part: obturator nerve
		Hamstring part: extends the thigh		Hamstring part: sciatic nerve (tibial division
	Biceps femoris	Extends the thigh	Perforating branches of the profunda femoris, inferior gluteal, and medial circumflex femoral arteries	Long head: sciatic nerve (tibial division) Short head: sciatic nerve (common fibular division)
	Gluteus maximus	Extends the flexed thigh, assists in external rotation, and abducts the thigh	Inferior gluteal arteries and superior gluteal arteries	Inferior gluteal nerve

(Continued)

Table 1.1 (*Continued*) Groups of muscles, function and neurovascular supply

Group of muscles	Muscle	Function	Blood supply	Innervation
	Semimembranosus	Extends the thigh	Perforating branch of the profunda femoris and the medial circumflex arteries	Sciatic nerve (tibial division)
	Semitendinosus	Extends the thigh	Perforating branch of the profunda femoris and the medial circumflex arteries	Sciatic nerve (tibial division)
Adductors	Adductor brevis	Adducts thigh at the hip, internally rotates the thigh, weak hip flexor	Profunda femoris, medial circumflex, and obturator arteries	Obturator nerve
	Adductor longus	Adducts and flexes the thigh, and helps internally the rotate thigh	Profunda femoris, medial circumflex arteries	Obturator nerve (anterior division)
	Adductor magnus	Adductor part: adducts, flexes, and internally rotates the thigh	Femoral, profunda femoris, and obturator arteries	Adductor part: obturator nerve
		Hamstring part: extends the thigh		Hamstring part: sciatic nerve (tibial division
	Gracilis	Adducts thigh, and flexes and internally rotates the leg	Profunda femoris artery, medial circumflex artery	Obturator nerve
	Pectineus	Adducts and flexes the thigh	Medial circumflex artery, obturator artery	Femoral nerve and occasionally anterior division of obturator nerve
Abductors	Gluteus maximus	Extends the thigh, assists in external rotation, and abducts the thigh	Inferior gluteal arteries and superior gluteal arteries	Inferior gluteal nerve
	Gluteus medius	Abducts and internally rotates the thigh, steadies the pelvis when standing only on that leg	Superior gluteal artery	Superior gluteal nerve
	Gluteus minimus	Abducts and internally rotates the thigh, steadies the pelvis when standing only on that leg	Main trunk and deep branch of the superior gluteal artery	Superior gluteal nerve
	Obturator internus	Externally rotates the extended thigh, abducts the flexed thigh	Internal pudendal and obturator arteries	Nerve to obturator internus
	Piriformis	Externally rotates the extended thigh, abducts the flexed thigh	Superior and inferior gluteal arteries, internal pudendal artery	Ventral rami of L5, S1, S2
	Sartorius	Abducts, externally rotates, and flexes the thigh	Femoral artery	Femoral nerve

Table 1.1 (*Continued*) Groups of muscles, function and neurovascular supply

Group of muscles	Muscle	Function	Blood supply	Innervation
Internal rotators	Gluteus medius	Abducts and internally rotates the thigh, steadies the pelvis when standing only on that leg	Superior gluteal artery	Superior gluteal nerve
	Gluteus minimus	Abducts and internally rotates the thigh, steadies the pelvis when standing only on that leg	Main trunk and deep branch of the superior gluteal artery	Superior gluteal nerve
	Tensor fasciae latae	Abducts, internally rotates, and flexes the thigh	Ascending branch of the lateral circumflex femoral artery	Superior gluteal nerve
External rotators	Gluteus maximus	Extends the thigh, assists in external rotation, and abducts the thigh	Inferior gluteal arteries and superior gluteal arteries	Inferior gluteal nerve
	Inferior gemellus	Externally rotates the extended thigh	Medial circumflex artery	Nerve to quadratus femoris
	Obturator externus	Externally rotates the thigh	Medial circumflex artery, obturator artery	Obturator nerve
	Obturator internus	Externally rotates the extended thigh, abducts the flexed thigh	Internal pudendal and obturator arteries	Nerve to obturator internus
	Piriformis	Externally rotates the extended thigh, abducts the flexed thigh	Superior and inferior gluteal arteries, internal pudendal artery	Ventral rami of L5, S1, and S2
	Quadratus femoris	Externally rotates the thigh	Medial circumflex artery	Nerve to quadratus femoris
	Sartorius	Abducts, externally rotates, and flexes the thigh	Femoral artery	Femoral nerve
	Superior gemellus	Externally rotates the extended thigh	Inferior gluteal and internal pudendal arteries	Nerve to obturator internus

    B. Posteriorly, the skin over the gluteal region is relatively thick. The gluteal fold is a horizontal skin crease that marks the junction of the inferior border of the gluteus maximus muscle as it crosses oblique to the crease. Asymmetry of the gluteal folds is pathognomonic for DDH, however may be an unreliable clinical sign for diagnosis.[13]

II. Bony Landmarks:

    A. Iliac crest:

        1. It has lateral prominence on both sides of the pelvis. It projects anteriorly to form the ASIS and posteriorly the posterosuperior iliac spine (PSIS).

        2. It is palpable in its entire length and has many curves: convex superiorly and concave at both the anterior and posterosuperior ends. The intermediate zone separates the inner and outer lips.

    B. Iliac tubercle:

        1. It has lateral projection of the outer lip of the iliac crest. It is approximately 5 cm behind the ASIS.

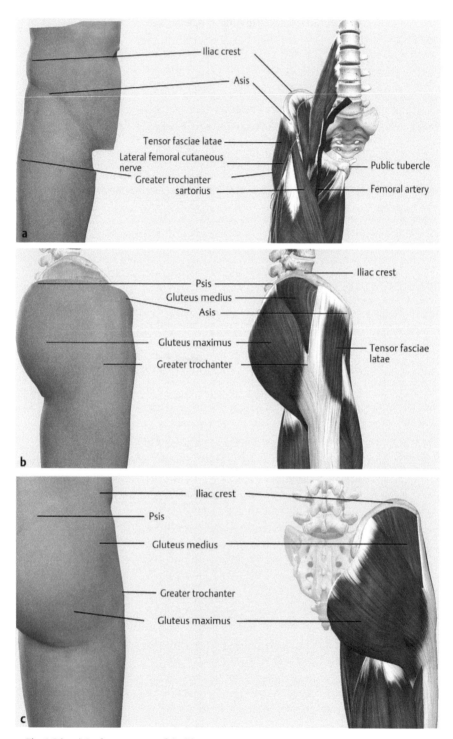

Fig. 1.6 (a–c) Surface anatomy of the hip.

    2. It provides attachment for the iliotibial tract. It lies at the level of L5 vertebrae.

C. ASIS:

    1. It projects from the iliac crest anterosuperiorly, bilateral.

    2. It is useful in measuring true leg length, acts as guide when identifying landmarks like the Roser–Nelaton line, measuring leg length, and quadriceps angle. The quadriceps angle is formed by a line connecting the ASIS to the mid-patella. The normal quadriceps angle is 140 degrees in men and 170 degrees in females. Higher quadriceps angle results in maltracking of the patella.[14]

    3. It provides attachment to the inguinal ligament and the sartorius muscle.

D. AIIS:

    1. It has interior prominence of the wing of the ilium below the ASIS.

    2. It borders the acetabular rim anteriorly and provides attachment to the iliofemoral ligament of the hip.

E. PSIS:

    1. It has a posterosuperior projection of the wing of the ilium.

    2. It provides attachment for the posterior sacroiliac ligaments.

F. Posteroinferior iliac spine:

    1. It has a posterior projection of the ilium below the PSIS.

    2. It is separated from the PSIS by a notch. This notch appears as dimples on the lower back of some individuals.

G. Ischial tuberosity:

    1. It has a posterior prominence on the superior ramus of the ischium.

    2. It bears the weight of the body in the sitting position.

    3. It lies beneath the gluteus maximus in the upright position but exposed in the sitting position.

    4. It provides attachment for the sacrotuberous ligament and the hamstring muscles: semimembranosus, semitendinosus, and biceps femoris.

H. Greater trochanter:

    1. It projects laterally and posteromedially on the femur, approximately 1 cm below the head of the femur.

    2. It has lateral and medial surfaces, and posterior, anterior, inferior, and superior borders.

    3. The posterior border is free and borders the trochanteric fossa posteriorly.

III. Muscular Landmarks:

A. Sartorius:

    1. It starts from the ASIS proximally and runs obliquely downward crossing the anterior thigh to attach to the medial border of the proximal tibia.

    2. The superior portion forms the lateral border of the femoral triangle.

    3. It inserts into the medial border of the proximal tibia with the gracilis and the semitendinosus via the pes anserinus.

B. Gluteus maximus:

1. It has an extensive origin from the posterior gluteal line, posterior sacrum, and the sacrotuberous ligament. It courses obliquely and laterally downward to insert into the greater trochanter and the iliotibial band.

2. It extends and abducts the hip joint.

C. Piriformis muscle:

1. It arises from the anterior of the sacrum, exits the pelvis through the greater sciatic notch dividing the notch into superior and inferior parts, and inserts into the greater trochanter.

2. The superior gluteal vessels and nerves exit the pelvis superior to the piriformis and the sciatic nerve exits inferior to the piriformis.

IV. Femoral Triangle:

A. It is marked by a triangular depression located superiorly on the anterior thigh.

B. It has three borders: adductor longus medially, sartorius laterally, and inguinal ligament superiorly.

C. The roof is formed by the fascia lata; the floor is formed by the iliopsoas laterally and the pectineus and the adductor longus medially.

D. It contents, medial to lateral, are as follows: deep inguinal lymph nodes, femoral vein, femoral artery, femoral sheath, and femoral nerve.

Surgical Approaches

Anterior Approach (Smith-Petersen) (Fig. 1.7)

I. The patient is placed in the supine position and a longitudinal skin incision starts approximately 3 cm distal and lateral to the ASIS; the incision continues along the tensor fasciae latae.[15]

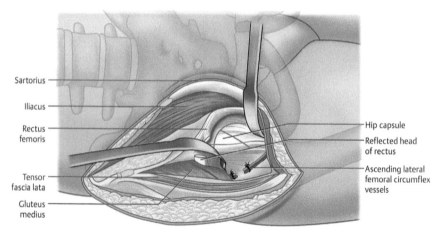

Fig. 1.7 Anterior Approach. (Source: Femoral Neck Fractures, In: Mullis B, Gaski G, eds. Synopsis of Orthopaedic Trauma Management. New York, NY: Thieme; 2020.)

II. Internervous planes between sartorius (femoral nerve) and tensor fasciae latae (superior gluteal nerve) are utilized. The lateral cutaneous nerve should be protected; the ascending branch of the lateral circumflex femoral artery traversing the anterior aspect of the hip, visible in the internervous plane, is cauterized.

III. The surrounding muscles are retracted and an anterior capsular incision is done along the neck to access the joint.

Anterolateral Approach (Watson Jones) (Fig. 1.8)

I. The patient is place in the supine or lateral position. Incision starts 2.5 cm posterior and distal to the ASIS and continues posteriorly toward the greater trochanter.[16]

II. The interval between the tensor fasciae latae is identified. The inferior branch of the superior gluteal nerve is identified and preserved. The vastus lateralis is reflected proximally 1 to 2 cm from the origin.

III. The retractors placed anteriorly, posteriorly, and inferiorly maximize joint visualization, and capsular incision exposes the joint.

Direct Lateral Approach (Hardinge)

I. The patient is placed in the supine position. Incision starts 5 cm proximal to the greater trochanter and ends 5 to 6 cm distal to the greater trochanter.[17]

II. The tensor fascia latae is incised to expose gluteus maximus. A retractor is used to protect the sciatic nerve from injury. The gluteus medius and vastus lateralis at the attachment to greater trochanter is split. Precaution is taken to preserve the superior gluteal nerve.

III. A **T**-shaped capsulotomy is made to optimize joint visualization.

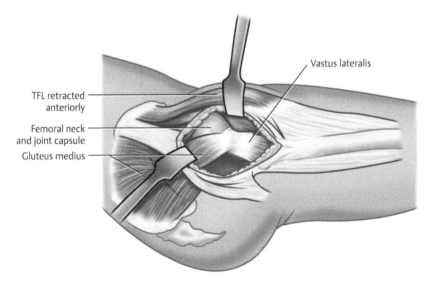

Vastus lateralis

TFL retracted anteriorly

Femoral neck and joint capsule

Gluteus medius

Fig. 1.8 The anterolateral approach. (Source: Femoral Neck Fractures, In: Mullis B, Gaski G, eds. Synopsis of Orthopaedic Trauma Management. New York, NY: Thieme; 2020.)

Posterolateral Approach

I.   The patient is placed in the lateral decubitus or prone position and outline all the bony landmarks: the greater trochanter and the PSIS. Incision starts posterior to the lateral side of the greater trochanter, continues downward 6 cm along the femoral axis; it is extended proximally toward the PSIS approximately 6 cm from the greater trochanter.[18]

II. The gluteal fascia and the tensor fascia latae are incised and the underlying gluteus maximus is bluntly divided. The posterior border of the gluteus medius is retracted using a 90-degree-angled thin Hohmann retractor. The exposed short external rotators are secured with nonabsorbable high-strength sutures before releasing their insertion. The released short external rotators form protection for the sciatic nerve.

III. The gluteus minimus is split from the capsule and retracted. Capsulotomy and full-thickness broad-based flap of the posterior hip capsule exposes the posterior aspect of the joint.

Modified Hueter Approach

I.   The patient is placed in the supine position on the orthopaedic extension table with perineal support of 10-cm diameter. Ipsilateral upper limb is placed on the chest and stabilized with a tape. Light traction is applied with the pelvis horizontally and balanced.

II. A 5- to 8-cm incision is made an inch lateral to the ASIS and extended obliquely downward toward the mid area of the external condyle.[19]

III. Intermuscular incision separates the space between tensor fascia lata and sartorius, taking precautions to preserve the femoral cutaneous nerve deep in the sartorius sheath.

IV. The superficial aponeurosis of the rectus femoris is incised longitudinally to expose the deep aponeurosis. The iliopsoas muscle is separated from the anterior side of the joint capsule.

V.   The intra-articular space is assessed by either capsulectomy or capsulotomy. The ideal site for femoral neck osteotomy is marked by the depression formed by the junction of the superior and inferior vastus lateralis capsular insertions.

VI. The prosthesis is set in place and operative limb reduced by returning the lower limb into a slightly upward-sloping plane while applying traction axially.

Hip Arthroscopy

It is a minimally invasive technique. It addresses intra-articular and extra-articular hip pathologies: labral tear, femoroacetabular impingement, greater trochanteric pain syndrome, piriformis syndrome, heterotopic ossification, and deep gluteal syndrome (**Fig. 1.9**).

I.   Supine approach:

   A. The patient is placed in the supine position on a modified fracture table. A perineal post is used and lateralized to the operative hip. The operative hip is placed in neutral abduction, neutral flexion–extension, and the foot is internally rotated.

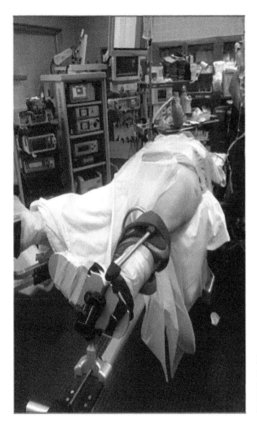

Fig. 1.9 Supine position for hip arthroscopy requires a perineal post lateralized to the operative side. The operative hip is placed in extension, approximately 25-degree abduction and neutral rotation.

Traction of 25 to 50 lbs is applied to distract the operative limb. Joint distraction creates a negative intracapsular pressure, the vacuum phenomenon. Prolonged traction time confers a risk of neuropraxia. Joint space is confirmed by fluoroscopic guidance (**Fig. 1.10**).

B. The ASIS, the greater trochanter, and the anterior and posterior borders of the femur are marked out. A line is drawn inferiorly from the ASIS to the patella while protecting the femoral neurovascular structures located medially.

C. Incisions are made anterolaterally, 1 cm anterior to tip greater trochanter, and longitudinal incision; relatively deep in skin and fascia.

D. Spinal needle is inserted into the joint under fluoroscopic supervision, nitinol wire is passed through, portal site is widened to transmit the cannula and scope, and the anterolateral portal is established.

E. Three standard portals:

1. The anterolateral portal penetrates the gluteus medius and enters the lateral aspect of the capsule at its anterior margin. The superior gluteal nerve is at risk of injury.

2. The anterior portal is located at the intersection of a line drawn inferiorly from the ASIS and a line bisecting across the superior margin of the greater

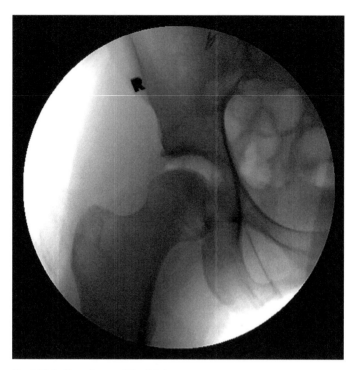

Fig. 1.10 An X-ray image of the joint space.

trochanter. It penetrates the sartorius and rectus femoris and enters the anterior capsule. The lateral cutaneous femoral cutaneous nerve is at risk of injury.

3. The posterolateral portal enters the capsule by penetrating the gluteus medius and minimus muscles. The sciatic and superior gluteal nerves are at risk of injury.

F. The mid-anterior portal is established under direct visualization using the same technique. Capsulotomy is made connecting both portals to access the joint space. Pincer morphology is corrected using a burr, the labrum is cleaned up and debrided, osteochondroplasty is done for cam morphology, and labral repair is done using anchors, fixing it to the acetabulum, occasionally utilizing a distal anterolateral portal.

G. The capsule may be closed using high-strength sutures.

II. Lateral approach:

A. In the lateral decubitus position, surfaces are marked (greater trochanter, ASIS) and fluoroscopic C-arm is centered over the trochanter to confirm hip positioning and anatomy.

B. The anterolateral portal is established: A Nitinol wire is passed through a spinal needle and skin incision is made with a no. 11 blade, passing the cannulated arthroscopic trocar and sheath over the wire into the joint. A 70-degree arthroscope is introduced.

C. The anterior and posterolateral portals are made using the same technique. The lateral cutaneous nerve is at risk of injury while establishing the anterior portal.

D. Capsulotomy is made along the femoral neck in line with the zona orbicularis fibers of the Iliofemoral ligament.

E. Pincer morphology is corrected using a burr, the labrum is cleaned up and debrided, osteochondroplasty is done for cam morphology, and labral repair is done using anchors, fixing it to the acetabulum.

F. The capsule may be closed using high-strength sutures.

References

1. Parvaresh KC, Pennock AT, Bomar JD, Wenger DR, Upasani VV. Analysis of Acetabular Ossification From the Triradiate Cartilage and Secondary Centers. J Pediatr Orthop 2018;38(3):e145–e150

2. Carton P, Filan D. Anterior Inferior Iliac Spine (AIIS) and Subspine Hip Impingement. Muscles Ligaments Tendons J 2016;6(3):324–336

3. Philippon MJ, Michalski MP, Campbell KJ, et al. An anatomical study of the acetabulum with clinical applications to hip arthroscopy. J Bone Joint Surg Am 2014;96(20):1673–1682

4. Harty M. Some aspects of the surgical anatomy of the hip joint. J Bone Joint Surg Am 1966;48(1):197–202

5. Hanson JA, Kapron AL, Swenson KM, Maak TG, Peters CL, Aoki SK. Discrepancies in measuring acetabular coverage: revisiting the anterior and lateral center edge angles. J Hip Preserv Surg 2015;2(3):280–286

6. Mannava S, Geeslin AG, Frangiamore SJ, et al. Comprehensive Clinical Evaluation of Femoroacetabular Impingement: Part 2, Plain Radiography. Arthrosc Tech 2017;6(5):e2003–e2009

7. Chosa E, Tajima N. Anterior acetabular head index of the hip on false-profile views. New index of anterior acetabular cover. J Bone Joint Surg Br 2003;85(6):826–829

8. Beck EC, Nwachukwu BU, Chahla J, et al. Patients With Borderline Hip Dysplasia Achieve Clinically Significant Outcome After Arthroscopic Femoroacetabular Impingement Surgery: A Case-Control Study With Minimum 2-Year Follow-up. Am J Sports Med 2019;47(11):2636–2645

9. Tönnis D, Heinecke A, Nienhaus R, Thiele J. [Predetermination of arthrosis, pain and limitation of movement in congenital hip dysplasia (author's transl)]. Z Orthop Ihre Grenzgeb 1979;117(5):808–815

10. Vleeming A, Schuenke MD, Masi AT, Carreiro JE, Danneels L, Willard FH. The sacroiliac joint: an overview of its anatomy, function and potential clinical implications. J Anat 2012;221(6):537–567

11. Alderink GJ. The sacroiliac joint: review of anatomy, mechanics, and function. J Orthop Sports Phys Ther 1991;13(2):71–84

12. Becker I, Woodley SJ, Stringer MD. The adult human pubic symphysis: a systematic review. J Anat 2010;217(5):475–487

13. Anderton MJ, Hastie GR, Paton RW. The positive predictive value of asymmetrical skin creases in the diagnosis of pathological developmental dysplasia of the hip. Bone Joint J 2018;100-B(5):675–679

14. Egund N, Ryd L. Patellar and Quadriceps Mechanism. Imaging of the Knee. Med Radiol (Berl); 2003:217–248

15. Patel RM, Stover MD. Smith-Petersen Approach to the Hip. Hip Arthroscopy and Hip Joint Preservation Surgery; 2015:379–85

16. Krismer M. Total Hip Arthroplasty: A Comparison of Current Approaches. European Instructional Lectures; 2009:163–75

17. Kelmanovich D, Parks ML, Sinha R, Macaulay W. Surgical approaches to total hip arthroplasty. J South Orthop Assoc 2003;12(2):90–94
18. Foran JRH, Valle CJD. Posterolateral Approach to the Hip. Hip Arthroscopy and Hip Joint Preservation Surgery; 2015:361–70
19. Laude F. Total hip arthroplasty through an anterior Hueter minimally invasive approach. Interact Surg 2006;1(1):5–11

Suggested Readings

Byrd TJW, Bedi A, Stubbs AJ. The Hip. AANA Advanced Arthroscopic Surgical Techniques. Thorofare, NJ: SLACK Inc.; 2016

Gray H. Anatomy of the Human Body New YorK, NY: Elsevier; 2015

Harty M. Some aspects of the surgical anatomy of the hip joint. J Bone Joint Surg Am 1966;48(1):197–202

Kelmanovich D, Michael L, Parks ML, Sinha R, Macaulay W. Surgical approaches to total hip arthroplasty. J South Orthop Assoc 2003;12(2):90–94

Kinov P. Arthroplasty—Update. London: InTech; 2013

Wright JM, Crockett HC, Sculco TP. Mini-incision for total hip arthroplasty. Orthop Spec Ed 2001;7(2):18–20

2 History and Physical Examination

Edward C. Beck, Brian R. Waterman, Gift Echefu, Jahanzeb Kaikaus, William H. Neal, Kyleen Jan, Alexander Newhouse, Shane J. Nho

History

Diagnosing Disorders of the Hip

I. Comprehensive history and physical examination are essential in evaluating the patient:

   A. They allow one to establish a preliminary differential diagnosis.

   B. They help determine course of the physical examination and special testing.

II. Presentation of hip pathologies can be broad and vague, requiring thorough investigation into the course of the disease process.

III. Pathologies arising from sites other than the hip such as knee or back may present as hip pain.[1]

IV. Characterizing the patient complaint:

   A. Symptoms of hip disease include pain, stiffness, deformity, mechanical (e.g., popping, snapping, locking, etc.), and limping.

V. Progression of degenerative hip disease:

   A. Typically, external rotation is the first motion to be lost:

      1. Patients will complain of difficulty putting their shoes on.[2]

   B. This is followed by loss of abduction/adduction.

   C. Flexion is generally well preserved until more advanced stages.

Mechanical Symptoms

I. Pain in the presence of locking, catching, or popping indicate better prognostic outcome:

   A. It implies a mechanical problem that is typically correctable.

   B. It is not a pathognomonic, injury-specific finding, as the hip can be completely normal.

II. Pain in the absence of other symptoms is a poorer prognostic indicator.

III. Characterize specific movements precipitating pain:

   A. Patient typically lacks symptoms in straight plane activity.

   B. Pain arises in direction change and twisting motions.

IV. Classic activities triggering symptoms:

   A. Sitting, particularly with excess flexion.

   B. Standing up from the seated position.

   C. Ascending or descending stairs.

   D. Entering/exiting automobile.

   E. Putting on shoes and socks involves rotation.

Physical Examination

Inspection

I. Assessment of gross appearance:
    A. Lesions, bruising, and visible trauma.
    B. Symmetry and pelvic obliquity.
    C. Atrophy.
    D. Visible signs of variable limb length.

II. Assessment of stance:
    A. Signs of abnormality:
        1. Slight flexion of the symptomatic hip with associated ipsilateral knee flexion.

III. Assessment of gait. The patient is asked to walk normally and in a toe-and-heel gait in the examination room.
    A. Normal gait:
        1. Gait is steady, even, and with equal stride length with normal trunk and pelvis control.
        2. Indication that legs are of equal length and motion is intact.
    B. Antalgic gait:
        1. A possible consequence of hip pain.
        2. The patient will alter position to avoid placing body weight over the affected hip.
    C. Short leg limp: seen in limb length discrepancy. During walking, the body lands onto the short leg and takes off with the long leg.
    D. Trendelenburg gait:
        1. It indicates abductor muscle weakness and inability to support pelvic weight.
        2. Unaffected hip shifts downward when the affected leg is in midstance of the gait cycle (**Fig. 2.1**).

Motion Assessment

I. Ensure the patient's pelvis remains stationary by keeping a hand on the antero-superior iliac spine.

II. Flexion:
    A. In the supine position and with the knee flexed, bend the patient's leg into the abdomen until resistance is met.
    B. Normal range is 120 to 135 degrees.

III. Extension:
    A. In the prone or upright position, draw the leg backward until pelvic movement is detected or resistance is met.
    B. Normal range is 20 to 30 degrees.

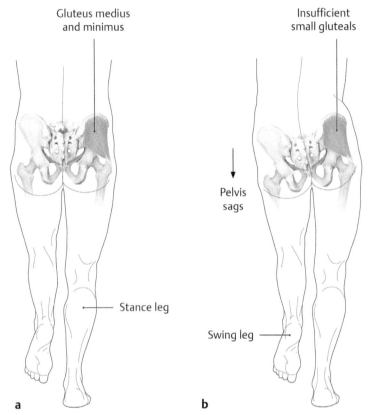

Fig. 2.1 (a) Normal gait, **(b)** Trendelemburg gait. (Source: Schuenke M, Schulte E, Schumacher U. General Anatomy and the Musculoskeletal System: Thieme Atlas of Anatomy. New York: Thieme; 2005. Illustrations by Voll M and Wesker K.)

IV.   Abduction:

    A. In the lateral decubitus position, place a hand on the iliac crest, and pull the leg away from midline until pelvic movement is detected or resistance is met.

    B. Normal range is 40 to 50 degrees.

V.   Adduction:

    A. It is assessed with the patient in the supine or lateral decubitus position, with the test leg resting on the table. The upper leg is abducted to 25 degrees with resistance hand placed on the distal medial femur of the test leg while the patient actively adducts.

    B. Normal range is 20 to 30 degrees.

VI.   Internal rotation:

    A. In the supine position, the knee and hip are both flexed at 90 degrees, and the leg is rotated outward while stabilizing the knee in position.

    B. Normal is 30 degrees. It is positive in femoroacetabular impingement (FAI) syndrome.

VII. External rotation:
   A. In the supine position, the knee and hip are both flexed at 90 degrees, and the leg is rotated inward while stabilizing the knee.
   B. Normal is 50 degrees.

Range of Motion Assessment

I.   Supine:
   A. Flex the hip with the knee extended.
   B. Pull the knee toward the chest while the opposite leg is kept straight.
   C. Move the leg medially and laterally while maintaining a straight knee.
   D. Side of the foot is placed on the opposite knee, moving the flexed knee toward the table.
II. Prone or standing:
   A. The straightened leg is swung behind the body to assess extension (**Fig. 2.2**).

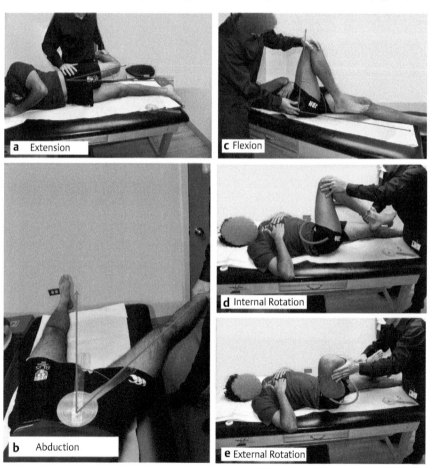

Fig. 2.2 (**a**) Hip flexion with straight knee. (**b**) Hip extension. (**c**) Hip flexion with knee flexed. (**d**) Abduction and adduction. (**e**) External rotation.

Special Signs and Tests

I. Straight leg raise:
    A. The examiner actively flexes the hip by raising the leg with the knee extended.
    B. Test is positive with back, leg, or buttock pain elicited at 60 degrees or less with radiation distal to the knee. Dorsiflexion at the ankle worsens pain and flexion at the knee or hip relieves the pain.
    C. Positive test indicates lumbosacral nerve root irritation and/or radiculopathy.[3]

II. Leg-length test:
    A. Ensure consistency in the angle between the limb and the pelvis. Note the height of the iliac crests.
    B. True leg length is measured from the anterosuperior iliac spine or the greater trochanter of the femur to the medial malleolus of the ipsilateral ankle with the patient in the supine position, using a tape measure.[4]
    C. Repeat the assessment with the patient going from lying to the sitting position. It is useful in excluding sacroiliac joint dysfunction or a fixed pelvic rotation, which can give the false impression of a leg-length discrepancy.
    D. In the case of shortening, determin e whether the discrepancy occurs above or below the trochanteric level.
    E. Variations above the trochanteric level are indicative of abnormality in the hip.
    F. Apparent leg length: umbilicus to the medial malleolus of the ipsilateral leg.
    G. In hip fractures, the affected leg appears shortened and externally rotated.

III. Allis' (or Galeazzi's) sign:
    A. It is used primarily for assessing developmental dysplasia of the hip.
    B. The patient is in the supine position and the knees are flexed with ankles touching the buttocks. If the knees are not level, then the test is positive, indicating a potential congenital hip malformation or apparent limb-length discrepancy.
    C. Positive test is indicative of hip dislocation and femoral or tibial structural defect.[5]

IV. Ludloff's sign:
    A. It is a test for iliopsoas tendinitis or bursitis.[6]
    B. Instruct the patient to assume a seated position with the feet hanging free of the examination table.
    C. Ask the patient to raise the affected leg from the table surface.
    D. The test is positive when a patient fails to raise the leg and there is associated swelling and ecchymosis in Scarpa's triangle.[6]

V. Ober's test (**Fig. 2.3**):
    A. Instruct the patient to lie on the side of the unaffected hip.
    B. Place one hand on the patient's pelvis for stability and grab the ankle with the other hand, maintaining a 90-degree angle of the knee.
    C. Abduct and extend the thigh. A positive sign occurs if the leg remains abducted.
    D. Positive test is indicative of iliotibial band tightness.[7]

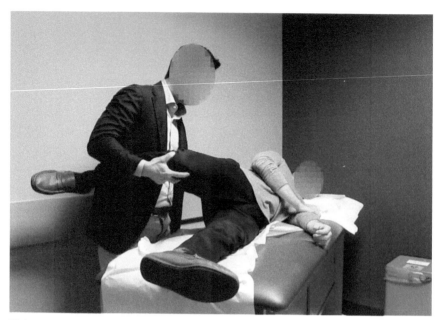

Fig. 2.3 Ober's test.

VI.   FABER (flexion, abduction, and external rotation) or Patrick's test

    A. Instruct the patient to lie supine.

    B. Grab the patient's ankle and flex the knee.

    C. Once the knee is bent, proceed to flex, abduct, externally rotate, and extend the hip. Apply downward pressure in order to further extend the hip. A positive sign is indicative of a coxa pathologic condition.

VII. Thomas's test:

    A. Instruct the patient to assume the supine position.

    B. Request that the patient flex the unaffected knee and pull the knee toward the abdomen. As the patient holds this position with both hands, examine the lower back posture and the affected leg.

    C. If the spine remains in lordosis and the affected leg does not remain flat on the table, a positive test is obtained, indicating hip flexion contracture.[9]

VIII. Stinchfield's test:

    A. The patient is in the supine position, with the leg raised off the table with knee in extension, against resistance at the shin.

    B. Presence of weakness or pain indicates iliopsoas or intra-articular hip pathology.[10]

IX.   Ely's test:

    A. With patient in the prone position, the knee is passively flexed to 120 to 130 degrees.

B. The pelvis coming off the examination table indicates tight rectus femoris muscle.[11]

X. FADIR (flexion, adduction, and internal rotation) test:

A. The patient is placed in the supine position and the examiner passively flexes patient's hip to 90 degrees; while holding the ipsilateral knee and ankle, the hip is adducted and internally rotated.

B. Pain is highly sensitive but not specific for diagnosis of FAI syndrome.[12]

XI. Gillet's test:

A. With patient in upright position, the examiner stands behind the patient and places each hand on the posterosuperior iliac spine with thumbs placed along the sacrum.

B. The patient is then asked to pull the knee to the chest while holding it in place with both hands. Each side is tested for comparison.

C. Inability of the sacrum to move posteriorly during hip and knee flexion indicates a positive test.[13]

XII. Fulcrum test:

A. Assessment is done with the patient in the sitting position with the lower legs off the examination table.

B. One arm is placed under the symptomatic thigh and the palm of the hand serves as a fulcrum.

C. The arm is then moved toward the proximal thigh while pressure is applied to the back of the knee.

D. In the setting of stress fracture, pressure on the dorsum of the knee produces sharp pain, often accompanied by apprehension.

XIII. Ortolani's tests:

A. It is performed on newborns and infants for assessment of developmental dysplasia of the hip.

B. The infant is placed in the supine position, with the hips and knees are flexed to 90 degrees. The examiner applies anterior pressure to the greater trochanters and the hips are abducted gently using the thumbs.

C. A "clunk" is present when the femoral head relocates anteriorly into the acetabulum and is indicative of posterior hip dislocation.

D. The test is done in conjunction with Barlow's maneuver and reduces the hip dislocation previously elicited.[14]

XIV. Barlow's maneuver:

A. It is an assessment of developmental dysplasia of the hip.

B. Infant hips are adducted and slight pressure applied on the anterior knee, directing the force posteriorly and reproducing posterior hip instability.

C. Posterior dislocation is indicative of developmental dysplasia of the hip.[15]

D. False-negative findings may be encountered if the hip is already in a subluxated or dislocated position.[15]

References

1. Byrd JW. Evaluation of the hip: history and physical examination. N Am J Sports Phys Ther 2007;2(4):231–240
2. Byrd JWT. Patient Selection and Physical Examination. Operative Hip Arthroscopy; 2013:7–32
3. Donatelli R. Evaluation of the Trunk and Hip CORE. Sports-Specific Rehabilitation; 2007:193–221
4. Sabharwal S, Kumar A. Methods for assessing leg length discrepancy. Clin Orthop Relat Res 2008;466(12):2910–2922
5. Noordin S, Umer M, Hafeez K, Nawaz H. Developmental dysplasia of the hip. Orthop Rev (Pavia) 2010;2(2):e19
6. Poultsides LA, Bedi A, Kelly BT. An algorithmic approach to mechanical hip pain. HSS J 2012;8(3):213–224
7. Willett GM, Keim SA, Shostrom VK, Lomneth CS. An Anatomic Investigation of the Ober Test. Am J Sports Med 2016;44(3):696–701
8. Kreder HJ. The Hip. Musculoskeletal Examination and Joint Injection Techniques; 2006:46–65
9. Fagerson TL, Babatunde OM, Safran MR. Hip Pathologies. Pathology and Intervention in Musculoskeletal Rehabilitation; 2016:651–691
10. Maslowski E, Sullivan W, Forster Harwood J, et al. The diagnostic validity of hip provocation maneuvers to detect intra-articular hip pathology. PM R 2010;2(3):174–181
11. Marks MC, Alexander J, Sutherland DH, Chambers HG. Clinical utility of the Duncan-Ely test for rectus femoris dysfunction during the swing phase of gait. Dev Med Child Neurol 2003;45(11):763–768
12. Griffin DR, Dickenson EJ, O'Donnell J, et al. The Warwick Agreement on femoroacetabular impingement syndrome (FAI syndrome): an international consensus statement. Br J Sports Med 2016;50(19):1169–1176
13. Grgić V. [The sacroiliac joint dysfunction: clinical manifestations, diagnostics and manual therapy]. Lijec Vjesn 2005;127(1-2):30–35
14. Ivkovic A, Bojanic I, Pecina M. Stress fractures of the femoral shaft in athletes: a new treatment algorithm. Br J Sports Med 2006;40(6):518–520, discussion 520
15. Dwyer NS. Congenital dislocation of the hip: to screen or not to screen. Arch Dis Child 1987;62(6):635–637

Suggested Readings

Byrd JWT. Evaluation of the hip: history and physical examination. N Am J Sports Phys Ther 2007;2(4):231–240

Magee DJ, Sueki D, Chepeha J. Orthopedic Physical Assessment Atlas and Video: Selected Special Tests and Movements. Philadelphia, PA: Saunders; 2011

Swartz MH. Textbook of Physical Diagnosis: History and Examination. Philadelphia, PA: Saunders/Elsevier; 2010

3 Radiographic Anatomy of The Hip

Gift Echefu, Brian R. Waterman, Edward C. Beck, Jahanzeb Kaikaus, Shane J. Nho

General Considerations

I.   Comprehension of the normal radiographic anatomy of the hip is helpful in the interpretation of hip pathology on radiographs (**Fig. 3.1**).

Plain Film Radiographs

I.   Primary imaging for adult hip. Routine: anteroposterior (AP) and lateral views. Specialized views: frog-leg lateral, anterior and posterior oblique (Judet's views), false profile, Ferguson's view (pelvic outlet), and the pelvic inlet view.[1]

II. Alignment is evaluated by visualization of symmetry. Important landmarks are as follow: iliopectineal line, ilioischial line of Kohler, Shenton's line, sourcil, teardrop sign, and acetabular floor.[2]

III. Evaluation of plain radiographs:

   A. AP pelvis and hip radiograph (**Figs. 3.1, 3.2**):

      1. Neutral alignment of the hip and pelvis is confirmed by measuring the distance from the sacrococcygeal junction to the superior symphysis pubis. Distance of 3 to 5 cm is considered normal.[3,4]

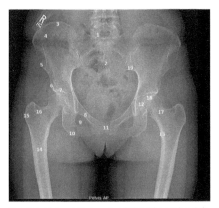

Fig. 3.1 Plain radiograph of the hip and pelvis (anteroposterior view). 1, the fifth lumbar vertebrae; 2, sacrum; 3, iliac crest; 4, ilium; 5, anterosuperior iliac spine; 6, anteroinferior iliac spine; 7, acetabulum; 8, superior pubic ramus; 9, obturator foramen; 10, ischial tuberosity; 11, pubic symphysis; 12, fovea; 13, lesser trochanter; 14, shaft of femur; 15, greater trochanter; 16, intertrochanteric crest; 17, neck of femur; 18, head of femur; 19, posteroinferior iliac spine.

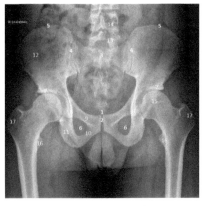

Fig. 3.2 Plain radiograph evaluation. 1, coccyx; 2, pubic symphysis; 3, sacrum; 4, sacroiliac joint; 5, iliac crests; 6, obturator foramen; 7, acetabular sourcil; 8, teardrop; 9, superior pubic ramus; 10, inferior pubic ramus; 11, ischial ramus; 12, ala of ilium; 13, fifth lumbar vertebrae; 14, fourth lumbar vertebrae; 16, lesser trochanter; 17, greater trochanter.

2. The pubic symphysis should be in line with the center of the sacrum. The symphyseal joint space should be ≤ 5 mm.

3. The sacroiliac joint widths should be equal. Normal sacroiliac joint appears as a thin white line. Sclerosis and joint space narrowing characterize sacroiliitis. Arcuate lines should be symmetrical; angular lines indicate sacral fracture.

4. Iliac crests should both be on the same level.

5. The obturator foramen should be symmetric bilaterally.

6. The acetabular walls: the posterior wall should be lateral to the anterior wall. In acetabular retroversion, anterior and posterior walls cross each other. Positive crossover sign indicates presence of femoroacetabular impingement or developmental dysplasia of the hip.

7. Iliopectineal line: this line extends posteriorly from the sacral promontory, arcuate line, and ends anteriorly at the pectineal line. It divides the pelvis into major (false) and minor (true) pelvis. Disruption indicates anterior column fracture (**Fig. 3.3**).

8. Ilioischial line: this line represents the posterior column. On each side, the line is drawn from the medial border of the iliac wing to the medial border of the ischium, ending at the ischial tuberosity (**Fig. 3.3**). Location of the femoral head medial to the pectineal line indicates acetabular bone loss or possible medial femoral head migration in the acetabulum.[5]

9. The sourcil should be clearly defined. Teardrop sign should be assessed: it marks the convergence of the pubis, the ischium, and the ilium. Asymmetry of the teardrop sign may indicate occult acetabular fracture.[5]

10. Shenton's line: this line is drawn from the inferomedial neck of the femur to the inferior border of the superior ramus (**Fig. 3.3**). A discontinuation of this line may indicate femoral neck fracture.[5]

11. The cortex of the femoral head and neck should be smooth and continuous with a normal trabecular pattern. Disruption may indicate a fracture.

12. The greater and lesser trochanters should be clearly visible and symmetric on both sides.

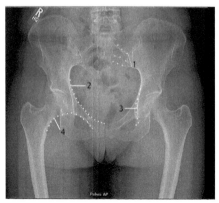

Fig. 3.3 Pelvic lines on anteroposterior plain radiograph. 1, sacral arcuate lines; 2, iliopectineal line; 3, ilioischial line; 4, Shenton's line.

IV. Pediatric plain radiograph:

   A. Assessment is done on AP and frog-leg lateral views of both pelvis (**Figs. 3.4, 3.5**). The pelvic bones are not fused and appear separated on radiographs. Knowledge of the patient's age is important in order to differentiate open epiphysis from fractures.

V. Two main features help distinguish male and female pelvis (**Fig. 3.6**):

   A. The pubic angle is obtuse in females and acute in males.

   B. The iliac crests appear flared in males and broad in females.

   VI. Lateral pelvis radiograph (**Fig. 3.7**):

   A. Cross-table view: this view provides visualization of the anterior and posterior aspects of the femoral neck, and the lateral aspect of the femoral head and the proximal femur.

   B. Femoral head, neck, and shaft; greater and lower trochanters and ischial tuberosity should be visible on the lateral view.

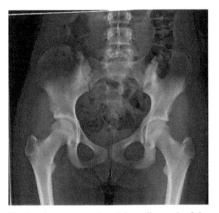

Fig. 3.4 Anteroposterior plain radiograph of the pediatric hip.

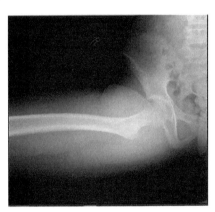

Fig. 3.5 Lateral plain radiograph of the hip.

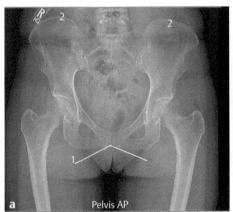

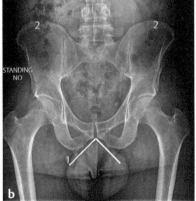

Fig. 3.6 Anteroposterior plain radiograph comparing female and male pelvis. (**a**) Female pelvis. Note the more obtuse pubic angle and broad iliac crests. (**b**) Male pelvis. Note the acute pubic angle and flared iliac crests. 1, pubic angle; 2, iliac crests.

C. The ischial tuberosity is posterior and aids in orienting the image.

D. Posteroinferior migration of the femoral head on the lateral view indicates posterior dislocation.

E. The femoral head and neck should be continuous. The femoral neck appears shorter and discontinuous in displaced fracture.

VII. Fat planes: visible on AP plain radiograph (**Figs. 3.8, 3.9**):

A. The gluteal fat stripe is represented by a line parallel to the upper part of neck of the femur. It is formed by fat between the gluteus minimus tendon and the ischiofemoral ligament. In hip joint effusion, the line is directed superiorly.

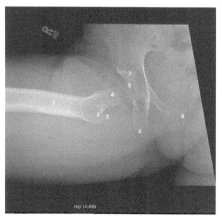

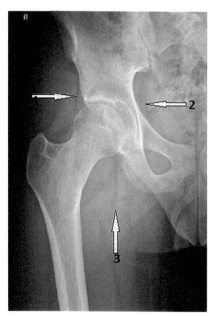

Fig. 3.7 Plain radiograph of the hip and pelvis frog-leg view. 1, lesser trochanter; 2, shaft of the femur; 3, greater trochanter; 4, neck for the femur; 5, head of the femur; 6, ischial tuberosity; 7, acetabulum; 8 pubic symphysis.

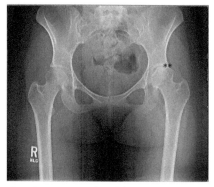

Fig. 3.8 Fat planes on anteroposterior plain radiograph. 1, gluteal fat stripe; 2, iliopsoas fat stripe; 3, obturator fat stripe.

Fig. 3.9 Anteroposterior plain radiograph osteoarthritis. The *asterisks* (**) indicate the narrow joint space characteristic of osteoarthritis.

B. The iliopsoas fat stripe is represented by a line that runs below the iliopsoas tendon.

C. The obturator fat stripe is a line that runs parallels to the iliopectineal line and is formed by the pelvic fat adjacent to the obturator internus muscle.

Computed Tomography

I.   Three-dimensional reconstruction of CT images (digital subtraction) provides the rotational profile of the acetabulum, the proximal femur, the posterior condylar axis, the tibial tubercle, and the tibial plafond.

II.   CT evaluation: assessment is done on axial CT and begins with investigation of the integrity of the obturator ring, iliac wings, ilioischial line, iliopectineal line, anterior and posterior columns, and anterior and posterior walls to rule out fracture (disruption indicates fracture; **Figs. 3.10, 3.11**).

Magnetic Resonance Imaging

I.   Structures (**Fig. 3.12**):

A.   Cartilage.

B.   Osseous structures:

1.   Femoral neck.

2.   Head.

3.   Acetabular rim.

4.   Anterosuperior iliac spine.

5.   Anteroinferior iliac spine.

6.   Pubic rami.

7.   Sacral ala.

C.   Soft tissue:

1.   Labrum.

2.   Ligament:

a.   Ligamentum teres femoris.

b.   Iliofemoral ligament.

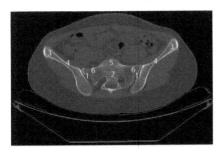

Fig. 3.10 Axial CT of the pelvis. 1, sacroiliac joint; 2, sacrum; 3, ala of ilium; 4, Iliac fossa; 5, sacral promontory; 6, lateral mass of the sacrum.

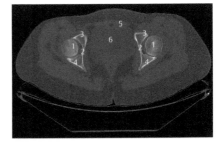

Fig. 3.11 Axial CT of the pelvis. 1, head of the femur; 2, acetabular floor; 3, anterior wall; 4, posterior wall; 5, rectus femoris; 6, urinary bladder.

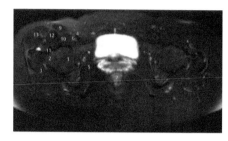

Fig. 3.12 MRI axial T2 hip and pelvis. 1, head of the femur; 2, neck of the femur; 3, greater trochanter; 4, femoral vein; 5, obturator internus; 6, femoral artery; 7, anus; 8, rectus abdominis; 9, sartorius; 10, iliacus; 11, iliofemoral ligament; 12, rectus femoris; 13, tensor fascia lata.

3. Iliopsoas.

4. Gluteus medius/minimus.

5. Tensor fascia lata and iliotibial band.

6. Piriformis.

7. Rectus femoris.

D. Neurovascular structures:

1. Sciatic nerve.

2. Femoral nerve/artery/vein.

Ultrasound

A. Provides visualization of possible intra-articular effusion/infection.

B. Pediatric indication in assessment of developmental dysplasia of the hip.[6]

C. Can be used for dynamic examination in cases of snapping hip.

References

1. Clohisy JC, Carlisle JC, Beaulé PE, et al. A systematic approach to the plain radiographic evaluation of the young adult hip. J Bone Joint Surg Am 2008;90(Suppl 4):47–66

2. Lim SJ, Park YS. Plain Radiography of the Hip: A Review of Radiographic Techniques and Image Features. Hip Pelvis 2015;27(3):125–134

3. Siebenrock KA, Kalbermatten DF, Ganz R. Effect of pelvic tilt on acetabular retroversion: a study of pelves from cadavers. Clin Orthop Relat Res 2003; (407):241–248

4. Courtney PM, Melnic CM, Howard M, Makani A, Sheth NP. A Systematic Approach to Evaluating Hip Radiographs–A Focus on Osteoarthritis. J Orthop Rheumatol 2014;2(1):7

5. Campbell SE. Radiography of the hip: lines, signs, and patterns of disease. Semin Roentgenol 2005;40(3):290–319

6. Kang YR, Koo J. Ultrasonography of the pediatric hip and spine. Ultrasonography 2017;36(3):239–251

Suggested Readings

Campbell SE. Radiography of the hip: lines, signs, and patterns of disease. Semin Roentgenol 2005;40(3):290–319

Courtney PM, Melnic CM, Howard M, Makani A, Sheth NP. A systematic approach to evaluating hip radiographs: a focus on osteoarthritis. J Orthopedics Rheumatol 2014; 2(1):7

4 Hip Imaging and Diagnostic Tests

Gift Echefu, Brian R. Waterman, Edward C. Beck, Kyleen Jan, Shane J. Nho

Imaging Modalities

General Considerations

I. Hip imaging modalities (**Table 4.1**):

A. Plain radiographs.

B. Ultrasound.

C. Computed tomography (CT).

D. Magnetic resonance imaging (MRI).

E. Scintigraphy.

Table 4.1 Comparison of different hip imaging techniques.

	Indications	Advantages	Limitations
Plain radiographs	• Osteoarthritis • Trauma (initial imaging) • Femoroacetabular impingement • Hip dysplasia • Hip fracture • Neoplasm • Dislocation	• Fast and easy to obtain • Convenient and relatively inexpensive	• Low soft-tissue resolution and accuracy • 30–40% bone loss required for detection • Contraindicated in pregnancy
CT	• Developmental disorders of acetabulum and femur (dysplasia, FAI) • Fractures of hip and pelvis • Bone tumors	• High bony detail • Multiplanar, with 3D reconstruction capabilities • Useful for radiographic guided procedures	• Risk of radiation exposure • Contraindicated in pregnancy • Poor soft-tissue contrast
MRI	• Labral tear • Tumors • AVN • Synovial proliferative disorders • Cartilage disorders • Muscle tear and bursitis (gluteal muscle tears, trochanteric bursitis)	• Noninvasive • High soft-tissue resolution and accuracy • No radiation • Multiplanar images • Operator independence	• Contraindicated in individuals wearing metallic objects • Expensive • Lower bony detail • Sedation for claustrophobic patients

(Continued)

Table 4.1 *(Continued)* Comparison of different hip imaging techniques.

	Indications	Advantages	Limitations
MRA	• Labral tear	• Noninvasive • No radiation • Operator independence	• Minimally invasive • Contrast allergy
Ultrasound	• Pediatric hip disorders (DDH) • Therapeutic imaging-guided injections and joint aspirations • Bursitis • Joint effusion • Functional causes of hip pain (e.g., snapping hip	• Fast and easy to obtain • Inexpensive • Noninvasive	• Operator dependence • Poor tissue contrast
Bone scintigraphy	• Infections • Stress fractures	• Early detection of stress fractures • Localizes infection	• Allergic reactions to radioactive substance • Contraindicated in pregnancy

Abbreviations: AVN, avascular necrosis; DDH, developmental dysplasia of the hip; FAI, femoro-acetabular impingement; MRA, magnetic resonance angiography

II.   Hip pain often indicates an underlying pathology. Pain may be primary or referred from spine, sacroiliac joint, pubic symphysis, or knee (**Fig. 4.1**).

III. Comprehensive history and physical examination will suggest possible clinical diagnosis and determine the appropriate confirmatory diagnostic tests.

IV.   Disease process, patient age, general health condition, and type of tissue involved (soft tissue or bone) can determine the imaging modality to be employed (**Table 4.2**).

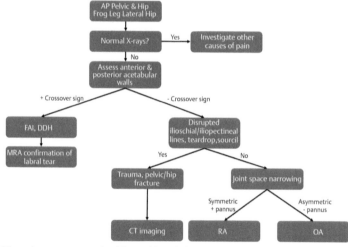

Fig. 4.1 Hip pain assessment algorithm. Abbreviations: AP, anteroposterior; DDH, developmental dysplasia of the hip; FAI, femoroacetabular impingement; RA, rheumatoid arthritis.

Table 4.2 Imaging for hip conditions.

Conditions	Plain radiograph	Ultrasound	CT	MRI	Bone scan
Trauma	✔*	✗	✔*	✔	✗
Avascular necrosis	✔	✗	✔	✔	✗
Fracture	✔*	✗	✔*	✔	✔ (stress)
Acetabular disorders	✔	✗	✔*	✗	✗
Degenerative disorders	✔*	✗	✗	✗	✔
Osteoporosis	✔	✗	✔	✗	✔*
Soft tissue disorders	✗	✔	✗	✔*	✗
Tumors	✔	✗	✔	✔*	✔

✔ = sensitive for condition.
✗ = low/no sensitivity for condition.
* = imaging of choice.

Plain Radiographs

I.   First-line imaging to evaluate hip complaints.

II.   Initial radiograph includes an anteroposterior and false profile view of the pelvis, as well as a frog-leg lateral or modified Dunn view of the symptomatic hip.[1,2]

III. Appropriate image examination and understanding of standard radiographic techniques are necessary for diagnostic accuracy.

IV.   Plain radiographic techniques:

A.   Anteroposterior (AP):

1.   AP hip radiographs may be taken in the supine or prone position.

2.   Images of both hips are taken on the same film. The X-ray tube projects toward the middle of a line from the pubic symphysis to the anterosuperior iliac spine of femur.

3.   AP view in supine position: feet in 15 degrees of internal rotation with both patellae.

4.   Femoral anteversion and flexion contracture may distort image magnification.[3]

5.   Imaging in patients with flexion contracture is done with the legs positioned perpendicularly to in a flexed position.

6.   AP oblique (Judet): hip should be in 45-degree oblique position. Anterior oblique (obturator oblique) positioning captures anterior column and posterior acetabular wall. Posterior oblique (iliac oblique) position captures the posterior column and anterior acetabular column. It is obtained for assessment of acetabular fracture.

7.   The coccyx and pubic symphysis must be in a straight line and in the midline of the image.

8. Distance from the superior border of the pubic symphysis and the sacro-coccygeal junction of 3 to 5 cm is considered normal.[4,5] Obturator foramen and wings of the ilium on both sides must be symmetric.

9. The lesser, greater trochanters and calcar femoris should be clearly visible.

10. Both patellae should be directed upward or limbs internally rotated by 10 degrees; this prevents the greater trochanter from overlapping with the femoral head.[3] This is important in fracture diagnosis.

11. Leg length, neck shaft angle, acetabular depth, acetabular inclination, acetabular coverage, acetabular version, and joint space are evaluated on the AP plain radiograph.

B. Lateral hip radiographs:

1. These are useful in the assessment of the femoral head–neck junction offset, the alpha angle (AA). Anterior femoral head–neck junction: In normal cases, the anterior and posterior concavities are symmetric. In cam deformity, it is convex anteriorly. Decreased head–neck offset is characterized by decrease in anterior concavity. Head–neck offset ratio and AA are used to determine the femoral head–neck junction.

2. Lateral hip radiographic views:

   a. Frog-leg lateral view:

      i. Both sides are shown on the same film. The knee is flexed to approximately 40 degrees in the supine position, with the hip externally rotated by 45 degrees.[3]

      ii. Image is taken with X-ray tube projecting to the middle of the line connecting the upper pubic symphysis and the anterior superior iliac spine.

      iii. It evaluates joint congruency, sphericity of femoral head, and femoral head–neck junction offset.

      iv. It is useful in diagnosis of femoroacetabular impingement syndrome (FAIS).

   b. Cross-table lateral view:

      i. Symptomatic limb is internally rotated by approximately 20 degrees in the supine position, while the opposing limb is flexed at the knee and hip.

      ii. The greater trochanter is positioned in such a way that the femoral head–neck junction is visible.

   c. False profile view:

      i. The foot of the symptomatic limb is placed parallel to the cassette, and then the pelvis is rotated approximately 65 degrees to the wall stand.

      ii. It evaluates the anterior coverage of the femoral head.

   d. Radiographic patterns of the pathologic and developmental conditions.

      i. Trauma.

Pelvic Fractures

I.   The Young and Burgess classification system categorizes pelvic fractures into types based on mechanism of injury (high-impact injuries).[6]

    A.   Anteroposterior compression (APC I–III): radiograph shows an open book fracture of the pubic ramus or symphysis.

    B.   Vertical shear (VS): radiograph shows fracture of the superior and inferior pubic rami with contralateral sacroiliac joint disruption/dislocation (bucket handle fracture or Malgaigne's fracture).

    C.   Lateral compression (LC I–III): radiograph shows unilateral anteroposterior compression injury with or without a contralateral compression injury (i.e., wind-swept pelvis fracture).

    D.   Combined pattern.

II. Duverney's fracture: fracture of the iliac wing is seen on plain radiograph.

III. Acetabular fractures: fractures are classified into anterior column, anterior acetabular rim, posterior column, posterior acetabular rim, transverse, posterior column and wall, transverse and posterior wall, anterior column, and posterior hemitransverse fractures based on the Judet and Letournel classification system (**Table 4.3**).

IV. CT is more sensitive in diagnosing pelvic fractures.[7]

Femoral Head Dislocation

I.   Anterior dislocation: the head of the femur is seen lying below to the acetabulum; the lesser trochanter appears more visible due to external rotation of the affected limb and disruption of Shenton's line is noted. Two radiographic features distinguish the superoanterior hip dislocation from the posterior hip dislocation.[8]

    A.   The head of the femur appears larger on the affected side.

    B.   The lesser trochanter is more visible in the anterior dislocation.

II. Posterior dislocation: radiograph reveals femoral head that is displaced posterior, superior, and lateral to the acetabulum. On AP plain radiograph, the lesser trochanter is obscured and the head of the femur of the affected limb appears smaller.

Femoral Neck Fractures

AP pelvis and lateral views are obtained. Neck fractures are classified as subcapital, transcervical, and basicervical fractures. On plain radiograph, the lesser trochanter appears more prominent, fracture plane appears sclerotic, and the bone trabeculae are disrupted and angulated. Subcapital fractures are the most common and are graded I to IV based on the Garden system.[9]

I.   Garden grade I: incomplete, nondisplaced fracture; medial trabeculae may demonstrate a greenstick fracture.

II. Garden grade II: complete, undisplaced fracture; no trabeculae displacement.

III. Garden grade III: partial displacement with complete fracture. The femoral head is in the varus position, with trabeculae disruption.

IV. Garden grade IV: characterized by complete, displaced fracture. The femoral head still remains in the acetabulum without trabeculae disruption.

Table 4.3 Radiographic findings in acetabular fractures

Type of fracture	Spur sign	Iliac wing fracture	Iliopectineal line disruption	Ilioischial line	Split pelvis?	Obturator ring fracture	fracture of posterior wall
Anterior column	No	Yes	Yes	No	Anteroposterior	Yes	No
Posterior column	No	No	No	Yes	Anteroposterior	Yes	No
Posterior wall	No	No	No	No	No	No	Yes
Anterior wall	No	No	Yes	No	No	No	No
Transverse	No	No	Yes	Yes	Superoposterior	No	No
Posterior column + posterior wall	No	No	No	Yes	Anteroposterior	Yes	Yes
Both-column	Yes	Yes	Yes	Yes	Anteroposterior	Yes	No
T-shaped?	No	No	Yes	Yes	Superoposterior	Yes	No
Transverse + posterior wall	No	No	Yes	Yes	Superoposterior	No	Yes

Nontraumatic Hip Conditions

I.   Arthritis:

    A.   Osteoarthritis: radiographic findings include concentric joint space narrowing, cyst formation, subchondral sclerosis, osteophytes, and superolateral subluxation of the femoral head.

    B.   Rheumatoid arthritis: plain radiograph shows symmetric or concentric joint space narrowing and erosion by pannus.

II. Acetabular developmental deformities:

    A.   Protrusio acetabuli: the medial acetabular wall is seen superior to the ilioischial line on the AP view. Associated with acetabular overcoverage defined as lateral center edge angle (LCEA) greater than or equal to 40 degrees.[10]

    B.   Coxa profunda: characterized by deep acetabular socket. Plain pelvic radiograph reveals the acetabular fossa lying medial to the ilioischial line.

    C.   Femoroacetabular impingement: plain radiographs are obtained initially to assess the joint and rule out other causes of hip pain (avascular necrosis [AVN], degenerative joint diseases). MRI or MR arthrography can subsequently be used to assess the integrity of the labrum, cartilage damage, and other pathologic signs of internal hip derangement.

       1.   Images include two views: AP pelvic view and cross-table lateral view of the proximal femur. The Dunn/Rippstein view (the patient is in 45 degrees of flexion) can be obtained for further evaluation of deformities of anterior femoral head–neck junction.

       2.   The AP view is obtained with the patient in the supine position and legs 15 degrees internally rotated. This compensates for femoral anteversion and provides visualization of the lateral femoral head–neck junction.

       3.   Pincer deformity: It is characterized by deep acetabulum, with overcoverage of the head of femur. The anterior acetabular rim is seen projecting laterally over the posterior rim (positive crossover sign). It is quantified with LCEA or the acetabular index. Normal range LCEA is 25 to 390, ≥ 40 Normal range LCEA is 25 to 39 degrees, with ≥40 degrees indicating acetabular overcoverage. Pincer deformity may be seen in the setting of acetabular retroversion, coxa profunda, and protrusio acetabuli.[10]

       4.   Cam deformity: the head of the femur loses it sphericity. Radiograph demonstrates reduced femoral head–neck junction offset (i.e., pistol grip deformity). Cam deformity is quantified by AA. AA is the angle formed between the femoral neck axis and a line from the center of the femoral head to the transition of the femoral head into the femoral neck. Normal value is less than 55 degrees, with evidence strongly associating 57 degrees as a cut off-value for cam impingement resulting in symptomatic hip pathology.[11]. Cam deformity may be seen in the setting of relative or absolute retroversion, coxa valga, coxa profunda, or protrusio acetabuli.

    D.   Acetabular dysplasia: diagnosis is done using the lateral center edge angle (LCEA) of Wiberg, which is determined by measuring the angle formed between a line drawn vertically from the center of the femoral head and a line from the center of the femoral head through the edge of the acetabulum. LCEA measuring

20 to 25 degrees indicates borderline hip dysplasia, while less than 20 degrees indicates dysplasia[12] (see **Table 4.1**).

E. DDH: radiographic signs are shallow acetabulum, acetabular sclerosis, loss of Shenton's line, femoral head migration above Hilgenreiner's line and lateral to Perkin's line, small capital femoral epiphysis, and delayed ossification of femoral head. LCEA measuring less than 20 degrees is indicative of DDH.[13]

III. Femoral stress fractures: plain radiographs have low sensitivity for stress fractures; CT confirms the presence of stress fractures. Later radiographic signs include graying of the cortex, sclerosis (linear and perpendicular to the trabeculae), and progressive periosteal reaction. MRI is more sensitive for evaluating femoral stress reaction or fractures.[14]

IV. Slipped capital femoral epiphysis (SCFE): assessed using AP and frog-leg views. Fracture is through the physis (Salter type I fracture). The femoral head migrates inferiorly and medially to the neck. The physis appears widened with loss of epiphyseal height on the AP view (**Fig. 4.2**).

V. Legg–Calvé–Perthes disease (LCPD): The Catterall classification groups the pathology into four stages based on radiographic findings. Plain radiograph has high sensitivity for detecting LCPD (**Fig. 4.3**; **Tables 4.4, 4.5**).[15]

A. Early signs: radiographic findings are subtle joint space widening, small joint effusion, small femoral epiphysis, femoral head sclerosis with sequestration and collapse, and failure of epiphyseal growth.

B. Late signs: coxa plana, loose bodies, radiolucent crescent line indicating subchondral fracture, fragmentation of the femoral head and femoral neck cysts, and coxa magna (wide and flat femoral head).

VI. Osteonecrosis: radiographs are normal in early stages. Based on radiographic findings, there are four stages (0–IV) based on Ficat classification.[16]

A. Stage 0: normal radiographic findings.

B. Stage I: loss of clarity and blurring of the trabeculae.

C. Stage II: femoral head sclerosis and cysts.

D. Stage III: crescent line, segmental flattening of the femoral head.

E. Stage IV: deformed femoral head, loss of articular cartilage, acetabular osteophytes, and osteoarthritis.

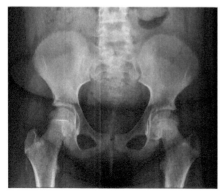

Fig. 4.2 Anteroposterior plain radiograph demonstrating slipped capital femoral epiphysis.

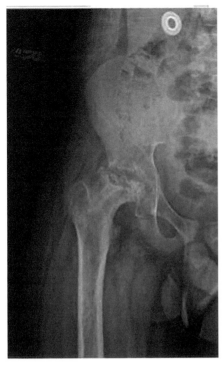

Fig. 4.3 Legg–Calvé–Perthes disease.

Table 4.4 Catterall classification of Legg–Calvé–Perthes disease

Catterall stages	Radiographic findings
Stage I	Early stage, normal radiographic findings
Stage II	Sclerosis ± cystic changes with preservation of the contour and of the femoral head
Stage III	Loss of structural integrity of the femoral head
Stage IV	Loss of structural integrity of the femoral head and acetabulum

Table 4.5 Modified Herring pillar classification of Legg–Calvé–Perthes disease

Group	Characteristics	Height maintained	Outcome
Group A	Lateral pillars with no disease involvement, no density changes	100%	Positive outcome
Group B	Pillars with disease involvement	>50%	Positive outcome
Group B/C	> 50% height + narrow column (2 to 3 cm width), > 50% height + poor ossification, 50% height + depressed compared to central pillar	>50%	Intermediate outcome
Group C	<50%	<50%	Poor prognosis

VII. Hip joint infections: MRI or, more commonly, ultrasound-guided aspirations offer superior sensitivity in cases of periarticular infections. Radiographic signs are increased teardrop distance (effusion) and displacement of the gluteus minimus fat stripe on the AP radiograph. Bone erosions and loss of joint space indicate chronic joint infection.

VIII. Paget's disease: plain radiographs show sclerosis of the iliopectineal and ishiopubic lines with cortical thickening and enlargement of the ischium and pubic rami.

IX. Synovial osteochondromatosis: multiple uniform size juxta-articular chondroid bodies, joint erosions, and scalloped femoral head may be seen on radiographs.

X. Tumors:

A. Simple bone cyst: plain radiograph shows well-defined centrally located lucent lesions with sclerotic margins. The endosteum appears thin without disruption of the cortex. Osseous septa may be seen as pseudotrabeculations on plain radiograph. Fracture in this setting appears as bony fragment in the cyst.

B. Fibrous dysplasia: plain radiograph shows ground-glass matrix and well-delineated lesions, and lucent or sclerotic margins (rind sign) may be present.

C. Osteochondroma: sessile or pedunculated lesion located in the metaphyseal area with an ossified core and a cartilage cap.

D. Chondrosarcoma: plain radiograph shows lytic lesions with intralesional calcifications, endosteal scalloping, cortical remodeling, thickening, and periosteal reaction.

E. Osteoid osteoma: small well-circumscribed and sclerotic lesion.

F. Osteosarcoma: radiograph shows evidence of medullary and cortical bone destruction, Codman's triangle, lamellated reaction (onion skin), wide zone of transition (moth-eaten appearance), remarkable periosteal reaction, sunburst appearance, and cloudlike chondroid lesions.

Computed Tomography

I. CT is performed in acute settings, after plain radiograph, especially where there is high suspicion of a fracture. It has high accuracy in characterizing matrix calcifications (bone tumors) and acute fractures.

II. It may be obtained with or without contrast. It is useful in radiographic-guided procedures (percutaneous instrumentation, bone and soft-tissue biopsy and aspiration procedures, and closed reduction of dislocations) and preoperative planning.

III. Radiation risk limits its use. CT is of minimal concern to claustrophobic patients and does not discriminate against patients with metallic implants, pacemakers, and the use of life-support equipment compared to MRI.

IV. 3D reconstruction of CT images offer effective characterization of location and extent of FAI deformities, acting as preoperative guide for proper bone resection.

V. Dual-energy CT (DECT): scans an area of the body at two different energies. It is useful in differentiating materials with similar densities (e.g., bone and iodine) and precise in differentiating soft-tissue masses.

VI. CT patterns of pathologic and developmental conditions:

A. Developmental conditions affecting bones of the hip are evaluated by CT; femoral and acetabular versions; FAIS.

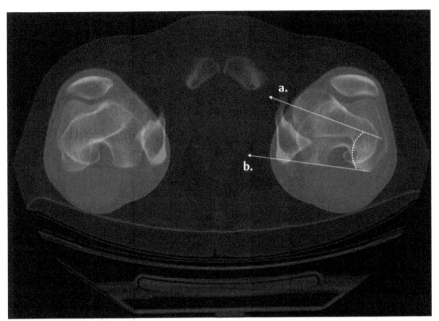

Fig. 4.4 Femoral version on axial CT. Femoral anteversion is performed by measuring the angle formed between the long axis of the femoral neck (**a**) and a line parallel to the dorsal aspect of the femoral condyles (**b**). Femoral anteversion is performed by measuring the angle formed between the long axis of the femoral neck and a line parallel to the dorsal aspect of the femoral condyles.

1. Femoral version: measured as the relationship of the axis of the femoral neck to the transcondylar axis of the distal femur. Normal values of anteversion are 5 to 25 degrees (**Fig. 4.4**).[17]

   a. Anteversion: femoral neck axis is oriented anteriorly in relation to the transcondylar femoral axis at the level of the knee. Values are 30 to 40 degrees at birth and 8 to 14 degrees in adults.[18] Females have a slightly higher femoral anteversion than males.[19] It is increased in DDH and FAI.

   b. Retroversion: femoral neck axis is oriented posteriorly and in relation to the transcondylar femoral axis at the level of the knee.

2. Acetabular version: measured as the angle between a line joining the anterior and posterior edges of the acetabulum and a line perpendicular to the line joining the posterior acetabular edges. Normal acetabulum is anteverted between 15 and 20 degrees; retroversion is defined by an angle less than 15 degrees (**Fig. 4.5**).[20]

3. FAI syndrome: 3D CT can provide better assessment of pincer and cam deformities. Femoral neck deformities (femoral retroversion and coxa vara) are reliably evaluated on the axial CT view of the neck.

B. Bone tumors: CT provides detailed assessment of bone tumors, especially matrix calcifications; chondroid calcification (punctate popcorn pattern on CT), osteoid mineralization, fibrous calcification (ground-glass-like appearance), nidus (osteoid osteoma). It is effective for evaluating cortical destruction by metastatic lesions.

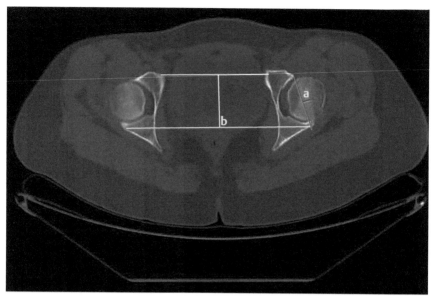

Fig. 4.5 Acetabular version measured as the angle between **(a)** a line joining the anterior and posterior edges of the acetabulum and **(b)** a line perpendicular to the line joining the posterior acetabular edges.

    C. Osteoarthritis: CT reveals joint space narrowing, subchondral cysts and sclerosis, and osteophyte formation.

    D. Fractures:

        1. Acetabular fractures. Axial CT and 3D reconstructed images provide excellent visualization of acetabular fractures.

            a. Anterior column fracture: on CT, superior pubic ramus is seen entering the inferior portion of the acetabulum.

            b. Posterior column fracture: displaced fracture appears to be separating the posterior column from the sciatic buttress.

            c. Anterior wall: fracture involves the anterior acetabular rim with no involvement of the anterior column.

            d. Both columns: iliopectineal and ilioischial lines appear disrupted. The spur sign (posterior displacement of the sciatic buttress of iliac wing fragment) is pathognomonic. Sciatic buttress appears separate from the acetabular roof.

            e. T-shaped fracture: obturator ring, and iliopectineal and ilioischial line disruption. The transverse component of the fracture is sagittally oriented and is medial and superior in relation to the acetabulum.

            f. Transverse fracture: fracture is best visualized on 3D reconstructed image. It has three forms: transtectal fracture (medial displacement of the femoral head and fracture fragment; juxtatectal fracture (fragment traverses inferior to the weight-bearing acetabular dome, at the junction of the articular surface and the cotyloid fossa; and infratectal fractures (fragment traverses the cotyloid fossa and the anterior and posterior horns of the acetabular articular surface).[21]

2. Stress fractures: CT and, to a greater extent, MRI, are highly sensitive in detecting stress fractures or stress reactions. Imaging shows sclerosis, new bone formation, periosteal reaction, and/or fracture line propagation.

Magnetic Resonance Imaging

I.   MRI provides excellent soft-tissue contrast and detailed evaluation of articular and physeal cartilage, synovium, subchondral bone. There is no risk of radiation as observed with CT. Multiplanar images of structures surrounding the hip can be obtained.

II.   Nonferromagnetic implants (e.g., titanium) permit better imaging.

III.   It is expensive and provides lower osseous detail than CT; claustrophobic patients may require be sedation.

IV.   Special indications and patterns of pathologic disorders:

A.   Labral tear: study reveals paralabral cysts, advanced cartilage lesions, and mucoid or cystic degeneration on T2. MRA has superior accuracy than MRI.

B.   Tumors: MRI provides distinction between reactive bone edema from tumor extension in malignancy and quantifies degree of tumor necrosis.

C.   Avascular necrosis: MRI is the most sensitive study (71–100%) for AVN. [22] Findings include areas of low intensities (edema) surrounded by hyperintense areas (blood). The "double line sign" seen on T2 is pathognomonic for AVN: hyperintense inner line between normal marrow and ischemic marrow.[22]

D.   SCFE: study reveals high signal in epiphysis and metaphysis with joint effusion on short tau inversion recovery (STIR). T1 shows metaphyseal displacement.

E.   Cartilage injuries and disorders: focal or global areas of degeneration and cartilage loss.

F.   Synovial proliferative disorders:

1.   Synovial chondromatosis: synovial thickening with intermediate-signal cartilaginous bodies and low-signal calcified bodies.

2.   Pigmented villonodular synovitis: low-signal hemosiderin deposits on T1- and T2-weighted images.

G.   Contraindications:

1.   Implanted hearing aid.

2.   Heart pacemakers.

3.   Insulin pumps.

4.   Neurostimulators.

5.   Intracranial metal clips or implants.

6.   Metallic bodies in the eye.

Magnetic Resonance Arthrography

I.   Imaging provides excellent diagnosis of labral tears.

II.   It is minimally invasive compared to arthroscopy.

III.   The procedure is carried out using diluted intra-articular gadolinium injection (0.0025 mmol/mL) with adequate joint distension and allows proper assessment of the labrum on fat-saturated T1 sequences.

IV.   Findings in labral tears include longitudinal, bucket handle tear patterns, labral detachment, and cartilage delamination.

Ultrasound

I.   Ultrasonography diagnoses tendonitis, bursitis, identifying joint effusions and functional causes of hip pain.

II.   It is especially useful for safely and accurately performing imaging-guided injections and aspirations around the hip.

III.   It is a subjective examination and accuracy depends on the dexterity of the sonographer. There is limited to soft-tissue diagnosis.

IV.   DDH: In infants (<6 months), ultrasound is the test of choice due to nonossified proximal femoral epiphysis.

V.   Ultrasonographic acetabular alpha angle is used in the assessment of DDH. It is formed between the acetabular roof and the vertical cortex of the ilium and thus reflects the depth of the bony acetabular roof. This is a similar measurement to the acetabular angle. Normal value is ≥60 degrees. A value less than 60 degrees suggests dysplasia of the acetabulum.[23]

Bone Scintigraphy

I.   It involves the use of small amounts of nontoxic, radioactive materials (e.g., technetium-99), usually injected into the bloodstream, inhaled, or swallowed.

II.   It identifies areas of active osteoblastic activity and localizes infections.

III.   Bone scan can detect early stress fracture not visualized on plain radiographs.[24]

References

1.   Uemura K, Atkins PR, Anderson AE, Aoki SK. Do Your Routine Radiographs to Diagnose Cam Femoroacetabular Impingement Visualize the Region of the Femoral Head-Neck Junction You Intended? Arthroscopy 2019;35(6):1796–1806
2.   Clohisy JC, Carlisle JC, Beaulé PE, et al. A systematic approach to the plain radiographic evaluation of the young adult hip. J Bone Joint Surg Am 2008;90(Suppl 4):47–66
3.   Lim SJ, Park YS. Plain Radiography of the Hip: A Review of Radiographic Techniques and Image Features. Hip Pelvis 2015;27(3):125–134
4.   Siebenrock KA, Kalbermatten DF, Ganz R. Effect of pelvic tilt on acetabular retroversion: a study of pelves from cadavers. Clin Orthop Relat Res 2003; (407):241–248
5.   Courtney PM, Melnic CM, Howard M, Makani A, Sheth NP. A Systematic Approach to Evaluating Hip Radiographs–A Focus on Osteoarthritis. J Orthop Rheumatol 2014;2(1):7
6.   Alton TB, Gee AO. Classifications in brief: young and burgess classification of pelvic ring injuries. Clin Orthop Relat Res 2014;472(8):2338–2342
7.   Cabarrus MC, Ambekar A, Lu Y, Link TM. MRI and CT of insufficiency fractures of the pelvis and the proximal femur. AJR Am J Roentgenol 2008;191(4):995–1001
8.   Mandell JC, Marshall RA, Weaver MJ, Harris MB, Sodickson AD, Khurana B. Traumatic Hip Dislocation: What the Orthopedic Surgeon Wants to Know. Radiographics 2017;37(7):2181–2201
9.   Kazley JM, Banerjee S, Abousayed MM, Rosenbaum AJ. Classifications in Brief: Garden Classification of Femoral Neck Fractures. Clin Orthop Relat Res 2018;476(2):441–445
10.   Chadayammuri V, Garabekyan T, Jesse MK, et al. Measurement of lateral acetabular coverage: a comparison between CT and plain radiography. J Hip Preserv Surg 2015;2(4):392–400

11. Barrientos C, Barahona M, Diaz J, Brañes J, Chaparro F, Hinzpeter J. Is there a patho-logical alpha angle for hip impingement? A diagnostic test study. J Hip Preserv Surg 2016;3(3):223–228

12. Beck EC, Nwachukwu BU, Chahla J, et al. Patients With Borderline Hip Dysplasia Achieve Clinically Significant Outcome After Arthroscopic Femoroacetabular Impingement Surgery: A Case-Control Study With Minimum 2-Year Follow-up. Am J Sports Med 2019;47(11):2636–2645

13. Byrd JW, Jones KS. Hip arthroscopy in the presence of dysplasia. Arthroscopy 2003;19(10):1055–1060

14. Tins BJ, Garton M, Cassar-Pullicino VN, Tyrrell PN, Lalam R, Singh J. Stress fracture of the pelvis and lower limbs including atypical femoral fractures-a review. Insights Imaging 2015;6(1):97–110

15. Ruiz Santiago F, Santiago Chinchilla A, Ansari A, et al. Imaging of Hip Pain: From Radiography to Cross-Sectional Imaging Techniques. Radiol Res Pract 2016;2016:6369237

16. Jawad MU, Haleem AA, Scully SP. In brief: Ficat classification: avascular necrosis of the femoral head. Clin Orthop Relat Res 2012;470(9):2636–2639

17. Hetsroni I, Dela Torre K, Duke G, Lyman S, Kelly BT. Sex differences of hip morphology in young adults with hip pain and labral tears. Arthroscopy 2013;29(1):54–63

18. Fabry G, MacEwen GD, Shands AR Jr. Torsion of the femur. A follow-up study in normal and abnormal conditions. J Bone Joint Surg Am 1973;55(8):1726–1738

19. Kate BR. Anteversion versus torsion of the femoral neck. Acta Anat (Basel) 1976;94(3):457–463

20. Maheshwari AV, Zlowodzki MP, Siram G, Jain AK. Femoral neck anteversion, acetabular anteversion and combined anteversion in the normal Indian adult population: A computed tomographic study. Indian J Orthop 2010;44(3):277–282

21. Bogdan Y, Dwivedi S, Tornetta P III. A surgical approach algorithm for transverse posterior wall fractures aids in reduction quality. Clin Orthop Relat Res 2014;472(11):3338–3344

22. Pierce TP, Jauregui JJ, Cherian JJ, Elmallah RK, Mont MA. Imaging evaluation of patients with osteonecrosis of the femoral head. Curr Rev Musculoskelet Med 2015;8(3):221–227

23. Graf R. The diagnosis of congenital hip-joint dislocation by the ultrasonic Combound treatment. Arch Orthop Trauma Surg 1980;97(2):117–133

24. Shammas A. Nuclear medicine imaging of the pediatric musculoskeletal system. Semin Musculoskelet Radiol 2009;13(3):159–180

Suggested Readings

Abd Elatif Drar HAE, Abd Elmoneim Dessouky Mohammed B, Abd Elaziz Mohammed Ali Z. The role of MRI in the evaluation of painful hip joint (MRI of hip joint). International Journal of Medical Imaging 2014;2(3):77–82

Byrd TJW, Bedi A, Stubbs AJ. The Hip: AANA Advanced Arthroscopic Surgical Techniques. Thorofare, NJ: SLACK Inc.; 2015

Herring JA, Kim HT, Browne R. Legg-Calve-Perthes disease. Part I: classification of radiographs with use of the modified lateral pillar and Stulberg classifications. J Bone Joint Surg Am 2004;86(10):2103–2120

Santiago FR, Santiago Chinchilla A, Ansari A, et al. Imaging of hip pain: from radiography to cross-sectional imaging techniques. Radiology Research and Practice 2016;2016:6369237

Tannast M, Siebenrock KA, Anderson SE. Femoroacetabular impingement: radiographic diagnosis: what the radiologist should know. AJR Am J Roentgenol 2007;188(6):1540–1552

Tönnis D. Normal values of the hip joint for the evaluation of X-rays in children and adults. Clin Orthop Relat Res 1976;(119):39–47

Weber AE, Jacobson JA, Bedi A. A review of imaging modalities for the hip. Curr Rev Musculoskelet Med 2013;6(3):226–234

5 Hip Biomechanics

Brian R. Waterman, Kyle Kunze, Edward C. Beck, Kyleen Jan, Shane J. Nho

General Considerations

Functional Anatomy

The hip joint is a multiaxial ball-and-socket joint that provides support and balance to the upper body during stance and gait. Soft tissues and osseous structures of the hip contribute to the equilibrium of forces that provide controlled hip motion.

I.   Stability of hip joint is provided by the articular surfaces of the acetabulum and the head of the femur alongside the ligaments, capsule, and labrum.

II. Hip joint orientation: the neck of the femur is angulated in the sagittal and coronal planes in relation to the shaft.

A. The femoral neck shaft angle is formed by the femoral shaft axis and a line drawn along the axis of the femoral neck through the center of the head of the femur. Normal angle is 120 to 135 degrees in adults, and can be 20 to 25 degrees greater at birth.[1]

B. The femoral anteversion is the orientation of the neck in relation to femoral condyles. Normal angle is 30 to 40 degrees at birth and 8 to 14 degrees in adults.[2]

III. Long axis of the acetabulum is directed forward, and has 15 to 20 degrees of anteversion with 45-degree inferior inclination.[3]

IV. Upper body weight is transmitted to the lower limb through the sacroiliac (SI) joint.

V.   The narrower femoral neck in relation to the head aids mobility of the lower limb.

Hip Joint Motions

There is high degree of congruency of the articulating surfaces. Motion between the femoral head and the acetabulum is mostly rotational with minimal or no translation. The pelvis contributes to the hip joint motion to (**Table 5.1**).[4]

I.   Normally, the hip joint moves an average of 120-degree flexion and 15-degree extension. In a position of 90 degrees and neutral adduction, internal rotation (FADIR) ranges from 30 to 40 degrees. External rotation ranges from 40 to 60 degrees. Normal hip abduction and adduction are 30 to 50 degrees and 20 to 30 degrees, respectively.[5]

II. Hip flexion is limited by the iliofemoral ligament, anterior capsule, and hip flexors. Hip extension puts soft-tissue structures of the hip under tension and limits internal and external rotation.

III. **Pelvic Motions**

A. Anterior pelvic rotation: it includes anterior movement of superior pelvis with the iliac crest tilting forward in a sagittal plane.

Table 5.1 Pelvic motion.

Pelvic motion	Left hip motion	Right hip motion
Anterior rotation	Flexion	Flexion
Posterior rotation	Extension	Extension
Right lateral rotation	Abduction	Adduction
Left lateral rotation	Adduction	Abduction
Right transverse rotation	External rotation	Internal rotation
Left transverse rotation	Internal rotation	External rotation

B. Posterior pelvic rotation: the superior pelvis moves backward and the iliac crest tilt backward in a sagittal plane.

C. Left lateral pelvic rotation: the left pelvis moves distally in relation to the right pelvis in the frontal plane and rotates downward.

D. Right lateral pelvic rotation: the right pelvis moves inferiorly in relation to the left pelvis in the frontal plane and rotates downward.

E. Left transverse pelvic rotation: in the horizontal plane, the pelvis rotates to the left; the right iliac crest moves anteriorly in relation to the left iliac crest; the iliac crest moves posteriorly.

F. Right transverse pelvic rotation: in the horizontal plane, the pelvis rotates to the body's right; the left iliac crest moves anteriorly in relation to the right iliac crest, which moves posteriorly.

IV. **Intrapelvic Motions**

There are three classes of intrapelvic motions:

A. Posteroanterior and anteroposterior rotations of the ilia in relation to the sacrum and the pubis.

B. Sacral movement in relation to the ilia. The SI motion occurs superiorly, inferiorly, anteriorly, and posteriorly, and axial rotation occurs about a transverse axis.

C. The sitting–standing changes that affect the relationship of the movement of the ilia in relation to each other and the sacrum.

Hip–Spine Kinematics

I. Flexion of the lumbar spine to 45 degrees relies on lumbar muscle activity, while flexion greater than 45 degrees requires pelvic rotation.[6] The spine contributes greatly to early stage of hip flexion and extension. Lateral flexion of the lumbar spine elicits ipsilateral hip abduction; contralateral hip adduction while twisting movement of the trunk is contributed mostly by the hip.

Lower Limb Axis

I. Mechanical axis of the femur: this is assessed by a line passing from the center of the femoral head to the center of the tibial plafond of the ankle joint. Normal is 3 degrees to the vertical axis.[7]

II. Anatomic axis of femur: this is assessed by a line drawn from the piriformis fossa to the center of the knee joint. It depends on the length of the femur; it increased in shorter femurs and decreased in longer femurs. Normal is 6° from mechanical axis and 9° from the vertical axis.

Gait

Normal gait is characterized by rhythmic, alternating propulsive, and retropulsive motions of the lower limbs. It comprises of double- and single-leg support patterns.

I. Gait cycle classification: gait cycle is a repetitive process that begins from heel strike to heel strike of a limb and includes the stance and swing phases.

A. Initial contact.

B. Loading response.

C. Mid-stance.

D. Terminal stance.

E. Preswing.

F. Initial swing.

G. Mid-swing.

H. Late swing.

II. Gait phases:

A. Stance phase: it begins with heel strike (the heel makes initial contact with the ground without the toes), followed by foot flat, mid-stance, and progresses to heel-off (terminal stance). The toe-off phase (propulsive phase) begins after the termination of the heel-off. This marks the end of the stance phase. The hip is adducted and internally rotated; the center of gravity is closer in line with the hip joint. This phase lasts approximately 60% of normal gait duration.[8]

B. Swing phase: the swing phase is between the toe-off phase and the heel strike phase. It begins right after the stance phase. In this phase, the hip is abducted and externally rotated. It makes up 40% of the normal gait cycle.[9] The pelvis rotates forward in the horizontal plane to about 8 degrees in the swing phase. Acceleration and deceleration phases are observed in the swing phase.

1. The acceleration phase extends from toe-off to mid-swing. The swing leg makes an accelerated forward movement that propels the body weight forward.

2. The deceleration phase extends from mid-swing to heel strike. It decreases the velocity of the forward body movement.

III. Gait cycle phases (**Table 5.2**):

A. Heel strike: it is the initial contact of a limb in motion. In this phase, the knee is in full extension with the hip slightly flexed to about 30 degrees.[10] The ankle goes from the neutral position to plantar flexion.

B. Foot flat: the foot is pronated with slight ankle plantar flexion, the hip is extended, and the knee is flexed to about 20 degrees.[10]

Table 5.2 Eight phases of the gait cycle

Phase of gait	Hip position	Muscles involved	Cycle duration (%)
Stance			
Initial contact	30-degree flexion	Gluteus maximus and hamstrings	0–2
Loading response	30-degree flexion, 5- to 10-degree adduction, 5- to 10-degree internal rotation	Hamstrings and gluteus maximus	0–10
Mid-stance	Neutral flexion–extension, neutral abduction–adduction	Gluteus medius, gluteus minimus, and tensor fascia lata	10–30
Terminal stance	10-degree extension	Iliacus	30–50
Preswing	0 degrees of flexion–extension	Iliacus and adductor longus	50–60
Swing			
Initial swing	20-degree flexion, 5-degree abduction	Rectus femoris, iliopsoas, gracilis, and sartorius	60–73
Mid-swing	20- to 30-degree flexion	Gracilis, iliopsoas, and sartorius	73–87
Terminal swing	30-degree flexion	Hamstrings and gluteus maximus	87–100

C. Mid-stance: In this phase, the body is supported on one leg. The hip moves from minimal flexion to extension, the knee returns from maximal flexion to extension, and the ankle is supinated and dorsiflexed. The body moves from force absorption at impact to force propulsion forward.

D. Heel-off: The heel leaves the floor and the body weight is dispersed over the metatarsal heads. The hip goes into hyperextension, and then flexion. The knee undergoes flexion followed by ankle supination and plantar flexion.

E. Toe-off: In this phase, the knee is flexed, the ankle undergoes plantar flexion, and the toe leaves the ground.

F. Early swing: The hip is slightly extended to 10 degrees, then 20-degree flexion with lateral rotation of the hip; the knee flexes to about 60 degrees; the ankle undergoes plantar flexion to dorsiflexion and then ends in the neutral position.[10]

G. Mid-swing: The hip is flexed to about 30 degrees, the ankle undergoes dorsiflexion, and the knee flexes to 60 degrees with 30-degree extension.

H. Late swing: In this phase, the hip undergoes 30-degree flexion, the knee is extended, and the ankle ends in the neutral position.

IV. Run cycle: This cycle is short with high ground reaction force and high velocity. There is just one stance phase in the run cycle. The float phase (feet off the ground) duration is increased.

Hip Joint Forces and Equilibrium

I. Static hip loading:

   A. The weight of the body, during standing, is borne on the legs, while the center of gravity is projected to the midline and force exerted on both hips.

   B. The weight of the body to the knees is borne equally on the femoral heads, and the resultant vectors are vertical.

   C. Little or no muscular force is required to maintain equilibrium.

II. Dynamic hip loading:

   A. Single-leg stance: Single-leg stance accounts for 60% of the gait cycle.[9] Three times the body weight is transmitted to the joint.

      1. Lower limb constitutes two-sixths of the body weight and the upper limbs and trunk constitute four-sixths of the body weight. In the single-leg stance, the stance leg carries five-sixths of total body weight. The effective center of gravity shifts distally and away from the supporting leg to produce a downward force that tilts the pelvis. The nonsupporting leg adds to the total body weight during the single-leg stance.

      2. The distally directed force exerts turning motion around the center of the femoral head on the stance leg. The body weight (K) provides the moment of the turning motion and the distance from the femur to the center of gravity forms the moment arm (a).

      3. The abductors of the supporting leg exert downward counterbalancing force with the hip joint acting as a fulcrum.

      4. Force exerted by the abductor muscles creates a moment around the center of the femoral head.

      5. The hip joint reaction force (JRF) is the total force generated within the hip joint in response to forces acting across the hip joint (**Fig. 5.1**).

         a. The JRF is determined by the body weight and the abductor force. It maintains the pelvis in equilibrium.

         b. The JRF is increased in slow gait, due to increased abduction force required to maintain the pelvis in equilibrium during stride.[11]

         c. The magnitude of JRF varies depending on the activity

            i. JRF is three times the weight of the body in the single-leg stance.

            ii. JRF is five times the body weight during walking and stair ascent.

            iii. JRF is 10 times the weight of the body while running.

         d. The JRF is reduced by deepening the acetabulum to centralize the femoral head, increasing the neck length and subsequent lateral reattachment of the trochanter.

      6. The magnitude and direction of the compressive forces are determined by the lever arm ratio (i.e., ratio between the weight of body moment arm and the abductor muscle moment arm) and the position of the center of gravity. Increasing the lever arm ratio also increases the abductor muscle force required for gait.

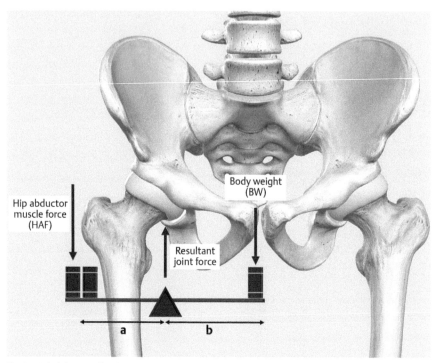

Fig. 5.1 Hip joint reaction force.

7. Variations in the osseous structures determine the magnitude of forces acting across the hip joints.[12]

   a. Individuals with short femoral neck have increased abductor demand and joint loading.

   b. Individuals with a wide pelvis structure have increased hip joint forces.

   c. Shortened lever arm that overpowers the abductors predisposes to a Trendelenburg gait or gluteal lurch.

8. The magnitude of the forces acting at the hip during walk is biphasic. The force across the acetabulum peaks at heel strike and at terminal stance of the gait cycle.

References

1. Daldrup-Link HE, Gooding CA. Essentials of Pediatric Radiology. Cambridge University Press; 2010
2. Fabry G, MacEwen GD, Shands AR Jr. Torsion of the femur. A follow-up study in normal and abnormal conditions. J Bone Joint Surg Am 1973;55(8):1726–1738
3. Wang RY, Xu WH, Kong XC, Yang L, Yang SH. Measurement of acetabular inclination and anteversion via CT generated 3D pelvic model. BMC Musculoskelet Disord 2017;18(1):373
4. Lewis CL, Laudicina NM, Khuu A, Loverro KL. The Human Pelvis: Variation in Structure and Function During Gait. Anat Rec (Hoboken) 2017;300(4):633–642
5. Roaas A, Andersson GB. Normal range of motion of the hip, knee and ankle joints in male subjects, 30-40 years of age. Acta Orthop Scand 1982;53(2):205–208

6. Lee SY. Muscle activities of the rectus abdominis and rectus femoris and their ratio during leg raises performed by healthy adults. J Phys Ther Sci 2015;27(3):549–550

7. Cherian JJ, Kapadia BH, Banerjee S, Jauregui JJ, Issa K, Mont MA. Mechanical, Anatomical, and Kinematic Axis in TKA: Concepts and Practical Applications. Curr Rev Musculoskelet Med 2014;7(2):89–95

8. Pirker W, Katzenschlager R. Gait disorders in adults and the elderly : A clinical guide. Wien Klin Wochenschr 2017;129(3-4):81–95

9. Umberger BR. Stance and swing phase costs in human walking. J R Soc Interface 2010;7(50):1329–1340

10. Shultz SJ, Houglum PA, Perrin DH. Examination of musculoskeletal injuries. 2nd ed. Champaign, IL: 2005

11. Giarmatzis G, Jonkers I, Wesseling M, Van Rossom S, Verschueren S. Loading of Hip Measured by Hip Contact Forces at Different Speeds of Walking and Running. J Bone Miner Res 2015;30(8):1431–1440

12. Byrne DP, Mulhall KJ, Baker JF. Anatomy & Biomechanics of the Hip. The Open Sports Medicine Journal 2010;4(1):51–57

Suggested Readings

Bowman KF, Fox J, Sekiya JK. A clinically relevant review of hip biomechanics. Arthroscopy 2010;26(8):1118–1129

Byrne DP, Mulhall KJ, Baker JF. Anatomy & biomechanics of the hip. The Open Sports Medicine Journal 2010;4:51–57

Polkowski GG, Clohisy JC. Hip biomechanics. Sports Med Arthrosc Rev 2010;18(2):56–62

6 Hip Pathomechanics

Brian R. Waterman, Edward C. Beck, Kyle Kunze, Gift Echefu, Shane J. Nho

General Considerations

I.   Alterations of bony structures of the hip (femoroacetabular impingement, hip dysplasia) alter the equilibrium of forces and contact areas of the articular surfaces resulting in instability.[1] Joint contact pressures are significantly increased in abnormal osseous morphology and dysplastic conditions, causing early onset hip osteoarthritis.[2,3]

II. Neck deformities:

A.   Coxa valga: the neck shaft angle is increased (normal value: 125 degrees; valgus > 135 degrees) on imaging.[4] As greater trochanter migrates distally, the abductor moment arm is increased with resultant increase in the joint reaction force.

B.   Coxa valga: the neck shaft angle is decreased (<120 degrees), the greater trochanter is at a higher level, and the abductor lever arm is reduced with resultant reduction in joint reaction force.[4]

C.   Femoral torsion: normal value is 10- to 15-degree anteversion in adults. Retroversion or anteversion greater than 15 degrees may result in changes in the position of the femoral head within the acetabulum, which may precipitate hip joint instability. Anteversion greater than 15 degrees results in greater internal rotation.[4] In-toeing is a compensatory gait mechanism seen in individuals with excessive anteversion, while out-toeing compensates for retroversion.

III. Pathomechanics and maneuvers of lower limb disorders:

A.   Weight gain increases the total compressive forces applied to the hip joint. Abductor muscle forces increase in reaction to the increased body weight. The increase in the joint reaction force may contribute to joint degeneration along with other factors.

B.   Limping reduces hip joint load by bringing the center of gravity closer to the moment arm of the femoral head. Limping entails lateral acceleration of body mass, deceleration during stance phase, and subsequent acceleration back to midline. Energy expenditure is increased and movement is less efficient.

C.   Cane walking: the abductor muscles and walking cane together produce a moment that is equal to the moment of the body weight. Cane reduces the joint force reaction because the cane–ground reaction force acts at a much larger distance from the center of the hip.

IV. Pathomechanic patterns of structural hip disorders:

A.   Hip dysplasia: individuals with hip dysplasia experience limitation in hip extension during walking, reduced net activity of the hip flexors in preswing phase, and compensatory increase in pelvic excursion.

B.   Femoroacetabular impingement (FAIS): limitations in all planes of motion. Individuals with symptomatic FAIS have diminished squat depth, external moments during hip flexion and external rotation, hip abduction, and pelvic frontal plane motion during the swing phase of walking. Abductor moment arm is reduced and joint reaction force is increased.[5,6]

V. Hip–spine syndrome: This refers to hip pathology in the setting of degenerative disease of the spine. Individuals with hip pathology show increased lumbar lordosis and sloping of the sacrum. Flexion contracture of the hip results in pelvic rotation and increases lumbar lordosis, consequently increasing loading of the lumbar facets and ligaments.[7] Individuals with unilateral degenerative disease of the hip have increased bend of the lumbar spine on the side of the joint disease and increased movement in the sagittal plane with decreased coronal plane movement.[8] Osseous deformities and soft-tissue pathology of the hip that limit hip motion can also increase compensatory lumbopelvic motion.[9]

VI. Gait pathomechanics: abnormal gait patterns may be adopted in compensation for injury to the lower extremity.

A. Osteoarthritis: individuals show loss of hip range of motion during gait and sagittal plane reversal motion as the hip goes into extension. The muscle force output is reduced and the hip joint reaction force is increased.

B. Hip contracture: individuals flex the hip during the stance phase, with marked posterior pelvic tilt and reduced stride length.

C. Hip abductor weakness: During the one-leg stance, gluteal muscles normally abduct the contralateral limb, preventing the pelvis from tipping toward the swing leg. Injury to the superior gluteal or obturator nerves results in weakness of the abductor muscles. Weak gluteus medius is unable to stabilize the unaffected pelvis. During the stance phase, the trunk leans over the affected side, while the unaffected pelvis drops. This is clinically seen as the Trendelenburg sign (see **Fig. 2.1**).

D. Antalgic gait: a compensatory gait pattern reflective of intra-articular or extra-articular hip pain. The duration of the stance phase is reduced in the affected limb with decrease in the swing phase of the unaffected limb. Body weight is shifted laterally to the unaffected limb.

E. Hamstring weakness: Hamstring muscles function normally to slow down the swing phase. Weakness causes the knee to snap into extension during the swing phase.

F. Gluteus maximus gait: the trunk leans backward during early stance phase; the center of gravity shift posterior to the hip to reduce demand on the hip extensors.

G. Psoatic gait: psoatic limp in patients with the Legg–Calvés–Perthes disease may be caused by weakness or reflex inhibition of the psoas major muscle. The affected leg moves in external rotation, flexion, and adduction. The limp may be accompanied by exaggerated trunk and pelvic movement.

H. Weak hip flexors: the lower extremity is unable to shorten for proper foot clearance off the floor; the unaffected pelvis rises during the swing phase elongating the limb to provide extra clearance for the affected leg.

I. Leg length discrepancy results in compensatory tilting of the pelvis to the shorter limb.

J. Scissors gait is the abnormal gait from hip adductor spasticity. During the swing phase, the trunk leans over the stance leg.

References

1. Yeung M, Memon M, Simunovic N, Belzile E, Philippon MJ, Ayeni OR. Gross Instability After Hip Arthroscopy: An Analysis of Case Reports Evaluating Surgical and Patient Factors. Arthroscopy 2016;32(6):1196–1204.e1

2. Buckwalter JA, Anderson DD, Brown TD, Tochigi Y, Martin JA. The Roles of Mechanical Stresses in the Pathogenesis of Osteoarthritis: Implications for Treatment of Joint Injuries. Cartilage 2013;4(4):286–294

3. Ferguson SJ, Bryant JT, Ganz R, Ito K. The influence of the acetabular labrum on hip joint cartilage consolidation: a poroelastic finite element model. J Biomech 2000;33(8):953–960

4. Yochum TR, Rowe LJ. Essentials of Skeletal Radiology. Lippincott Williams & Wilkins; 2004

5. Ng KC, Lamontagne M, Labrosse MR, Beaulé PE. Hip Joint Stresses Due to Cam-Type Femoroacetabular Impingement: A Systematic Review of Finite Element Simulations. PLoS One 2016;11(1):e0147813

6. Samaan MA, Schwaiger BJ, Gallo MC, et al. Abnormal Joint Moment Distributions and Functional Performance During Sit-to-Stand in Femoroacetabular Impingement Patients. PM R 2017;9(6):563–570

7. Czaprowski D, Stoliński Ł, Tyrakowski M, Kozinoga M, Kotwicki T. Non-structural misalignments of body posture in the sagittal plane. Scoliosis Spinal Disord 2018;13:6

8. Thurston AJ. Spinal and pelvic kinematics in osteoarthrosis of the hip joint. Spine 1985;10(5):467–471

9. Saltzman BM, Louie PK, Clapp IM, et al. Assessment of Association Between Spino-Pelvic Parameters and Outcomes Following Gluteus Medius Repair. Arthroscopy 2019;35(4):1092–1098

Suggested Readings

Gotlib A. The hip joint: a manual of clinical biomechanics and pathomechanics. J Can Chiropr Assoc 1982;26(1):37–38

Grimaldi A, Mellor R, Hodges P, Bennell K, Wajswelner H, Vicenzino B. Gluteal tendinopathy: a review of mechanisms, assessment and management. Sports Med 2015;45(8):1107–1119

Redmond JM, Gupta A, Nasser R, Domb BG. The hip-spine connection: understanding its importance in the treatment of hip pathology. Orthopedics 2015;38(1):49–55

Sotirow B. [Biomechanics and pathomechanics of the hip joint in the sagittal plane]. Pol Orthop Traumatol 1981;46(4):374–379

7 Implant Biology

Brian R. Waterman, Edward C. Beck, Gift Echefu, Jahanzeb Kaikaus, Shane J. Nho

General Considerations

Cartilage Repair Biology

I. Biologic injections are indicated for focal and diffuse chondral disease of the hip.

   A. Hyaluronic acid (HA): intra-articular injection of HA reduces pain and inflammation.[1] HA binds to receptors on the cluster determinant 44 (CD44), intracellular adhesion molecule-1 (ICAM-1), and the receptor for hyaluronate-mediated motility (RHAMM) to effect anti-inflammatory and chondrogenic changes.

   B. Platelet-rich plasma (PRP): peripheral blood undergoes centrifugation to produce concentrated sample of platelets. Endogenous (calcium chloride) or exogenous activators cause the release of plasma contents (growth factors, proteins, and chemokines). These factors may promote healing, reduce pain, and suppress inflammation. However, preparation techniques and compositions vary widely, which may lead to the inconsistent efficacy observed in the literature.[2]

   C. Bone marrow concentrates (BMCs): mesenchymal stem cells (MSCs) are isolated from BMCs. MSCs are chondrogenic, anti-inflammatory, and very effective as early as the first few weeks. Use of stem cell therapy for hip osteoarthritis and chondral defects is still in its infancy, offering promising short term results.[3]

II. Microfracture: This is a single-step procedure used to treat chondral defect with full-thickness outer bridge grade 3 or 4 defect and no minimal evidence of osteoarthritis (Tonnis grade ≤ 1).[4] Small puncture holes are created at the site of the chondral damage deep enough to allow for bone marrow bleed through the holes, which promotes healing. Fibrin adhesive is used to secure the chondral flap if applicable.

III. Autologous chondrocyte transplantation (ACT): this is a two-stage cartilage repair procedure. Viable chondrocytes are extracted from an individual, cultured, and then implanted. Indications include chondral defects ≥ 3 cm^2 with focal, full-thickness outer bridge grade 3 or 4 defect and no minimal evidence of osteoarthritis (Tonnis grade ≤ 1).

IV. Autologous matrix-induced chondrocytes (AMIC) is a single-step procedure that recreates hyaline cartilage. Indications for AMIC are chondral defects ≥3cm^2 with focal, full-thickness outer bridge grade 3 or 4 defect and no minimal evidence of osteoarthritis (Tonnis grade ≤ 1).

V. Osteochondral graft: the indication is subchondral plate involvement >0.5 cm^2 thickness. The procedure includes surgical hip dislocation, femoral or acetabular lesion debridement completely exposing the subchondral bone, and finally the defect is packed with bone graft.

Implant Prosthesis

Hip implants for total hip arthroplasty consists of three parts: acetabular cup, femoral component, and the articular interface.

I.   Acetabular cup: the part that fits into the acetabulum. Cups come as one-piece shells (monobloc) or modular.

   A. One-piece shells: shells are either metal or ultra-high-molecular-weight poly-ethylene (UHMWPE). The metal cup is held in place by metal coating and UHM-WPE requires cement fixation.

   B. Modular cups consist of a metal shell and liner. The outer part of the shell has porous coating for friction fitting. Two types of porous coating; foam metal and sintered beads, form friction fittings, which are designed to mimic the trabec-ulae of cancellous bone. Implant stability is determined by insertion force, un-der-rimming, and bone growth into the porous coating.[5]

II. Femoral component: implant stem is fitted into the femur. The femoral head is attached to the stem. Stem fixation methods consist of cemented and uncemented fixations.

   A. Cemented stems use acrylic bone cement to form mantle between the bone and stem. In uncemented stems, fixation is achieved by bone remodeling around the implant.

   B. Femoral stems may be monolithic or modular. Modular components have vari-able head dimensions and neck orientations that permit variability in leg length, offset, and version.

III. Articular interface: it fits between the femoral head and the acetabular compo-nents. Interface size is determined by the outside diameter of the head or the in-side diameter of the socket.[5]

Hip Replacement Implant Materials

Implant materials may be metal, polyethylene, or ceramic. The type of material used depends on the activity level and age; all ceramic hip joint may be used for very active or relatively young patients.[6]

I.   Metal ball and metal liner: metal-on-metal bearings (stainless steel or cobalt chro-mium alloy) have potential for bone loss and inflammation and are now rarely used.[7]

II. Metal ball and polyethylene liners: the metal ball is made of cobalt chrome. Highly cross-linked polyethylene liners are more durable and superior to the earlier tra-ditional polyethylene liners.[8]

III. Ceramic balls and ceramic liners have more wear potential compared to ceramic balls and polyethylene liners.[9]

IV. Ceramic ball and polyethylene liner: ceramic heads are hard and have ultrasmooth surfaces, with less wear rates and superior scratch resistance.[9]

Types of Hip Implants and Fixation

I.   Fixed-bearing implants: the femoral stem is inserted into the shaft of the femur; a ball replaces the head of femur and a shell lines the acetabulum. Fixation is achieved by cement or by bone ingrowth (cementless fixation).

II.   Hybrid total hip implant: it consists of one component (cup or stem) fixed without cement, while the other component is fixed with cement.

III. Mobile-bearing total hip implant: it uses a mobile-bearing design that fits into the acetabular shell. This fitting system offers the hip joint two points of articulation. The liner is able to move in the fitted acetabular shell to provide multidirectional movement and increase range of motion (RoM).[10]

IV.   Total hip implant fixation (cemented or cementless): it may be either a cemented or a cementless fixation. Polymethyl methacrylate (PMMA) acrylic polymer is used in cemented fixation.

Hip Implant Biomechanics

Flexibility of hip implants depends on type of material and cross-sectional geometry. Implant stability is contributed by component design and alignment, soft-tissue function, and tension.

I.   RoM: it is influenced by the size of the head of the femur, position of the femur in relation to the pelvis, and the geometry of the stem taper, not by the individual's active or passive RoM. The true RoM is achieved by the orientation of the implant components. Occasionally, during motion the head of the femur impinges on the acetabulum. Repetitive impingement with daily activities culminates in subluxation or dislocation.

II.   Component orientation: improper component positioning reduces the effective jumping distance and directly affects implant wear, friction, and risk of dislocation. Anteversion greater than 15 degrees and cup inclination greater than 50 degrees often result in malpositioning in large metal on metal bearings. Shorter femoral prostheses have less lever arm: if joint reaction force is greater than the load capacity of the bone, the implant may migrate into varus orientation or result in calcar fracture.

Implant–Bone Interface Biology

Implant materials are modified to prevent damage to the surrounding cells. Implant-mediated periprosthetic osteolysis and aseptic loosening are complications of hip arthroplasty. UHMWPE, ceramics, and metals are materials used for gliding surfaces and they provide low friction. Constant artificial joint gliding culminates in periprosthetic osteolysis and debris from implants. Abnormal implant motion, wear-mediated osteolysis, and altered mechanical loading are predisposing factors to osteolysis.[11]

I.   Implant motion: abnormal implant motion as a result of inadequate fixation may lead to osteolysis or component migration.

II.   Altered mechanical loading: arthroplasty alters hip joint load distribution and direction. Femoral stem redistributes stress from the proximal femur to the diaphyseal cortex. This redistribution leads to stress shielding of proximal femur and bone resorption. Bone resorption often stabilizes, but may progress to loosening or osteolysis.

III. Wear-mediated osteolysis: the particulate debris generated by wear of the implant migrate into surrounding bone (effective joint space) and induce cellular response. Implant debris and cement particles are phagocytosed by body macrophages, inducing macrophage-mediated foreign body reaction in the surrounding tissues. This inflammatory response weakens the surrounding connective tissues and contributes to periprosthetic osteolysis.

References

1. Bowman S, Awad ME, Hamrick MW, Hunter M, Fulzele S. Recent advances in hyaluronic acid based therapy for osteoarthritis. Clin Transl Med 2018;7(1):6
2. Kuffler DP. Differing efficacies of autologous platelet-rich plasma treatment in reducing pain following rotator-cuff injury in a single patient. J Pain Res 2018;11:2239–2245
3. McIntyre JA, Jones IA, Han B, Vangsness CT Jr. Intra-articular Mesenchymal Stem Cell Therapy for the Human Joint: A Systematic Review. Am J Sports Med 2018;46(14):3550–3563
4. Domb BG, Gupta A, Dunne KF, Gui C, Chandrasekaran S, Lodhia P. Microfracture in the Hip: Results of a Matched-Cohort Controlled Study With 2-Year Follow-up. Am J Sports Med 2015;43(8):1865–1874
5. Michel A, Bosc R, Meningaud JP, Hernigou P, Haiat G. Assessing the Acetabular Cup Implant Primary Stability by Impact Analyses: A Cadaveric Study. PLoS One 2016;11(11):e0166778
6. Jeffers JR, Walter WL. Ceramic-on-ceramic bearings in hip arthroplasty: state of the art and the future. J Bone Joint Surg Br 2012;94(6):735–745
7. Silverman EJ, Ashley B, Sheth NP. Metal-on-metal total hip arthroplasty: is there still a role in 2016? Curr Rev Musculoskelet Med 2016;9(1):93–96
8. Kurtz SM, Gawel HA, Patel JD. History and systematic review of wear and osteolysis outcomes for first-generation highly crosslinked polyethylene. Clin Orthop Relat Res 2011;469(8):2262–2277
9. Wang S, Zhang S, Zhao Y. A comparison of polyethylene wear between cobalt-chrome ball heads and alumina ball heads after total hip arthroplasty: a 10-year follow-up. J Orthop Surg Res 2013;8:20
10. De Martino I, Triantafyllopoulos GK, Sculco PK, Sculco TP. Dual mobility cups in total hip arthroplasty. World J Orthop 2014;5(3):180–187
11. Abu-Amer Y, Darwech I, Clohisy JC. Aseptic loosening of total joint replacements: mechanisms underlying osteolysis and potential therapies. Arthritis Res Ther 2007;9(Suppl 1):S6

Suggested Readings

Chahla J, Lapradre RF, Mardones R, Huard J, Phillippon MJ, Mei-Dan O, Garirido CP. Biological therapies for cartilage lesions in the hip: a new horizon. Orthopedics 2016;39(4):e715–e723
Makhni EC, Stone AV, Ukwuani GC, et al. A critical review: management and surgical options for articular defects in the hip. Clin Sports Med 2017;36(3):573–586
Morlock MM, Bishop N, Huber G. Biomechanics of Hip Arthroplasty. In: Knahr K, eds. Tribology in Total Hip Arthroplasty. Berlin: Springer; 2011

8 Hip Instability

Brian R. Waterman, Kamran Movassaghi, Edward C. Beck, Gift Echefu, Shane J. Nho

Biomechanics

Hip Joint Stability

Hip joint stability is maintained by the relationship between the static osseous structures (acetabulum and the head of the femur), soft tissues (capsule, ligaments, and labrum) of the hip joint, and surrounding hip musculature.

I. Acetabulum:

    A. It approximately creates a hemisphere that allows approximately 170 degrees of femoral head coverage.[1]

    B. It is oriented with 40 to 45 degrees of lateral inclination and 18 to 21 degrees of anteversion allowing for greater posterior coverage.[2]

II. Proximal femur:

    A. The head is considered as two-thirds of a sphere, while the neck is inclined superiorly 130 degrees relative to shaft and 10 degrees anteverted relative to the femoral transcondylar axis.[3]

    B. The coxa valga and coxa anteversion are associated with hip instability.

III. Soft-tissue structures contribute the static and dynamic stabilizers of the hip.

    A. Static stabilizers: these are the labrum, capsuloligamentous complex (iliofemoral ligament, pubofemoral ligament, ischiofemoral ligament, zona orbicularis), and the ligamentum teres.

        1. Labrum:

            a. It is in continuity with the bony acetabular rim.

            b. It provides stability to the hip by increasing the acetabular volume by 20% and the acetabular surface area by 25%.[4]

            c. It increases the intra-articular negative hydrostatic fluid pressure, causing a "suction cup" effect.

            d. It more evenly distributes stresses placed on the hip.

        2. Capsuloligamentous complex:

            a. Iliofemoral ligament:

                i. It is the strongest ligament of the body.

                ii. It runs from the anteroinferior iliac spine to the femoral neck creating a fan-shaped "Y" at insertion proximally and distally along the intertrochanteric line; it takes a spiral trajectory across anterior side of the capsule.

                iii. It is taut in extension and external rotation and resists anterior translation.

b. Pubofemoral ligament:

i. It has its origination on the iliopectineal eminence of the superior pubic ramus, courses inferoposteriorly, and wraps under the femoral head; it blends with the ischiofemoral ligament with no bony femoral attachment.

ii. It limits external rotation in hip extension and hyperabduction.

c. Ischiofemoral ligament:

i. It has a broad triangular origin on the ischial acetabular margin and spirals superolaterally to insert at the base of the greater trochanter.

ii. It restricts internal rotation (in flexion and extension) and posterior translation.

d. Zona orbicularis:

i. This is formed by confluent fibers from the medial arms of the iliofemoral ligament and the pubofemoral ligament that run longitudinally in parallel with the femoral neck; it encircles the femoral neck creating the narrowest part of the capsule.

ii. It resists axial distraction; helical orientation of capsuloligamentous fibers creates "screw-home" effect when the hip is in extension.

e. Ligamentum teres:

i. It has a pyramidal shape and originates from the acetabular notch and inserts into the fovea capitis of the femur; it has a great length variability.

ii. It is taut in hip adduction, flexion, and external rotation; it the least stable position of the hip.

iii. Its role in hip stability is controversial.

B. Dynamic stabilizers: these include the iliopsoas, iliocapsularis, rectus femoris, gluteus minimus, and the gluteus medius. The iliocapsularis is the greatest contributor to hip stability in this group.

Etiology

Traumatic

I.   Pathomechanism:

High-impact trauma with can cause injury to the soft tissues and/or the osseous structures of the hip.

A. Posteriorly directed forces through the knee with hip flexed and in neutral adduction may result in pure hip dislocation, subluxation, or, more commonly, fracture-dislocation.

B. Anteriorly directed forces on externally rotated and extended hip can cause anterior hip instability.

C. Repetitive microtrauma is seen in sports requiring continuous hip joint rotation and axial loading.

Atraumatic

I. Pathomechanism:
   A. Repetitive hip joint rotation and axial loading in the setting of anatomic abnormalities of the hip result in damage to the soft-tissue stabilizers of the hip.
   B. Connective tissue disorders such as Ehler–Danlos syndrome, Marfan's syndrome, and osteogenesis imperfecta confer the risk of developing microinstability.
   C. Iatrogenic instability may present as a postoperative complication in patients without prior history of instability.

II. Causes of atraumatic hip instability:
   A. Bony abnormalities: conflicts due to abnormal osseous morphology may lead to subluxation or dislocation of the hip, often with repetitive injury to the adjacent soft-tissue stabilizers.
       1. Developmental dysplasia of the hip (DDH).
       2. Femoroacetabular impingement (FAI): CAM or pincer impingement.
       3. Legg–Calvés–Perthes disease.
       4. Acetabular retroversion.
   B. Connective tissue disorders: abnormalities in the formation of collagen can result in capsuloligamentous insufficiency and laxity.
       1. Down's syndrome.
       2. Ehlers–Danlos syndrome.
       3. Marfan's syndrome.
       4. Benign hypermobility syndrome.
   C. Iatrogenic: unrepaired capsulotomy, overzealous acetabular rim resection, or component malposition during prior hip surgery may predispose to secondary hip instability.
       1. Total hip arthroplasty.
       2. Open hip procedures (hip dislocations required trochanteric osteotomy and capsulotomy).
       3. Hip arthroscopy without capsular repair.
   D. Idiopathic:
       1. Generalized laxity.
       2. Subclinical connective tissue disorder.
       3. Borderline and hip dysplasia.
   E. Extra-articular causes of hip instability:
       1. Pelvic malalignment (e.g., ankylosing spondylitis; instability is due to increased pelvic tilt classically with increased risk of anterior instability).
       2. Iliopsoas tendinitis.
       3. Abductor/gluteal insufficiency.
       4. Sacroiliitis.
       5. AIIS (anteroinferior iliac spine) impingement with prior rectus avulsion or proximal injury.

Diagnosis

History

I.   Patients often present with complaints of hip pain and apprehension or subjective feeling of the hip giving way during certain at-risk activities (rising from seated position, rolling over in bed).

   A.   Insidious onset and gradually worsening symptoms without a specific precipitating event is more characteristic of atraumatic causes of instability.

   B.   Pain most often reported in the inguinal fold or anterolateral hip.

   C.   Posterior instability can present as posterior hip/buttock pain. This typically occurs with rise from seated position or position of sleep (adduction, IR [internal rotation]), or with anterior impingement that permits levering out of the head.

   D.   History of clicking, locking, and giving way should be investigated.

   E.   Attention should be given to symptoms elicited by activities with repetitive hip rotation, axial loading, or the extremes of motion.

   F.   Any previous ipsilateral hip injuries or surgeries should be noted.

   G.   Patients with hip dislocation should be immediately identified based on substantial symptoms and difficulty with weight bearing.

II. Medical and family history should be explored for connective tissue disorders and hypermobility.

III. Referred pain from the sacroiliac joint and/or lumbar spine with radicular symptoms can be confused with primary hip pathology and should be ruled out.

Physical Examination

I.   If the patient is ambulatory, gait and posture should be initially inspected to identify limp.

II. Active and passive range of motion (ROM) of the hip should be evaluated and compared against unaffected side.

   A.   Painful, audible, or visible popping of the hip during movement from flexion to extension is among the most obvious signs, and it may indicate labral pathology, intra-articular loose body, or snapping of the iliopsoas tendon or the iliotibial band.

III. The patient should be evaluated for signs of generalized ligamentous laxity using the Beighton–Horan criteria, which is scored on a scale from 0 to 9.[5]

   A.   One point is annotated if there is hyperextension of each elbow beyond 10 degrees (maximum, 2), hyperextension of the knee (2), excessive passive dorsiflexion (>90 degrees) of the fifth metacarpophalangeal joint (2), passive flexion of both thumbs to the forearm (2), and ability to rest the palms and hands flat on the floor during trunk forward flexion with the legs straight (1).

   B.   Scores ≥4 indicate general joint hypermobility.

IV. Hip strength should be evaluated and attention to the lumbosacral spine, abdomen, and knee is required to rule out associated pathology.

V.   Hip should be assessed for signs of frank instability:

  A.   Posteriorly dislocated hip typically shows a flexed, internally rotated, adducted, and shortened limb.

  B.   In anterior dislocation, the hip is usually externally rotated, extended, and abducted.

VI. Specific tests should be performed to assess for more subtle hip stability, with the goal of reproducing corresponding patient symptoms.

  A.   Anterior impingement test[6] (**Fig. 8.1**):

    1.   The patient lies supine while the examiner flexes the patient's hip to 90 degrees and then places the hip in 25-degree adduction. The examiner then medially rotates the hip to end range. The test is positive if pain is reproduced in the anterior hip.

    2.   It may also be used to diagnose FAI, acetabular retroversion, and labral tear.

  B.   Posterior impingement test[7] (**Fig. 8.2**):

    1.   The patient lies supine and the examiner places the patient's hip in extension and external rotation.

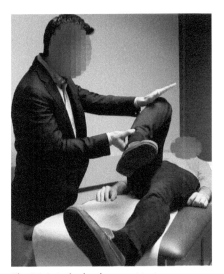

Fig. 8.1 Anterior impingement test.

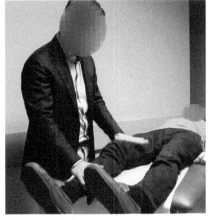

Fig. 8.3 Log roll test.

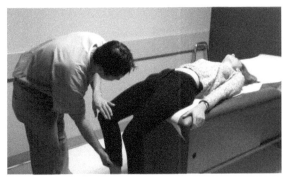

Fig. 8.2 Posterior impingement test.

    2. Discomfort or apprehension signifies positive finding and implies posterior impingement.

C. Log roll test/dial test[8] (**Fig. 8.3**):

    1. The patient lies supine in the neutral position and the examiner internally rotates the limb. The limb is then released and allowed to externally rotate. The test is positive when patient's limb passively rotates greater than 45 degrees from vertical in the axial plane and lacks a mechanical end point.

    2. Positive test indicates anterior capsular laxity or iliofemoral ligament insufficiency.

D. Anterior apprehension test/hyperextension–external rotation test[9]:

    1. The patient lies supine with buttocks just to the edge of the examination table. The patient holds one knee with hip in flexion, while the affected lower extremity is then extended and externally rotated. Positive test reproduces anterior hip pain and/or apprehension.

    2. Maneuver stresses the anterior hip capsules. Positive test indicates anterior labral lesion or anterior instability.

E. Posterior apprehension test[10]:

    1. The patient lies in the supine position with the affected hip in 90 degrees of flexion, adduction, and internal rotation with a posteriorly directed, downward force applied on the knee. Positive test reproduces pain and/or apprehension.

    2. Positive test indicates posterior labral lesion or posterior instability.

F. Prone external rotation test:

    1. The patient lies prone. The affected hip is maximally externally rotated with anteriorly directed pressure on posterior greater trochanter to translate femoral head anteriorly. Positive test reproduces pain.

G. Abduction–extension–external rotation test[11]:

    1. The patient is placed in the lateral decubitus position with the affected side up, abducted to 30 degrees and externally rotated. Anteriorly directed pressure is placed on the posterior greater trochanter and the leg is slowly extended from 10 degrees of flexion to full extension. Positive test reproduces patient symptoms.

    2. Positive test indicates anterior labral lesion or anterior instability.

H. Thomas' test for hip flexion iliopsoas contracture and Ober's test for iliotibial band tightness can also be positive as the muscles try to stabilize an unstable hip.[11]

Imaging

I. The objective of radiological assessment is to screen for risk factors for joint instability.

A. Plain radiographs including the anteroposterior (AP) view of the pelvis and the lateral view of the hip should be obtained initially to rule out trauma and any osseous abnormality.[12]

    1. Evaluate for concentric reduction of the hip joint. Assess for fractures and incarcerated or intra-articular bony fragments.

    2. Lateral center-edge angle of Wiberg should be used to assess appropriate acetabular coverage of the femoral head and rule out hip dysplasia (normal > 25 degrees).

    3. Abnormalities in the femoral head–neck offset may imply FAI.

    4. Retroversion of the acetabulum can be suggested by posterior wall sign and/or ischial spine sign (seeing ischial spines on the AP pelvis).

    5. Degenerative changes should be noted.

B. Computed tomography is useful in evaluation of traumatic instability and slight dysplasia.

    1. Small nondisplaced fractures of the acetabulum can be missed by plain radiograph. CT is routinely done following traumatic or atraumatic hip dislocation and subsequent reduction.

C. Magnetic resonance imaging allows for detailed evaluation of soft-tissue abnormalities, such as labral pathology, cartilage defects, or capsuloligamentous deficiency or attenuation.

Diagnostic Intra-articular Injection

I. Injection test with local anesthetic can be used to confirm the intra-articular origin of pain.[13] Injection is often performed under radiographic guidance (e.g., ultrasound, fluoroscopy). If pain is of intra-articular origin, majority of symptoms dramatically improve.

Treatment

I. Presentation following acute traumatic event with hip dislocation should prompt reduction to reduce risk of worsening chondral injury or avascular necrosis. Immediate postreduction imaging is important to confirm concentric reduction and stability throughout a ROM is necessary to assess the integrity of the joint and risk for recurrent instability.

II. Conservative:

A. Nonsurgical treatment is the first line of management in atraumatic instability.

    1. The patient should be enrolled in an activity modification module.

    2. Physical therapy should be initiated; focus should be on strengthening the lower back, core abdominal muscles, and hip stabilizers, primarily the hip external rotators and abductors.

    3. Anti-inflammatory medication and intra-articular injections help alleviate pain and existing inflammatory process.

    4. Patient progress should be reviewed after 6 weeks of physical therapy and activity modification. Persistent pain and symptoms should then be managed with surgical intervention.

III. Surgical:

A. Acute surgery is required if entrapped bony fragments from the posterior acetabular wall are noted after closed reduction of a dislocated hip.

B. Open hip surgery: this provides enhanced visualization and access. It requires proper capsular management.

C. Hip arthroscopy: minimally invasive evaluation and repair of soft-tissue sta-bilizers of the hip (labral tears, capsular plications, ligamentum teres tears) are necessary to restore joint stability. It is considered the first-line treatment when intra-articular pathology is accessible with standard surgical technique. Several forms of capsular management techniques exist and include the following:

1. Arthroscopic capsular closure by approximation of the capsular leaflets.

2. Arthroscopic capsular plication by overlapping of capsular leaflets.

3. Arthroscopic thermal capsulorrhaphy: hip capsular volume is reduced with the use of thermal energy by laser or radiofrequency. Used less frequently in practice.

D. Bony realignment procedures: these are more invasive and include acetabular osteotomy and derotational femoral osteotomy. This is usually required in patients with severe acetabular dysplasia or retroversion.

IV. Postoperative rehabilitation[14]:

A. ROM immediately in hip brace that prevents external rotation, extension beyond neutral, and abduction beyond 20 degrees.

B. Ambulation in brace using crutches with only 30% of weight on the affected hip at 4 weeks; this should gradually increase to full weight bearing over the next 2 weeks.

C. At 6 weeks, ROM restrictions are lifted with the goal of full ROM by 3 months.

D. Return to full activity is allowed at between 4 and 6 months.

References

1. Köhnlein W, Ganz R, Impellizzeri FM, Leunig M. Acetabular morphology: implications for joint-preserving surgery. Clin Orthop Relat Res 2009;467(3):682–691
2. Court-Brown C, McQueen M, Swiontkowski MF, Ring D, Friedman SM, Duckworth AD. Musculoskeletal Trauma in the Elderly. 2016
3. Toogood PA, Skalak A, Cooperman DR. Proximal femoral anatomy in the normal human population. Clin Orthop Relat Res 2009;467(4):876–885
4. Tan V, Seldes RM, Katz MA, Freedhand AM, Klimkiewicz JJ, Fitzgerald RH Jr. Contribution of acetabular labrum to articulating surface area and femoral head coverage in adult hip joints: an anatomic study in cadavera. Am J Orthop 2001;30(11):809–812
5. Beighton P, Horan F. Orthopaedic aspects of the Ehlers-Danlos syndrome. J Bone Joint Surg Br 1969;51(3):444–453
6. Hananouchi T, Yasui Y, Yamamoto K, Toritsuka Y, Ohzono K. Anterior impingement test for labral lesions has high positive predictive value. Clin Orthop Relat Res 2012;470(12):3524–3529
7. Frank RM, Slabaugh MA, Grumet RC, Virkus WW, Bush-Joseph CA, Nho SJ. Posterior hip pain in an athletic population: differential diagnosis and treatment options. Sports Health 2010;2(3):237–246
8. Byrd JW. Evaluation of the hip: history and physical examination. N Am J Sports Phys Ther 2007;2(4):231–240
9. Shu B, Safran MR. Hip instability: anatomic and clinical considerations of traumatic and atraumatic instability. Clin Sports Med 2011;30(2):349–367
10. Kalisvaart MM, Safran MR. Microinstability of the hip-it does exist: etiology, diagnosis and treatment. J Hip Preserv Surg 2015;2(2):123–135

11. Kivlan BR, Carroll L, Burfield A, Enseki KR, Martin RL. Length Change of the Iliofemoral Ligament during Tests for Anterior Microinstability of the Hip Joint: A Cadaveric Validity Study. Int J Sports Phys Ther 2019;14(4):613–622
12. Mannava S, Geeslin AG, Frangiamore SJ, et al. Comprehensive Clinical Evaluation of Femoroacetabular Impingement: Part 2, Plain Radiography. Arthrosc Tech 2017;6(5):e2003–e2009
13. Kraeutler MJ, Garabekyan T, Fioravanti MJ, Young DA, Mei-Dan O. Efficacy of a non-im-age-guided diagnostic hip injection in patients with clinical and radiographic evidence of intra-articular hip pathology. J Hip Preserv Surg 2018;5(3):220–225
14. Malloy P, Gray K, Wolff AB. Rehabilitation After Hip Arthroscopy: A Movement Control-Based Perspective. Clin Sports Med 2016;35(3):503–521

Suggested Readings

Bolia I, Chahla J, Locks R, Briggs K, Philippon MJ. Microinstability of the hip: a previously unrecognized pathology. Muscles Ligaments Tendons J 2016;6(3):354–360
Boykin RE, Anz AW, Bushnell BD, Kocher MS, Stubbs AJ, Philippon MJ. Hip instability. J Am Acad Orthop Surg 2011;19(6):340–349
Dangin A, Tardy N, Wettstein M, May O, Bonin N. Microinstability of the hip: a review. Orthop Traumatol Surg Res 2016;102(8S):S301–S309
Dumont GD. Hip instability: current concepts and treatment options. Clin Sports Med 2016;35(3):435–447
Kalisvaart MM, Safran MR. Microinstability of the hip-it does exist: etiology, diagnosis and treatment. J Hip Preserv Surg 2015;2(2):123–135
Kraeutler MJ, Garabekyan T, Pascual-Garrido C, Mei-Dan O. Hip instability: a review of hip dysplasia and other contributing factors. Muscles Ligaments Tendons J 2016;6(3):343–353
Shu B, Safran MR. Hip instability: anatomic and clinical considerations of traumatic and atraumatic instability. Clin Sports Med 2011;30(2):349–367
Smith MV, Sekiya JK. Hip instability. Sports Med Arthrosc Rev 2010;18(2):108–112
Slikker W III, Van Thiel GS, Chahal J, Nho SJ. Hip instability and arthroscopic techniques for complete capsular closure and capsular plication. Oper Tech Sports Med 2011;20(4):301–309

Section II

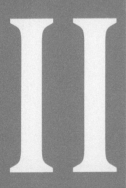

9 Pelvic Fractures

Joshua D. Harris, Robert A. Jack II

Introduction

Pelvic Ring Fractures

I. Mechanism of injury: high-energy blunt trauma[1,2]:
   A. Motorcycle collision.
   B. Auto-pedestrian collision.
   C. Fall.
   D. Motor vehicle collision.
   E. Crush injury.

II. Associated with other high-energy injuries:
   A. Chest/thoracic injury.
   B. Long bone fracture.
   C. Reproductive organ injury.
   D. Head injury.
   E. Abdominal injury.
   F. Spine fracture.

III. Mortality rate:
   A. 10–50%.[3–8]
   B. Hemorrhage is leading cause.[9–11]
   C. Associated with[12]:
      1. Systolic BP less than 90 on presentation.
      2. Age older than 60 years.
      3. Increased injury severity scale (ISS): an anatomical scoring system providing overall score for patients with multiple injuries, based on assignment of an Abbreviated Injury Scale (AIS) score to each of six body regions—score range 3 to 75.
         a. Head and neck.
         b. Face.
         c. Chest.
         d. Abdomen.
         e. Extremity.
         f. External.
      4. Need for greater than 4 U of pure red blood cells.

Acetabular Fractures

I.   Mechanism of injury: bimodal:
   A.   High energy in young patients.
   B.   Low energy in elderly patients.[13]
   C.   May be seen with concomitant hip dislocation (**Fig. 9.1**).
II. Associated injuries (up to 50% of patients)[14–17]:
   A.   Extremity injury: 35%.
   B.   Head injury: 19%.
   C.   Chest injury: 18%.
   D.   Nerve palsy: 13%.
   E.   Abdominal injury: 8%.
   F.   Genitourinary injury: 6%.
   G.   Spine injury: 4%.
III. Fracture pattern defined by[18]:
   A.   Force vector.
   B.   Position of the femoral head (hip position).
   C.   Bone mineral density.

Anatomic Considerations

Pelvic Ring (Fig. 9.2)

I.   Osteology:
   A.   Sacrum and two innominate bones.
   B.   Stability dependent on strong surrounding ligamentous structures.
   C.   Displacement with obligatory disruption of ring in minimum of two places.

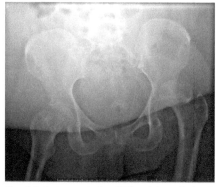

Fig. 9.1 Anteroposterior (AP) pelvis radiograph demonstrating a posterior left hip dislocation with associated posterior wall acetabulum fracture.

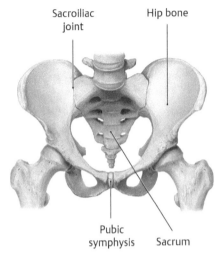

Sacroiliac joint

Hip bone

Pubic symphysis   Sacrum

Fig 9.2 The pelvic girdle and pelvic ring. Anterosuperior view. The pelvic girdle consists of the two hip bones (coxal bones). The SI joint and the cartilaginous pubic symphysis unite the bony parts of the pelvic girdle with the sacrum to form a stable ring called the pelvic ring (indicated by color shading). It allows very little mobility, because stability throughout the pelvic ring is an important prerequisite for transmitting the trunk load to the lower limbs. (Source: Schuenke M, Schulte E, Schumacher U. Thieme Atlas of Anatomy. General Anatomy and Musculoskeletal System. 2nd edition, ©2014, Thieme Publishers, New York. Illustrations by Voll M and Wesker K.)

II. Ligaments (**Fig. 9.3**):

    A. Anterior symphyseal (resist external rotation):

    B. Pelvic floor:

        1. Sacrospinous ligaments (resist external rotation).

        2. Sacrotuberous ligaments (resist shear and flexion).

    C. Posterior sacroiliac (SI) complex: most important for stability:

        1. Anterior SI ligaments (resist external rotation).

        2. Interosseous SI (resist anteroposterior [AP] translation).

        3. Posterior SI (resist cephalad–caudad translation).

        4. Iliolumbar (resist external and internal rotation).

III. Neurovascular structures (**Fig. 9.4**):

    A. Lumbosacral plexus.

    B. Internal iliac vessels.

    C. Numerous neurovascular structures intimately associated with posterior pelvic ligaments.

Acetabulum

I. Osteology:

    A. Based on two-column theory (**Fig. 9.5**):

        1. Acetabulum supported by two columns of bone.

        2. Inverted Y configuration.

        3. Anterior column:

            a. Anterior ilium.

            b. Anterior wall and dome.

            c. Iliopectineal eminence.

            d. Lateral superior pubic ramus.

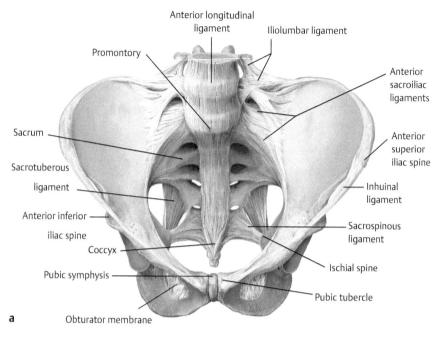

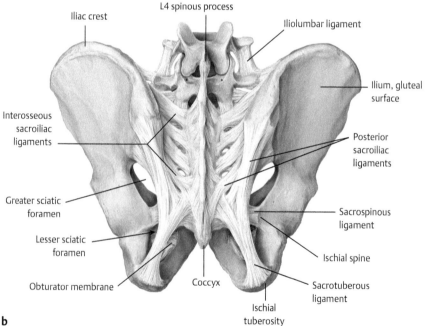

Fig. 9.3 (a, b) Ligaments of the male pelvis. (Source: Schuenke M, Schulte E, Schumacher U. Thieme Atlas of Anatomy. General Anatomy and Musculoskeletal System. 2nd edition, ©2014, Thieme Publishers, New York. Illustration by Karl Wesker/Markus Voll.)

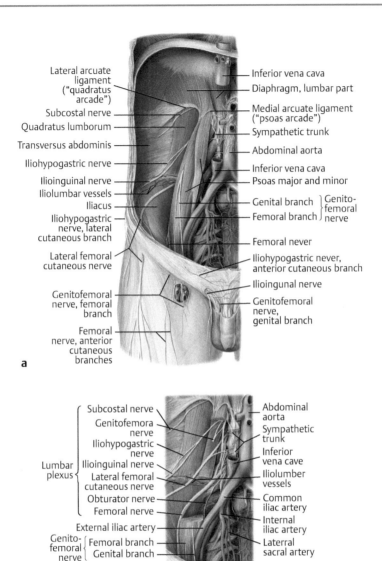

Lateral arcuate ligament ("quadratus arcade")
Subcostal nerve
Quadratus lumborum
Transversus abdominis
Iliohypogastric nerve
Ilioinguinal nerve
Iliolumbar vessels
Iliacus
Iliohypogastric nerve, lateral cutaneous branch
Lateral femoral cutaneous nerve
Genitofemoral nerve, femoral branch
Femoral nerve, anterior cutaneous branches

Inferior vena cava
Diaphragm, lumbar part
Medial arcuate ligament ("psoas arcade")
Sympathetic trunk
Abdominal aorta
Inferior vena cava
Psoas major and minor
Genital branch ⎱ Genito-femoral nerve
Femoral branch ⎰
Femoral never
Iliohypogastric never, anterior cutaneous branch
Ilioingunal nerve
Genitofemoral nerve, genital branch

a

Subcostal nerve
Genitofemora nerve
Iliohypogastric nerve
Lumbar plexus { Ilioinguinal nerve
Lateral femoral cutaneous nerve
Obturator nerve
Femoral nerve
External iliac artery
Genito-femoral nerve { Femoral branch
Genital branch

Abdominal aorta
Sympathetic trunk
Inferior vena cave
Iliolumber vessels
Common iliac artery
Internal iliac artery
Lateral sacral artery

b

Fig. 9.4 Neurovascular structures on the anterior side of the posterior trunk wall. (a) Lumbar fossa on the right side after removal of the anterior and lateral trunk wall, the intra- and retroperitoneal organs, the peritoneum, and all the fasciae of the trunk wall. The inferior vena cava has been partially removed. (b) Lumbar fossa with the lumbar plexus of the right side after removal of the superficial layer of the psoas major. (Source: Schuenke M, Schulte E, Schumacher U. Thieme Atlas of Anatomy. General Anatomy and Musculoskeletal System. 2nd edition, ©2014, Thieme Publishers, New York. Illustrations by Voll M and Wesker K.)

4.   Posterior column:

   a.   Quadrilateral surface.

   b.   Posterior wall and dome.

    c. Ischial tuberosity.

    d. Greater and lesser sciatic notches.

II.   Vascular structures:

   A. Obturator artery and vein.

   B. Corona mortis:

    1. Anastomosis of the external iliac and internal iliac vessels.

    2. At risk during injury and operative intervention.

Classification

Pelvic Ring

I.   Young–Burgess Classification (**Table 9.1; Fig. 9.6**).[19]

II.   Tile classification (**Table 9.2**).[20]

Acetabulum

I.   Letournel classification (**Table 9.3**).[15,16,18,21,22]

History and Examination

Information from Emergency Medical Transport Professionals

I.   Mechanism of injury.

II.   Level of consciousness:

   A. Glasgow Coma Scale (score range 3–15; eye opening, verbal, and motor responses).

III. Initial physical examination.

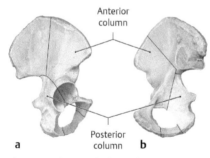

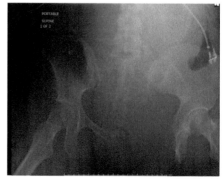

Fig. 9.5 Column principle of the hip bone. (a) Lateral and (b) medial views. (Source: Schuenke M, Schulte E, Schumacher U. Thieme Atlas of Anatomy. General Anatomy and Musculoskeletal System. 2nd edition, ©2014, Thieme Publishers, New York. Illustrations by Voll M and Wesker K.)

Fig. 9.6 Anteroposterior (AP) pelvis radiograph of an APC (anteroposterior compression) III injury.

Table 9.1 Young–Burgess classification system of pelvic ring injuries

Type	Description
Anterior posterior compression (APC)	
APC I	Symphysis widening <2.5 cm
APC II	Symphysis widening >2.5 cm, anterior SI joint diastasis. Posterior SI ligaments intact, disruption of sacrospinous and sacrotuberous ligaments
APC III	Disruption of anterior and posterior SI ligaments. Disruption of sacrospinous and sacrotuberous ligaments
Lateral compression (LC)	
LC type I	Oblique or transverse ramus fracture and ipsilateral anterior sacral ala compression fracture
LC type II	Rami fracture and ipsilateral posterior ilium fracture dislocation (crescent fracture)
LC type III	Ipsilateral lateral compression and contralateral APC (windswept pelvis)
Vertical shear	
Vertical shear	Posterior and superior displacement of the hemipelvis

Abbreviation: SI, sacroiliac.

Table 9.2 Tile classification system of pelvic ring injuries

Type	Description
A: rotationally and vertically stable	
A1	Fracture not involving the ring (avulsion or iliac wing)
A2	Stable or minimally displaced fracture of the ring
A3	Transverse sacral fracture
B: rotationally unstable, vertically stable	
B1	Open book injury (external rotation)
B2	Lateral compression injury (internal rotation)
B2-1	Anterior ring displacement through the ipsilateral rami
B2-2	Anterior ring displacement through the contralateral rami
B3	Bilateral
C: rotationally and vertically unstable	
C1	Unilateral
C1-1	Iliac fracture
C1-2	Sacroiliac fracture-dislocation
C1-3	Sacral fracture
C2	Bilateral with one side type B and one side type C
C3	Bilateral with both sides type C

Table 9.3 Letournel classification system for acetabulum fractures

Type	Notes	Frequency
Elementary		
Posterior wall	Most common	25%
Posterior column	Detachment of ischioacetabular segment from the innominate bone	3–5%
Anterior wall	Rare	1–2%
Anterior column	Anterior border of the innominate bone displaced from the intact ilium	3–5%
Transverse	Only elementary fracture to involve both columns	5–19%
Associated		
Associated both column	Acetabulum is completely separate from axial skeleton. "Spur sign" on obturator oblique	23%
Transverse and posterior wall	Transverse component may be transtectal, juxtatectal, or infratectal	20%
T-shaped	T portion is an inferior vertical fracture	7%
Anterior column/wall and posterior hemitransverse	75% will involve anterior column and not wall	7%
Posterior column and posterior wall	Only associated fracture that does not involve both columns	3–4%

Initial Assessment

I.   Airway.
II.   Breathing.
III. Circulation.
IV.   Disability/neuro status.
V.   Exposure and environment.

Symptoms

I.   Pain.
II.   Inability to bear weight.

Physical Examination

I.   Inspection:
   A. Abnormal lower extremity positioning:
      1. External rotation of one or both extremities.
      2. Leg length shortening.
   B. Skin:
      1. Degloving injury (Morel–Lavalée).
      2. Flank hematoma.

II.   Palpation:
   A.   Evaluate for crepitus.
   B.   Test pelvis stability with gentle lateral compressive or rotational force.
III. Neurological examination:
   A.   Lower extremity motor examination.
   B.   Lower extremity sensory examination.
   C.   Rectal examination.
IV.   Vascular examination:
   A.   Palpate and/or Doppler dorsalis pedis and posterior tibial arteries.
V.   Urogenital examination:
   A.   Scrotal/labial or perineal hematoma.
   B.   Blood at urethral meatus.
   C.   Traumatic laceration of perineum.
   D.   Hematuria.
   E.   Vaginal/rectal examination for open fracture.

Diagnostic Imaging

Radiographs

I.   AP pelvis (**Fig. 9.7**).
II.   Pelvic ring injuries:
   A.   Inlet radiograph:
      1.   Beam directed 45 degrees caudad.
   B.   Outlet radiograph:
      1.   Beam directed 45 degrees cephalad.
   C.   Flamingo view—more useful in chronic setting, rather than acute:
      1.   Standing single-leg stance AP view useful for evaluating pubic symphysis instability.
III. Acetabulum injuries—Judet's views:
   A.   Iliac oblique (**Fig. 9.8**):
      1.   Beam directed 45 degrees oblique toward noninjured side.
   B.   Obturator oblique (**Fig. 9.9**):
      1.   Beam directed 45 degrees oblique toward injured side.

Computed Tomography (Fig. 9.10)

I.   Routine for evaluation of pelvic ring or acetabulum fractures.
II.   Defines comminution, marginal impaction, and rotation.
III. Identifies loose bodies.
IV.   Three-dimensional reconstruction.

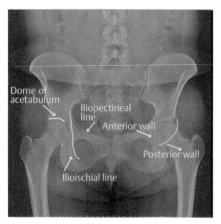

Fig. 9.7 Normal anteroposterior (AP) pelvis radiograph with radiographic markers.

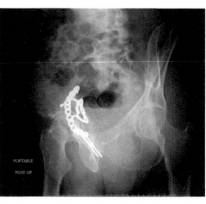

Fig. 9.8 Iliac oblique radiograph showing a patient who underwent open reduction and internal fixation of a right both-column acetabulum fracture.

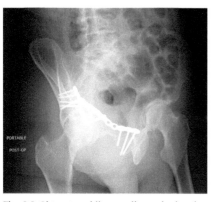

Fig. 9.9 Obturator oblique radiograph showing a patient who underwent open reduction and internal fixation of a right both-column acetabulum fracture.

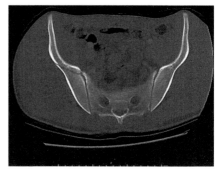

Fig. 9.10 An axial computed tomography (CT) scan showing a right-sided lateral compression 2 (LC-2) injury.

Treatment

Pelvic Ring Injuries

I.   Initial management:

 A. Stabilization and resuscitation:

  1. Appropriate immobilization should be applied to spine and extremities.

  2. Transfuse pure red blood cells and fresh frozen plasma in 1:1 ratio as needed.

  3. Twenty-four to 36 hours of observation in the intensive care unit for potential rapid deterioration from internal hemorrhage.

 B. Pelvic binder or sheet:

  1. Initial management of an unstable pelvic ring injury.[23,24]

  2. Decreases intrapelvic volume.

  3. Center over greater trochanters.

4. Tape ankle together if necessary to prevent external rotation.

5. A sheet can be cut prior to operative fixation without removing completely.

II. Nonoperative:

    A. Indications: mechanically stable pelvic ring injuries:

        1. LC1.

        2. APC1.

        3. Isolated pubic ramus fractures.

        4. Postpartum symphyseal widening less than 4 cm.

III. Operative:

    A. External fixation:

        1. Indications:

            a. Ring injuries with external rotation component.

            b. Continued blood loss in unstable patient.

        2. Contraindications:

            a. Acetabulum fracture.

            b. Ilium fracture.

    B. Open reduction and internal fixation:

        1. Indications:

            a. Open fracture.

            b. Displacement with rotation of hemipelvis.

            c. Symphyseal diastasis greater than 2.5 cm.

            d. SI joint diastasis greater than 1 cm.

            e. Sacral fracture with displacement.

            f. Postpartum diastasis greater than 6 cm.

        2. Technique:

            a. Anterior ring stabilization (**Figs. 9.11** and **9.12**):

                i. Superior plate.

                ii. Pfannenstiel incision.

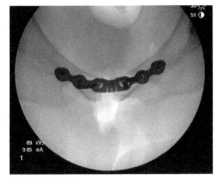 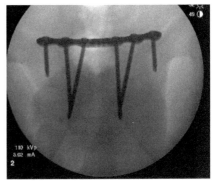

Fig. 9.11 Intraoperative fluoroscopy image in the inlet view showing pubic symphysis open reduction and internal fixation.

Fig. 9.12 Intraoperative fluoroscopy image in the outlet view showing pubic symphysis open reduction and internal fixation.

b. Posterior ring stabilization:

i.   Iliosacral screws: safe zone through S1 vertebral body and use inlet/outlet fluoroscopy for placement.

ii. Anterior SI screws.

iii. Posterior SI plating.

Acetabulum Fractures

I.   Initial management:

A. Skeletal traction:

1.   Unstable fractures.

2.   Involving weight-bearing dome.

3.   Subluxating or dislocating femoral head.

II. Nonoperative:

A. Indications[25]:

1.   Patient factors:

a. High operative risk.

b. Morbid obesity.

c. Late presentation.

2.   Fracture characteristics:

a. Minimally displaced (<2 mm).

b. Less than 20% involvement of posterior wall fracture:

i.   Examination under anesthesia to determine stability.

c. Femoroacetabular joint congruity.

B. Protocol:

1.   Toe-touch weight bearing[26,27]:

a. Less joint reactive forces than non-weight-bearing.

2.   Activity as tolerated with walker.

III. Operative:

A. Open reduction and internal fixation (**Fig. 9.13**):

1.   Indications:

a. Patient factors:

i.   Acute injury.

ii. Physiologically stable.

iii. No local infection.

b. Fracture characteristics:

i.   Acetabular dome displacement greater than 2 mm.

ii. Unstable fracture pattern.

iii. Posterior wall fracture greater than 40%.

iv. Marginal impaction.

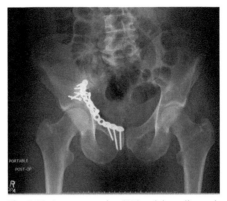

Fig. 9.13 Anteroposterior (AP) pelvis radiograph demonstrating plate and screw fixation of a right both-column acetabulum fracture.

    v. Intra-articular loose body.

    vi. Irreducible fracture-dislocation.

  c. Approach[22]:

    i. Kocher–Langenbeck:

      1. Posterior wall,

      2. Posterior column,

      3. Transverse,

      4. Posterior column and posterior wall,

      5. Transverse and posterior wall, and

      6. **T**-shaped (infra- or juxtatectal).

    ii. Ilioinguinal:

      1. Anterior wall,

      2. Anterior column,

      3. Transverse (infra- or juxtatectal),

      4. Interior wall/column and posterior hemitransverse, and

      5. Both columns.

    iii. Iliofemoral: anterior wall and anterior column.

    iv. Extended iliofemoral:

      1. Transverse (transtectal)

      2. Transverse (transtectal) and posterior wall, and

      3. Both columns.

    v. Combined: **T**-shaped and both columns.

    vi. Stoppa: medial wall.

B. Percutaneous fixation with column screws:

  1. Antegrade (iliac wing to ramus).

  2. Retrograde (ramus to iliac wing).

  3. Posterior column screw.

C. Total hip arthroplasty:
  1. Indications:
    a. Elderly patients with significant comminution or poor bone mineral density.
    b. Preexisting arthritis.

Complications

Pelvic Ring Injuries

I.   Urogenital[28]:
  A. Posterior urethral tear.
  B. Bladder rupture.
II.   Chronic instability:
  A. Rarely seen in nonoperative cases.
  B. Use pain during weight bearing as sign of instability.
  C. Mechanical symptoms.
III. After operative intervention:
  A. Neurologic injury:
    1. L5 nerve root injury if SI screw perforates anterior cortex.
    2. Lateral femoral cutaneous nerve injury after external fixation.
  B. Hardware failure.
  C. Nonunion.

Acetabulum Fractures

I.   Posttraumatic degenerative joint disease[15,18,29]:
  A. Quality of fracture reduction is the main determinant.
  B. Higher risk with greater than 1 mm of displacement.
II.   Heterotopic ossification[30,31]:
  A. Reported in up to 90% of patients after acetabular fracture surgery.
  B. Up to 50% have greater than 20% loss of hip range of motion.
  C. Increased incidence with extensile approach.
III. Osteonecrosis of femoral head:
  A. Associated with fracture dislocation injury patterns.
  B. May also be caused by malreduced fractures.[15,18]
IV.   Intra-articular hardware placement.
V.   Venous thromboembolism.
VI.   Abductor weakness.

References

1. Adams JE, Davis GG, Alexander CB, Alonso JE. Pelvic trauma in rapidly fatal motor vehicle accidents. J Orthop Trauma 2003;17(6):406–410
2. Demetriades D, Karaiskakis M, Toutouzas K, Alo K, Velmahos G, Chan L. Pelvic fractures: epidemiology and predictors of associated abdominal injuries and outcomes. J Am Coll Surg 2002;195(1):1–10
3. Gillila M, Ward R, Barton R, Miller P, Duke J. Factors affecting mortality in pelvic fractures. J Trauma Inj Infect Crit Care 1982;22(8):691–693</jrn>
4. Looser KG, Crombie HD Jr. Pelvic fractures: an anatomic guide to severity of injury. Review of 100 cases. Am J Surg 1976;132(5):638–642
5. Monahan PR, Taylor RG. Dislocation and fracture-dislocation of the pelvis. Injury 1975;6(4):325–333
6. Reynolds B, Balsano N, Reynolds F. Pelvic fractures. J Trauma Inj Infect Crit Care 1973;13(11):1011–1014</jrn>
7. Riska EB, von Bonsdorff H, Hakkinen S, Jaroma H, Kiviluoto O, Paavilainen T. External fixation of unstable pelvic fractures. Int Orthop 1979;3(3):183–188
8. Rothenberger D, Velasco R, Strate R, Fischer R, Perry J. Open pelvic fracture. J Trauma: Inj Infect Crit Care 1978;18(3):184–187</jrn>
9. Tile M. Acute pelvic fractures: II. Principles of management. J Am Acad Orthop Surg 1996;4(3):152–161
10. Karadimas EJ, Nicolson T, Kakagia DD, Matthews SJ, Richards PJ, Giannoudis PV. Angiographic embolisation of pelvic ring injuries. Treatment algorithm and review of the literature. Int Orthop 2011;35(9):1381–1390
11. Manson TT, Nascone JW, Sciadini MF, O'Toole RV. Does fracture pattern predict death with lateral compression type 1 pelvic fractures? J Trauma 2010;69(4):876–879
12. Smith W, Williams A, Agudelo J, et al. Early predictors of mortality in hemodynamically unstable pelvis fractures. J Orthop Trauma 2007;21(1):31–37
13. Rommens PM, Wagner D, Hofmann A. Fragility fractures of the pelvis. JBJS Rev 2017;5(3):1
14. Kregor PJ, Templeman D. Associated injuries complicating the management of acetabular fractures: review and case studies. Orthop Clin North Am 2002;33(1):73–95, viii
15. Matta J. Fracture of the acetabulum: accuracy of reduction and clinical results in patients managed operatively within three weeks after the injury. Orthop Trauma Dir 2011;9(2):31–36 </jrn>
16. Moed BR, WillsonCarr SE, Watson JT. Results of operative treatment of fractures of the posterior wall of the acetabulum. J Bone Joint Surg Am 2002;84(5):752–758
17. Moed BR, Yu PH, Gruson KI. Functional outcomes of acetabular fractures. J Bone Joint Surg Am 2003;85(10):1879–1883
18. Letournel E, Judet R. Fractures of the Acetabulum. Berlin: Springer-Verlag; 1993
19. Burgess AR, Eastridge BJ, Young JW, et al. Pelvic ring disruptions: effective classification system and treatment protocols. J Trauma 1990;30(7):848–856
20. Tile M. Acute pelvic fractures: I. Causation and classification. J Am Acad Orthop Surg 1996;4(3):143–151
21. Borrelli J Jr, Goldfarb C, Catalano L, Evanoff BA. Assessment of articular fragment displacement in acetabular fractures: a comparison of computerized tomography and plain radiographs. J Orthop Trauma 2002;16(7):449–456, discussion 456–457
22. Bucholz R, Court-Brown C, Green D, Heckman J, Rockwood C, Tornetta P. Rockwood and Green's Fractures In Adults. Philadelphia, PA: Wolters Kluwer Health/Lippincott Williams & Wilkins; 2010
23. Croce MA, Magnotti LJ, Savage SA, Wood GW II, Fabian TC. Emergent pelvic fixation in patients with exsanguinating pelvic fractures. J Am Coll Surg 2007;204(5):935–939, discussion 940–942
24. Routt ML Jr, Falicov A, Woodhouse E, Schildhauer TA. Circumferential pelvic antishock sheeting: a temporary resuscitation aid. J Orthop Trauma 2002;16(1):45–48

25. Tornetta P III. Non-operative management of acetabular fractures. The use of dynamic stress views. J Bone Joint Surg Br 1999;81(1):67–70
26. Rubin G, Monder O, Zohar R, Oster A, Konra O, Rozen N. Toe-touch weight bearing: myth or reality? Orthopedics 2010;33(10):729
27. Lewis CL, Sahrmann SA, Moran DW. Anterior hip joint force increases with hip extension, decreased gluteal force, or decreased iliopsoas force. J Biomech 2007;40(16):3725–3731
28. Watnik NF, Coburn M, Goldberger M. Urologic injuries in pelvic ring disruptions. Clin Orthop Relat Res 1996;(329):37–45
29. Mayo K. Open reduction and internal fixation of fractures of the acetabulum. results in 163 fractures. Clinical Orthopaedics and Related Research 1994;305(1):31–37
30. Bosse MJ, Poka A, Reinert CM, Ellwanger F, Slawson R, McDevitt ER. Heterotopic ossification as a complication of acetabular fracture. Prophylaxis with low-dose irradiation. J Bone Joint Surg Am 1988;70(8):1231–1237
31. Mears D, Rubash H. Pelvic and Acetabular Fractures. Thorofare, NJ: Slack; 1986

10 Intracapsular Hip Fractures

Carlos J. Meheux, Luis F. Pulido-Sierra

Femoral Head Fractures

Introduction

I.   Associated with hip dislocations[1–4]:
  A.   True orthopaedic emergency.
  B.   Shear type fractures.
  C.   Indentation or crush type.[5]
II.   Anatomy and blood supply to the femoral head[6]:
  A   Medial femoral circumflex artery (MFCA).
  B.   The MFCA branches from the deep femoral artery:
    1.   Five constant branches: superficial, ascending, acetabular, descending, deep.
  C.   The deep branch supplies the blood to the femoral head:
    1.   Perforates the posterior capsule.
    2.   Proximal to the superior gemellus.
    3.   Distal to the tendon of the piriformis.
  D.   Terminates in the posterolateral retinacular branches:
    1.   Covered by synovium.
    2.   Enters the femoral head: 2 to 4 mm lateral to the bone–cartilage junction.
  E.   Anastomosis of the inferior gluteal artery and the MFCA:
    1.   Inferior border of the piriformis.
    2.   Constant anastomosis.
    3.   Must be preserved with surgical approaches.

Mechanism

I.   High-energy motor vehicle collision (84%)[7]:
  A.   Posterior hip dislocation:
    1.   Twelve percent are associated with femoral head fractures.
    2.   Axial load with hip flexed and adducted.
    3.   Knee to dashboard.[8]
  B.   Associated injuries in hip dislocation and femoral head fractures:
    1.   Acetabular fracture.[8]
    2.   Femoral neck fracture.
    3.   Femoral shaft fracture.

4. Ipsilateral knee injuries (25%)[8]:
   a. Meniscus tear (22%).
   b. Bone marrow edema (33%).
   c. Knee effusion (37%).
   d. Cruciate ligament injury (25%).
   e. Collateral ligament injury (21%).
   f. Periarticular knee fracture (15%).
5. Sciatic nerve injury (10–23%)[9-12]:
   a. Peroneal division.
   b. Sixty to 70% recover.[13]
6. Pelvis, abdomen, chest, head, and spine injuries.

Diagnosis

I. History:
    A. Limited.
    B. High-energy trauma.
II. Physical examination:
    A. ATLS (Advanced Trauma Life Support):
       1. Prioritize (life, limb, function).
       2. Primary survey:
          a. Airway and cervical spine control.
          b. Breathing and ventilation.
          c. Circulation and hemorrhage.
          d. Disability.
          e. Exposure.
       3. Secondary survey:
          a. History.
          b. Head to toe examination.
          c. Extremity:
             i. Posterior dislocation: Hip position[14]: Flexed, adducted, and internally rotated.
             ii. Anterior dislocation: Hip position[15]: abducted, externally rotatated, flexed (inferior or obturator, and extended - superior or pubic), vascular examination. neurologic examination: motor and sensory to lower extremity and always before and after reduction attempts.
III. Imaging:
    A. Plain radiographs:
       1. Supine anteroposterior (AP) pelvis:
          a. Routine imaging in polytrauma.

      b. Symmetric femoral heads.

      c. Femoral head fragment in acetabular fossa.

      d. Femoral neck.

      e. Limb position.

      f. Pelvic ring injury:

          i. Inlet and outlet views.

          ii. CT scan.

      g. Acetabular fractures:

          i. Judet's views (iliac and obturator oblique).

          ii. CT scan.

2. Cross-table lateral:

    i. Orthogonal imaging.

B. CT:

    1. Frequently performed in polytrauma patients:

      a. Chest, abdomen, pelvis.

      b. Cervical, thoracic, and lumbar spine.

    2. Prereduction CT:

      a. Should not delay hip reduction.

      b. Indicated in irreducible dislocation.

    3. Postreduction evaluation:

      a. Always CT scan following closed reduction.

      b. Multicut detector, high-collimation, 1- to 2-mm cuts.

      c. Evaluation:

          i. Concentric reduction.

          ii. Intra-articular loose bodies.

          iii. Femoral head fracture: size and location.

          iv. Acetabular fractures:

             a. Posterior wall fracture.

          v. Femoral neck.

Classifications

I. Pipkin[17] (**Fig. 10.1**):

  A. Femoral head fracture with posterior hip dislocations:

    1. Type I:

      a. Fracture below the fovea.

      b. Fracture outside the weight-bearing joint area.

    2. Type II:

      a. Fracture cranial to the fovea.

      b. Fracture within the weight-bearing joint area.

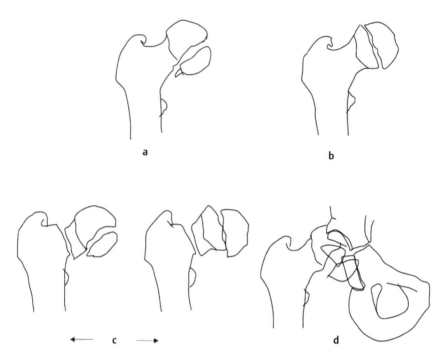

Fig. 10.1 The Pipkin classification system of femoral head fractures with posterior hip dislocations. The relationship to the fovea determines the type of fractures in types I and II (**a, b**). Type I fractures are caudal to the fovea. Type II fractures are cranial to the fovea and are usually in the weight-bearing zone. Type III (**c**) fractures are associated with a femoral neck fracture. Type IV (**d**) fractures are associated with additional acetabular fractures.

     3. Type III:

         a. Associated ipsilateral femoral neck fracture.

     4. Type IV:

         a. Associated ipsilateral acetabular fracture.

II.   Orthopaedic Trauma Association (OTA):

    A. 31-C, articular fracture head[18]:

        1. 31-C1, split fracture (Pipkin types I–II):

        2. 31-C2, with depression.

        3. 31-C3, with femoral neck fracture.

Treatment

I.   Nonoperative[15,19]:

    A. Emergent closed reduction.

    B. Touchdown weight bearing for 4 weeks.

    C. Knee immobilizer or hip abduction brace.

  D. Indications:
    1. Pipkin type I with articular incongruity of 1 mm or less.
    2. Pipkin type II without articular incongruity.
    3. No interposed fragment.
    4. Concentrically reduced joint.
    5. Patients that are unable to tolerate surgery.
II. Surgical treatment:
  A. Open reduction and internal fixation (ORIF)[19]:
    1. Indications:
        a. Pipkin type I with greater than 1 mm articular incongruity.
        b. Pipkin type II with any displacement.
        c. Pipkin types III and IV.
        d. Interposed fragment.
        e. Nonconcentrically reduced joint.
    2. Surgical approaches:
        a. Smith–Peterson approach.
        b. Trochanteric flip osteotomy.
        c. Surgical hip dislocation.
        d. Transgluteal approaches.
        e. Arthroscopic-assisted percutaneous fixation.
    3. Method of fixation:
        a. Mini or small fragment screws[20]:
           i. Cancellous biosabsorble.
           ii. Herbert screw fixation.
           iii. Countersunk screws.
        b. Pelvis reconstruction plate.
    4. Pipkin type III fractures:
        a. Femoral head and neck ORIF.
        b. Hip arthroplasty:
           i. Elderly.
           ii. Comminution.
    5. Pipkin type IV:
        a. Femoral head and acetabulum ORIF.
        b. Restore acetabular stability.
    6. Rehabilitation:
        a. Immediate mobilization.
        b. Touchdown weight bearing with two crutches:
           i. Six to 8 weeks: isolated femoral head fixation.
           ii. Eight to 12 weeks: femoral neck or acetabulum.

   B. Prosthetic replacement[19]:
      1. Total hip arthroplasty:
         a. Active.
         b. Longer life expectancy.
      2. Hemiarthroplasty:
         a. Older patient.
         b. Limited mobility.
      3. Indications:
         a. Pipkin type III in the elderly.
         b. Evidence of advanced hip arthritis.

Complications

I.   Posttraumatic arthritis (20%)[21]:
   A. Osteochondral lesion:
      1. Larger size.
      2. Weight-bearing location.
      3. Comminution.
   B. Acetabulum or femoral head bone loss.
   C. Incongruent reduction:
      1. Soft-tissue interposition.
      2. Incarcerated bone fragment.

II. Avascular necrosis (AVN; 12%)[22]:
   A. Hip dislocations with associated femoral head fractures:
      1. High-energy trauma disrupts vascular supply.
      2. Delay in treatment.
      3. Iatrogenic injury:
         a. Closed reduction.
         b. Surgical approaches: i. Preferable anterior or trochanteric flip.

III. Heterotopic ossification (6–64%)[9,11,12,23–25]:
   A. Muscle and soft-tissue injury:
      1. Mechanism of trauma.
      2. Surgical exposure.
   B. Acetabular fracture (Pipkin type IV):
   C. Associated head injury.

IV. Malunion.[26]

V. Hip instability.

Femoral Neck Fractures

Introduction

I.   Epidemiology:
  A. Higher in patients older than 70 years.[27]
  B. Common in the elderly patients.
  C. Uncommon in young patients.
  D. Osteoporosis major risk factor:
    1. Risks increases with decreasing bone mass.
    2. More common in women.
    3. Bone density in the proximal femur declines with age.
    4. Low bone mineral density:
      a. Chronic diseases:
        i. Hypothyroidism.
        ii. Rheumatoid arthritis.
      b. Menopause.
      c. Tobacco use.
      d. Alcohol use.
      e. Medications:
        i. Corticosteroids.
        ii. Seizure medications.
II. Anatomy:
  A. Osseous[28,29]:
    1. Femoral neck shaft angle is approximately 130 ± 7 degrees.
    2. Femoral neck anteversion is approximately 10 ± 7 degrees.
    3. Femoral head diameter varies between 40 and 60 mm.
  B. Vascular[6]:
    1. MFCA:
      a. Lateral epiphyseal branch.
      b. Main blood supply to the femoral head.
    2. Lateral femoral circumflex:
      a. Inferior metaphyseal branch.

Mechanism of Injury

I.   Young adults:
  A. High-energy trauma.
  B. Axial load.

II.   Elderly:
    A. Low-energy trauma.
    B. Fall from height.

III.   Femoral neck stress fractures:
    A. Pathologic:
        1. Rheumatoid arthritis.
        2. Osteoporosis.
        3. Postcam osteoplasty (either arthroscopic or open).
    B. Nonpathologic:
        1. Overuse injury caused by repeated submaximal stress[30]:
            a. Long distance runners.
            b. Military recruits.
        2. One to 7.2% of all stress fracture injuries.[30]
        3. Associated with coxa vara.
        4. Low risk:
            a. Inferomedial aspect of the femoral neck.
            b. Compression type.
            c. Lower risk of delayed union.
        5. High risk:
            a. Superolateral aspect of the femoral neck.
            b. Tension type.
            c. Higher risk of delayed union.
            d. Long-distance runners.
            e. Radiographs are negative in up to 80%.[31]

Diagnosis

I.   History:
    A. Groin pain.
    B. Nonambulatory.
    C. Mechanism of injury:
        1. High energy versus low energy.
    D. Preinjury:
        1. Level of activity.
        2. Ambulatory status.
        3. Cognitive status.
    E. Prior fragility fractures:
        1. Prior hip pain.

    F. Pain in other locations.

    G. Comorbidites:

       1. Prognosis.

II. Physical examination:

    A. Extremity[32]:

       1. Shortened.

       2. Externally rotated.

       3. Slightly flexed at the hip.

    B. Assess for associated injuries.

    C. Neurovascular examination.

    D. Skin.

III. Imaging:

    A. Plain radiographs:

       1. AP pelvis:

          a. Fracture pattern.

          b. Displacement.

       2. Cross-table lateral:

          a. Posterior head displacement.

       3. Do not perform frog leg laterals:

          a. Risk to displace nondisplaced fractures.

    B. CT:

       1. Multicut detector, high-collimation, 1- to 2-mm cuts.

       2. Evaluate posterior head displacement.

       3. Non displaced femoral neck fractures:

          a. Unable to get MRI.

          b. High-energy femoral shaft fracture.

    C. MRI:

       1. Test of choice in occult femoral neck fractures.

       2. Test of choice in femoral neck stress fractures:

          a. High sensitivity: 86 to 100%.[33]

          b. High specificity: 100%.[33]

Classification Systems

I. Garden's classification[34] (**Fig. 10.2**):

    A. AP pelvis.

    B. Poor interobserver agreement.

    C. Four types based on degree of displacement:

       1. Type I:

          a. Incomplete.

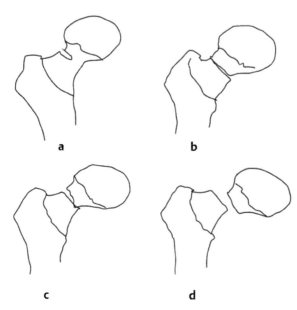

Fig. 10.2 The Garden classification of femoral neck fractures. Type I (**a**) is incomplete or valgus impacted. Type II (**b**) is complete and nondisplaced. Type III (**c**) is a complete fracture, partially displaced in varus alignment. Type IV (**d**) is completely displaced.

      b. Valgus impacted.

      c. Nondisplaced.

  2. Type II:

      a. Complete.

      b. Nondisplaced.

  3. Type III:

      a. Complete.

      b. Varus alignment.

      c. Functionally considered as displaced.

  4. Type IV:

      a. Completely displaced.

 D. Nondisplaced versus displaced for practical purposes.

II. Pauwels' classification (**Fig. 10.3**):

 A. AP pelvis.

 B. High-energy femoral neck fracture.

 C. Three types based on the fracture angle from the horizontal plane:

  1. Shear versus compression at fracture site.

  2. Type I:

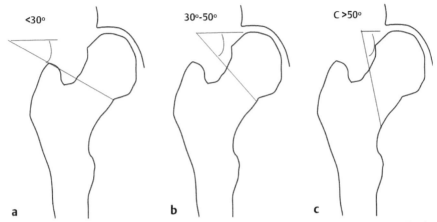

Fig. 10.3 The Pauwels classification of femoral neck fractures. This system is based on the angle for the fracture from the horizontal plane. Type I (**a**) is more horizontal with an angle less than 30 degrees. Type II (**b**) is between 30 and 50 degrees. Type III (**c**) is more vertical with an angle greater than 50 degrees.

        a. Less than 30 degrees.

        b. Compression forces predominate across fracture site.

    3. Type II:

        a. Thirty to 50 degrees.

    4. Type III:

        a. Greater than 50 degrees.

        b. Shear forces predominate across fracture site.

III.   OTA[18]:

   A. Research purposes.

   B. 31-B extraarticular fracture, neck:

      1. 31-B1 subcapital, with slight displacement.

      2. 31-B2 transcervical.

      3. 31-B3 subcapital, displaced, nonimpacted.

Treatment

I.   Nonoperative treatment[32]:

   A. Very ill patient.

   B. Unacceptable surgical risks.

   C. Low-risk and nonpathologic femoral neck stress fractures:

      1. Compression medial neck fractures.

      2. Toe-touch weight bearing for 8 weeks.

II.   Surgical treatment[32]:

   A. Indicated for most femoral neck fractures:

      1. Decreases morbidity and mortality.

2. Facilitates patient mobilization.

3. Improves patient outcomes.

4. Urgent or emergent surgery:

   a. Surgical emergency:

     i. High energy.

     ii. Displaced fracture.

     iii. Young patient.

B. Nondisplaced femoral neck fractures:

   1. In situ internal fixation[35-37]:

     a. Cannulated screws:

       i. Cancellous partially threaded screws.

       ii. 6.5-, 7.0-, and/or 7.3-mm screws.

       iii. Inverted triangle configuration.

       iv. Three screws:

         1. Inferior:

           a. Start proximal to lesser trochanter and

           b. Lower the risk of subtrochanteric fracture;

         2. Anterosuperior.

         3. Posterosuperior.

       v. Within 5 mm of subchondral bone.

       vi. Washer for poor osteoporotic bone.

       vii. Four screws (**Fig. 10.4**):

         1. Posterior neck comminution and

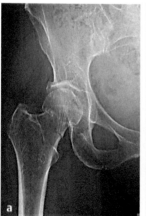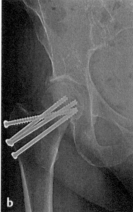

Fig. 10.4 (a) Vertically oriented and nondisplaced femoral neck fracture. The fracture angle is greater than 50 degrees (Pauwels III). **(b)** Healed fracture following in situ cannulated screw fixation. A fourth horizontally aligned screw was used.

2. Horizontal screw for Pauwels III:

   a. Antishear.

b. Sliding hip screw:

   i. Pauwels III.

   ii. Basicervical femoral neck fractures:

      1. Derotational screw.

   iii. Tip apex distance less than 25 mm.

   iv. Higher risk of AVN.

2. Displaced femoral neck fractures:

   a. Surgical treatment is determined by the following:

      i. Patient:

         1. Age,

         2. Activity level,

         3. Life expectancy, and

         4. Medical comorbidities.

      ii. Fracture:

         1. Location,

         2. Orientation, and

         3. Comminution.

   b. Treatment options:

      i. Closed ORIF[35–37]:

         1. Young adults,

         2. Elderly nonambulatory unfit for arthroplasty,

         3. Acceptable reduction criteria:

            a. Neck shaft angle 130 to 150 degrees;

            b. Anteversion 0 to 15 degrees;

            c. Valgus angulation up to 15 degrees;

         4. Unacceptable reduction:

            a. Varus angulation;

            b. Retroversion;

            c. Higher risks—nonunion, AVN, and hardware failure;

         5. Approach for open reduction:

            a. Anterior—Heuter, Smith–Peterson, and separate incision for fixation;

            b. Anterolateral.

      ii. Hemiarthroplasty[35–38] (**Fig. 10.5**):

         1. Indications:

            a. Elderly patient;

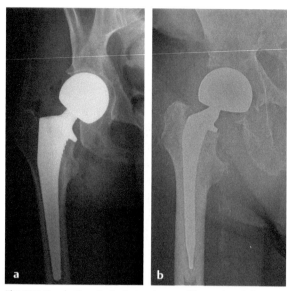

Fig. 10.5 Hemiarthroplasty for treatment of femoral neck fracture. **(a)** Uncemented hemiarthroplasty with unipolar femoral head. **(b)** Cemented hemiarthroplasty with bipolar femoral head.

    b. Low demand;

    c. Demented;

2. Approach:

    a. Anterior;

    b. Anterolateral;

    c. Posterior—higher dislocation rate;

3. Method of fixation:

    a. Cemented—risk of fat/cement embolism;

    b. Uncemmented—risk of fracture;

4. Unipolar versus bipolar heads:

    a. No difference on dislocation rate;

    b. Higher cost with bipolar heads.

iii. Total hip arthroplasty (THA)[35–38] (**Fig. 10.6**):

1. Indications:

    a. Older patient;

    b. Active and high demand;

    c. Preceding hip pain and arthritis;

2. increased use of THA over hemiarthroplasty;

3. Advantages over hemiarthroplasty:

    a. Better pain scores;

    b. Better function scores;

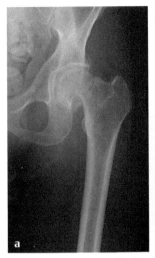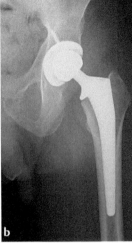

Fig. 10.6 (a) Completely displaced femoral neck fracture. **(b)** Left uncemented total hip arthroplasty.

    4. Disadvantages over hemiarthroplasty:
      a. Dislocation risk;
      b. Longer surgical time;
      c. Increased blood loss;
    5. Approach: same as hemiarthroplasty;
    6. Cemented and uncemented femoral fixation.
  iv. Hip resection "Girdlestone":
    1. Failed surgical treatment;
    2. Painful hip:
      a. Low-demand patient;
      b. Poor reconstruction candidate.

Complications

I.   AVN of the femoral head:
   A. Six months from injury.
   B. Collapse 1 to 2 years from surgery:
     1. Displaced fractures (20–30%).[39,40]
     2. Nondisplaced fractures (15%).[39,40]
II.   Nonunion:
   A. Younger, high energy, and displaced fractures (10–30%)[39,40]:
     1. Vertical fractures.
     2. Varus collapse.
   B. Elderly nondisplaced (5%).[39,40]

III. Impaired mobility:

    A. Elderly: 1 year after hip fracture:

        1. Fifty percent fail to regain preinjury level of mobility.[39,40]

        2. Physical and mental condition.

        3. Loss of independent living.

IV. Medical complications[41]:

    A. Deep vein thrombosis.

    B. Pulmonary embolism.

    C. Delirium.

    D. Pulmonary complications.

V. Mortality:

    A. Elderly: 1-year mortality rate of 20 to 30%.[39,41]

    B. Risk factors:

        1. General anesthesia.

        2. Delayed surgical intervention:

            a. More than 72 hours after injury.

        3. Anemia.

        4. Prior femoral neck fracture.

        5. Multiple comorbidities.

VI. Arthroplasty complications:

    A. Lower reoperation rates compared to ORIF.[39,42,43]

    B. Dislocation.

    C. Periprosthetic fractures.

    D. Mortality:

        1. Thirty-day mortality of 2.4%.[44,45]

        2. Six times higher than elective THA.[46]

References

1. Asghar FA, Karunakar MA. Femoral head fractures: diagnosis, management, and complications. Orthop Clin North Am 2004;35(4):463–472

2. Upadhyay SS, Moulton A, Burwell RG. Biological factors predisposing to traumatic posterior dislocation of the hip. A selection process in the mechanism of injury. J Bone Joint Surg Br 1985;67(2):232–236

3. Kozin SH, Kolessar DJ, Guanche CA, et al. Bilateral femoral head fracture with posterior hip dislocation. Orthop Rev Suppl 1994;20–24

4. Meislin RJ, Zuckerman JD. Case report: bilateral posterior hip dislocations with femoral head fractures. J Orthop Trauma 1989;3:353–361

5. Brumback RJ, Kenzora JE, Levitt LE, et al. Fractures of the femoral head. Proceedings of the Hip Society, 1986. St. Louis, MO: C.V. Mosby; 1987:181–206

6. Seeley MA, Georgiadis AG, Sankar WN. Hip vascularity: a review of the anatomy and clinical implications. J Am Acad Orthop Surg 2016;24(8):515–526

7. Christopher F. Fractures of the head of the femur. Arch Surg 1926;12:1049–1061

8. Schmidt GL, Sciulli R, Altman GT. Knee injury in patients experiencing a high-energy trau-matic ipsilateral hip dislocation. J Bone Joint Surg Am 2005;87(6):1200–1204

9. Roeder LF Jr, DeLee JC. Femoral head fractures associated with posterior hip dislocation. Clin Orthop Relat Res 1980;147:121–130

10. Epstein HC. Posterior fracture-dislocations of the hip; long-term follow-up. J Bone Joint Surg Am 1974;56(6):1103–1127

11. Marchetti ME, Steinberg GG, Coumas JM. Intermediate-term experience of Pipkin fracture-dislocations of the hip. J Orthop Trauma 1996;10(7):455–461

12. Kloen P, Siebenrock KA, Raaymakers E, Marti RK, Ganz R. Femoral head fractures revisited. Eur J Trauma 2002;28:221–233

13. Cornwall R, Radomisli TE. Nerve injury in traumatic dislocation of the hip. Clin Orthop Relat Res 2000;377:84–91

14. Funsten RV, Kinser P, Frankel CJ. Dashboard dislocation of the hip: a report of twenty cases of traumatic dislocation. J Bone Joint Surg 1938;20:124–132

15. Foulk DM, Mullis BH. Hip dislocation: evaluation and management. J Am Acad Orthop Surg 2010;18(4):199–209

16. Dussault RG, Beauregard G, Fauteaux P, Laurin C, Boisjoly A. Femoral head defect following anterior hip dislocation. Radiology 1980;135(3):627–629

17. Pipkin G. Treatment of grade IV fracture-dislocation of the hip. J Bone Joint Surg Am 1957;39-A(5):1027–1042, passim

18. Marsh JL, Slongo TF, Agel J, et al. Fracture and dislocation classification compendium - 2007: Orthopaedic Trauma Association classification, database and outcomes committee. J Orthop Trauma 2007;21(10, Suppl):S1–S133

19. Droll KP, Broekhuyse H, O'Brien P. Fracture of the femoral head. J Am Acad Orthop Surg 2007;15(12):716–727

20. Prokop A, Helling HJ, Hahn U, Udomkaewkanjana C, Rehm KE. Biodegradable implants for Pipkin fractures. Clin Orthop Relat Res 2005;(432):226–233

21. Paus B. Traumatic dislocations of the hip; late results in 76 cases. Acta Orthop Scand 1951;21(2):99–112

22. Dreinhöfer KE, Schwarzkopf SR, Haas NP, Tscherne H. Isolated traumatic dislocation of the hip. Long-term results in 50 patients. J Bone Joint Surg Br 1994;76(1):6–12

23. Swiontkowski MF, Thorpe M, Seiler JG, Hansen ST. Operative management of displaced femoral head fractures: case-matched comparison of anterior versus posterior approaches for Pipkin I and Pipkin II fractures. J Orthop Trauma 1992;6(4):437–442

24. Hougaard K, Thomsen PB. Traumatic posterior fracture-dislocation of the hip with fracture of the femoral head or neck, or both. J Bone Joint Surg Am 1988;70(2):233–239

25. Lang-Stevenson A, Getty CJ. The Pipkin fracture-dislocation of the hip. Injury 1987;18(4):264–269

26. Sontich JK, Cannada LK. Femoral head avulsion fracture with malunion to the acetabulum: a case report. J Orthop Trauma 2002;16(1):49–51

27. American Academy of Orthopaedic Surgeons. Management of Hip Fractures in the Elderly. 2014. Available at: http://www.aaos.org/research/guidelines/HipFxGuideline.pdf. Accessed August 21, 2017

28. Reikerås O, Høiseth A. Femoral neck angles in osteoarthritis of the hip. Acta Orthop Scand 1982;53(5):781–784

29. Reikerås O, Bjerkreim I, Kolbenstvedt A. Anteversion of the acetabulum and femo-ral neck in normals and in patients with osteoarthritis of the hip. Acta Orthop Scand 1983;54(1):18–23

30. Robertson GAJ, Wood AM. Lower limb stress fractures in sport: optimising their management and outcome. World J Orthop 2017;8(3):242–255

31. Greaney RB, Gerber FH, Laughlin RL, et al. Distribution and natural history of stress fractures in U.S. Marine recruits. Radiology 1983;146(2):339–346

32. Roberts KC, Brox WT, Jevsevar DS, Sevarino K. Management of hip fractures in the elderly. J Am Acad Orthop Surg 2015;23(2):131–137

33. National Clinical Guideline Centre. The Management of Hip Fracture in Adults. London: National Clinical Guideline Centre; 2011. Available from: https://www.nice.org.uk/guidance/cg124. Accessed August 21, 2017
34. Barnes R, Brown JT, Garden RS, Nicoll EA. Subcapital fractures of the femur. A prospective review. J Bone Joint Surg Br 1976;58(1):2–24
35. Probe R, Ward R. Internal fixation of femoral neck fractures. J Am Acad Orthop Surg 2006;14(9):565–571
36. Ye CY, Liu A, Xu MY, Nonso NS, He RX. Arthroplasty versus internal fixation for displaced intracapsular femoral neck fracture in the elderly: systematic review and meta-analysis of short- and long-term effectiveness. Chin Med J (Engl) 2016;129(21):2630–2638
37. Florschutz AV, Langford JR, Haidukewych GJ, Koval KJ. Femoral neck fractures: current management. J Orthop Trauma 2015;29(3):121–129
38. Rogmark C, Leonardsson O. Hip arthroplasty for the treatment of displaced fractures of the femoral neck in elderly patients. Bone Joint J 2016;98-B(3):291–297
39. Carpintero P, Caeiro JR, Carpintero R, Morales A, Silva S, Mesa M. Complications of hip fractures: a review. World J Orthop 2014;5(4):402–411
40. Lu-Yao GL, Keller RB, Littenberg B, Wennberg JE. Outcomes after displaced fractures of the femoral neck. A meta-analysis of one hundred and six published reports. J Bone Joint Surg Am 1994;76(1):15–25
41. Sciard D, Cattano D, Hussain M, Rosenstein A. Perioperative management of proximal hip fractures in the elderly: the surgeon and the anesthesiologist. Minerva Anestesiol 2011;77(7):715–722
42. Orwig DL, Chan J, Magaziner J. Hip fracture and its consequences: differences between men and women. Orthop Clin North Am 2006;37(4):611–622
43. Blomfeldt R, Törnkvist H, Ponzer S, Söderqvist A, Tidermark J. Comparison of internal fixation with total hip replacement for displaced femoral neck fractures. Randomized, controlled trial performed at four years. J Bone Joint Surg Am 2005;87(8):1680–1688
44. Brauer CA, Coca-Perraillon M, Cutler DM, Rosen AB. Incidence and mortality of hip fractures in the United States. JAMA 2009;302(14):1573–1579
45. Zuckerman JD. Hip fracture. N Engl J Med 1996;334(23):1519–1525
46. Le Manach Y, Collins G, Bhandari M, et al. Outcomes after hip fracture surgery compared with elective total hip replacement. JAMA 2015;314(11):1159–1166

11 Extracapsular Hip Fractures

Carlos J. Meheux, Luis F. Pulido-Sierra

Introduction

Incidence and Etiology

I. Intertrochanteric femur fractures:

    A. Increasing incidence and will likely approach 500,000 per year by 2040.[1]

    B. More common in women older than 65 years of age.

    C. About one-third of women reaching the age of 90 years will sustain a hip fracture.[2]

    D. Patients with osteoporosis are at increased risk for intertrochanteric femur fractures.

    E. Increased incidence of falls in the elderly population.

        1. Multifactorial:

            a. Postural and gait disturbances.

            b. Decreased visual and hearing acuity.

            c. Usage of one (or multiple) disorienting medications.

    F. Associated fractures include the following:

        1. Distal radius.

        2. Proximal humerus.

        3. Spine.

        4. Ribs.

        5. Pubic rami.

    G. Young patients:

        1. High-energy mechanisms:

            a. Usually have grossly displaced fractures.

            b. Reverse obliquity.

            c. Subtrochanteric extension.

    H. Pathologic fractures from metastasis.

II. Subtrochanteric femur fractures:

    A. Asymmetric age- and gender-related bimodal distribution:

        1. High-energy mechanism:

            a. Young patients.

            b. Mostly males.

            c. Usually motor vehicle accidents.

            d. Fall from heights.

            e. Penetrating trauma.

    2. Low-energy mechanism:

      a. Elderly patients.

      b. Mostly females.[3]

      c. Falls.

      d. Pathologic fractures:

        (i) Atypical fractures.

        (ii) Bisphosphonate use greater than 3 to 5 years.

B. Associated injuries involving other extremities:

    1. Commonly seen in high-energy mechanisms.[3]

C. Subtrochanteric femur fracture can result from prior surgery:

    1. Screw fixation of ipsilateral femoral neck fracture:

      a. Screw starting point distal to the lesser trochanter.

    2. Core decompression and vascularized free fibula autografting for avascular necrosis of the femoral head:

      a. Lateral cortical defect is below the lesser trochanter.

D. Pathologic fractures from bisphosphonate use or metastasis.

Anatomy

Intraosseous Scaffold of Trabecular Bone Supports Femoral Head and Neck (Fig. 11.1)

I. Primary compressive group:

  A. Dense cancellous bone.

II. Secondary compressive, tensile, and greater trochanter groups:

  A. Oriented along stress lines in the lateral femoral neck.

  B. Relative paucity of trabecular scaffolding in the central area also called Ward's triangle.[4]

III. Changes in the trabecular pattern affects bone density.

Numerous Muscle Attachments to the Intertrochanteric Area

I. Brings rich and abundant blood supply.

II. Very conducive to fracture healing.

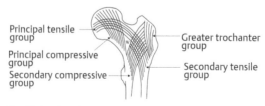

Fig. 11.1 Trabecular groups and Ward's triangle of the proximal femur.

Muscular Forces Dictate Direction of Displacement

I. Iliopsoas:

    A. Pulls on its insertion at the lesser trochanter.

II. Abductors and external rotators:

    A. Act through their attachments at the greater trochanter.

    B. Leads to shortened and externally rotated extremity in displaced fractures, especially intertrochanteric femur fractures with subtrochanteric extensions or subtrochanteric femur fractures.

Classification Systems

Intertrochanteric Femur Fractures[5]

I. Stable fracture:

    A. Posteromedial cortex:

        1. Fractured in only one place.

    B. Lateral cortex: intact.

    C. Obliquity: standard.

    D. Withstands axial loads:

        1. Without displacement after anatomic reduction.

II. Unstable fracture:

    A. Posteromedial cortex:

        1. Large fragment or comminuted.

    B. Lateral cortex:

        1. Fracture below the vastus ridge.

    C. Obliquity:

        1. May be standard or reverse.

    D. Fracture collapses with axial loading after reduction.

Subtrochanteric Femur Fractures

I. Russel–Taylor classification[6] (**Fig. 11.2**):

    A. Type IA:

        1. Does not involve piriformis fossa.

        2. Does not involve lesser trochanter.

    B. Type IB:

        1. Does not involve piriformis fossa.

        2. Involves less trochanter,

    C. Type IIA:

        1. Involves piriformis fossa.

        2. Does not involve lesser trochanter.

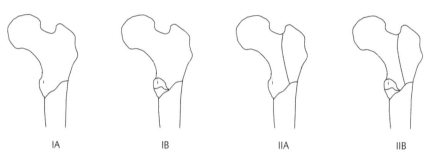

IA   IB   IIA   IIB

Fig. 11.2 Russell–Taylor classification of subtrochanteric femur fractures. In type I fractures, the piriform-is fossa remains intact and in type II fractures, the piriformis fossa is involved. In subtype A fractures, the lesser trochanter is not involved and in subtype B fractures, the lesser trochanter is involved.

     D. Type IIB:

        1. Involves the piriformis fossa.

        2. Involves the lesser trochanter.

Diagnosis

I.   History:

    A. Elderly patient:

       1. Most commonly a slip and fall mechanism.

         a. Preexisting pain may indicate pathologic lesion or arthritis.

       2. Evaluate for other injuries, including the following:

         a. Femoral shaft.

         b. Proximal humerus.

         c. Distal radius.

         d. Ankle.

         e. Knee.

       3. Evaluate preexisting medical condition:

         a. Preinjury functional status.

    B. Young patients:

       1. High-energy mechanism:

         a. Fracture likely involves the subtrochanteric region.

II. Physical examination:

    A. Extremity:

       1. Short and externally rotated.

       2. Local ecchymosis:

         a. Posterolateral aspect of the trochanteric area.

    B. Inspect pressure points for possible skin breakdown:

       1. Sacrum.

       2. Buttocks.

       3. Heel.

    C. Examine other extremities for occult injuries.

    D. Neurovascular examination of the extremity.

III. Imaging:

    A. Plain radiographs:

        1. Anteroposterior (AP) radiographs of the pelvis:

           a. Apply gentle traction and internal rotation to the affected extremity.

        2. Cross-table lateral view of the hip.

        3. Orthogonal views of the femur (AP and lateral radiographs):

           a. Evaluate for subtrochanteric fractures.

           b. Extension of intertrochanteric fractures.

           c. Other femur fractures.

           d. Presence of implants in the femur.

        4. Radiographs of contralateral hip and femur:

           a. Can aid with preoperative planning.

        5. Evaluate radiographs for:

           a. Osteopenia.

           b. Metastasis.

           c. Cortical irregularities.

    B. Computed tomography (CT) scans:

        1. Frequently performed in polytrauma patients:

           a. Chest, abdomen, pelvis.

           b. Cervical, thoracic, and lumbar spine.

        2. Delineate more complex fractures.

    C. Magnetic resonance imaging (MRI):

        1. High suspicion for occult fracture.

        2. Plain films are negative.

Treatment

I. Nonoperative treatment:

    A. Pain control:

        1. Indications:

           a. Unable to tolerate surgery due to medical condition.

           b. Intertrochanteric and subtrochanteric femur fractures.

    B. Skeletal or skin traction:

        1. Indications:

           a. Unable to tolerate surgery due to medical condition.

           b. Intertrochanteric and subtrochanteric femur fractures.

   2. Treatment:
       a. Skeletal traction:
           (i) Steinmann pin to distal femur or proximal tibia.
       b. Skin traction:
           (i) Apply soft padding to ankle.
       c. Apply 10 to 15 lb of traction.
II.   Operative:
   A. Sliding hip screw[7] (**Fig. 11.3**):
       1. Indications:
           a. Stable intertrochanteric femur fractures.
       2. Treatment:
           a. Position supine on a fracture table.
           b. Reduce fracture with gentle traction and internal rotation under fluoroscopy.
           c. Lateral approach to the proximal femur.
           d. Starting at the level of the lesser trochanter:
               (i)   Insert guide pin into neck and head.
               (ii) Aim for the apex of the femoral head.
               (iii) Tip–apex distance.
           e. Measure length and ream appropriately.
           f. Insert lag screw:
               (i) Tip–apex distance (**Fig. 11.4**):
                   (1) goal—less than 25 mm;
                   (2) greater than 25 mm—high failure rates.[8]
           g. Apply plate with barrel and apply screws to plate.
   B. Short cephalomedullary nail:
       1. Indications:
           a. Intertrochanteric femur fractures.
       2. Treatment:
           a. Position supine on a fracture table.

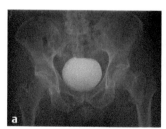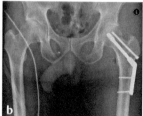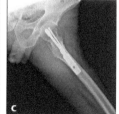

Fig. 11.3 (**a**) Anteroposterior (AP) view of the pelvis of a 68-year-old man with left intertrochanteric femur fracture. (**b, c**) AP view of the pelvis and lateral view of the left hip of the same patient after fixation with a sliding hip screw.

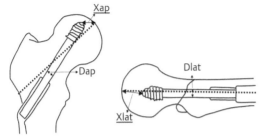

Fig. 11.4 Tip–apex distance (TAD) is the sum of the distance in millimeters from the tip of the lag screw to the apex of the femoral head on the anteroposterior view (Xap) and the lateral view of the hip (Xlat), after correction has been made for magnification. Correction for magnification can be performed as the original described using the known diameter of the lag screw used (Dtrue).

TAD = (Xap x [Dtrue/ Dap]) + (Xlat x [Dtrue / Dlat])

TAD = (Xap + Xlat (once corrected for magnification)

b. Reduce fracture with gentle traction and internal rotation under fluoroscopy.

c. Percutaneous approach to proximal femur for nailing.

d. Identify proper starting point under fluoroscopy:

(i) Tip of the trochanter on the anteroposterior view of the hip.

(ii) In line with the femoral neck on the lateral view.

e. Insert guide pin into proximal femur and ream over guide pin.

f. Insert nail.

g. Use guide on nail-inserting jig to insert lag screw and distal locking screw:

(i) Insert lag screw such that the tip–apex distance is ≤25 mm.

(ii) Use fluoroscopy for guidance.

C. Long cephalomedullary nail:

1. Indications:

a. Intertrochanteric femur fractures (**Fig. 11.5**):

(i) Stable.

(ii) Unstable.

b. Subtrochanteric femur fractures[9] (**Fig. 11.6**).

c. Pathologic pertrochanteric femur fractures.

2. Treatment:

a. Position supine on a fracture table.

b. Can position lateral on a radiolucent table:

(i) Displaced subtrochanteric femur fractures.

(ii) Lateral position helps with fracture reduction.

c. Reduce fracture with aid of fluoroscopy:

(i) May need to do provisional reduction with pins, clamps, wires, or other devices.

(ii) May need to do an open reduction depending on the complexity of the fracture:

(1) Lateral approach to proximal femur.

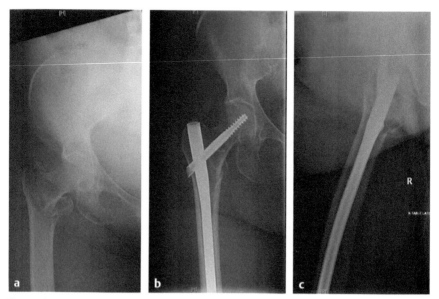

Fig. 11.5 (**a**) Anteroposterior (AP) view of the right hip showing an intertrochanteric femur fracture in a 63-year-old woman after a fall. (**b**) AP view of the right hip after cephalomedullary nail placement. (**c**) Lateral view of the right hip after cephalomedullary nail placement.

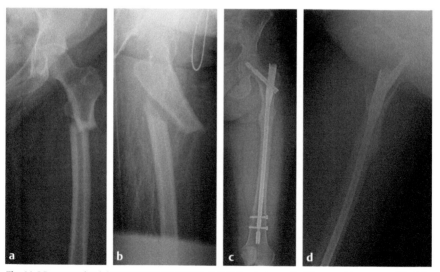

Fig. 11.6 Preoperative (**a**) anteroposterior (AP) and (**b**) lateral views of a 59-year-old woman with right atypical subtrochanteric femur fracture associated with bisphosphonate use. The patient was treated successfully with a left long cephalomedullary nail fixation. Postoperative (**c**) AP and (**d**) lateral femur radiographs at 3 months from surgical treatment. The patient also received teriparatide injections, calcium, and vitamin D.

    d. Percutaneous approach to proximal femur for nailing.

    e. Identify proper starting point under fluoroscopy:

       (i) Tip of the trochanter on the anteroposterior view of the hip;

      (ii) In line with the femoral neck on the lateral view.

    f. Insert guide pin into the proximal femur and ream over the guide pin.

    g. Insert ball-tip guidewire into the femoral canal and aim for the distal femur:

       (i) Measure the length of the guidewire in the femur to determine the length of the nail.

    h. Ream over ball-tip guidewire to prepare canal:

       (i) Over-ream by 1.5 to 2 mm to allow for easy insertion of the nail.

    i. Insert nail.

    j. Use guide on nail-inserting jig to insert lag screw:

       (i) Insert lag screw such that the tip–apex distance is ≤25 mm.

      (ii) Use fluoroscopy for guidance.

    k. Apply distal interlocking screw(s) under fluoroscopic guidance.

D. Prosthetic replacement:

   1. Not a primary treatment option for extracapsular hip fractures:

    a. Greater trochanter:

       (i) Difficulty with greater trochanter fixation.

      (ii) Success and stability of endoprosthesis rely on the greater trochanter.

    b. Conversion hip arthroplasty is successful after failed primary open reduction and internal fixation techniques.

   2. Indications:

    a. Elderly:

       (i) Preexisting symptomatic degenerative arthritis.

      (ii) Pathologic fractures.

     (iii) Open reduction and internal fixation (ORIF) likely to fail:

        (1) Comminution.

    b. Type of endoprosthesis:

       (i) Cemented hemiarthroplasty:

        (1) Calcar replacement prosthesis.

        (2) Proximal femoral replacement.

Complications

I.   Loss of fixation and implant failure:

   A. Screw cutout:

    1. Tip–apex distance greater than 25 mm:

    a. Higher and accumulative incidence.

II. Nonunion:

    A. Higher incidence with displaced fractures.

III. Malunion:

    A. Nonanatomic reduction during fixation.

    B. Inadequate fixation.

IV. Infection.

V. Fracture around the implant:

    A. Higher incidence with short cephalomedullary nails.

VI. Anterior perforation of the distal femur:

    A. Mismatch of the radius of curvature of the implant (longer) and femur (shorter).

References

1. Cummings SR, Phillips SL, Wheat ME, et al. Recovery of function after hip fracture. The role of social supports. J Am Geriatr Soc 1988;36(9):801–806
2. Cummings SR, Kelsey JL, Nevitt MC, O'Dowd KJ. Epidemiology of osteoporosis and osteoporotic fractures. Epidemiol Rev 1985;7:178–208
3. Bergman GD, Winquist RA, Mayo KA, Hansen ST Jr. Subtrochanteric fracture of the femur. Fixation using the Zickel nail. J Bone Joint Surg Am 1987;69(7):1032–1040
4. Griffin JB. The calcar femorale redefined. Clin Orthop Relat Res 1982; (164):211–214
5. Koval K, Zuckerman J. Intertrochanteric fractures. In: Buchholz R, Heckman J, eds. Rockwood and Green's Fractures in Adults. 6th ed. Philadelphia, PA: Lippincott Williams & Wilkins; 2005
6. Russell TA. Subtrochanteric fractures of the femur. In: Browner B, Jupiter J, Levine A, et al., eds. Skeletal Trauma: Basic Science, Management and Reconstruction. 3rd ed. Philadelphia, PA: Elsevier Science; 2002:1832–1878
7. Kaplan K, Miyamoto R, Levine BR, Egol KA, Zuckerman JD. Surgical management of hip fractures: an evidence-based review of the literature. II: intertrochanteric fractures. J Am Acad Orthop Surg 2008;16(11):665–673
8. Baumgaertner MR, Curtin SL, Lindskog DM. Intramedullary versus extramedullary fixation for the treatment of intertrochanteric hip fractures. Clin Orthop Relat Res 1998;(348):87–94
9. Lundy DW. Subtrochanteric femoral fractures. J Am Acad Orthop Surg 2007;15(11):663–671

12 Pediatric Hip Fractures

Joshua D. Harris, Robert A. Jack II

Introduction

Proximal Femur Fractures

I. "Hip fractures" account for less than 1% of all pediatric fractures.[1,2]
II. Mechanism of injury:
    A. High-energy trauma (75–80%)
    B. Breech delivery.
III. High rate of complications due to age-dependent challenging blood supply.

Acetabular Fractures

I. Comprise 1 to 15% of pediatric pelvic fractures.[3]
II. Triradiate cartilage injuries (below age 12–14 years) can cause growth arrest and deformities.
III. Often lower energy than adult fractures.
IV. Associated with femoral head fractures and dislocations.

Pelvic Ring Fractures[4]

I. Result of high-energy trauma
II. Commonly motor vehicle collision or automobile–pedestrian collision.
III. Differences from adult fractures:
    A. Lateral compression injuries greater than anteroposterior (AP) injuries.
    B. Higher rate of single ring break than adults.
    C. Increased plasticity.
    D. More robust and absorbent cartilage.
    E. Sacroiliac (SI) joint and pubic symphysis are more elastic:
        1. Different injury patterns.
        2. Prior to triradiate closure: bone weaker than ligament, resulting in isolated pubic rami or iliac wing fracture, rather than pelvic ring disruption.
    F. Thickened periosteum stabilizes fractures.
    G. Lower rate of hemorrhage:
        1. Smaller blood vessels.
        2. Higher capacity for vasoconstriction.
        3. Lower likelihood of "open book" injuries.

Pelvic Avulsion Fractures[5-7]

I. Result of low-energy trauma.

II. Tendon is disrupted from origin or insertion during explosive exercises:

   A. Eccentric contraction of muscle causing traction injury to cartilaginous apophysis.

   B. Sprinting.

   C. Jumping.

III. Multiple origins/insertions (**Fig. 12.1**):

   A. Ischial tuberosity avulsion: hamstring (semimembranosus superolaterally and conjoint semitendinosus/biceps femoris inferomedially) or adductors.

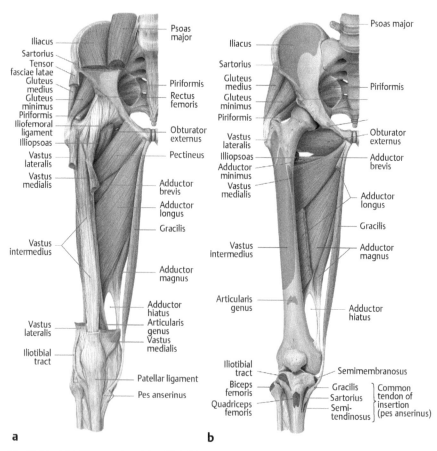

Fig. 12.1 (a, b) 1. The muscles of the thigh, hip, and gluteal region. (**a**) Shows anterior superficial and (**b**) shows anterior deep. The origins and insertions of the muscles are indicated by color shading (red = origin; blue = insertion). (Source: Schuenke M, Schulte E, Schumacher U. Thieme Atlas of Anatomy. General Anatomy and Musculoskeletal System. 2nd edition. ©2014, Thieme Publishers, New York. Illustrations by Voll M and Wesker K.)

B. Anterior inferior iliac spine (AIIS) avulsion: direct head of the rectus femoris.

C. Anterior superior iliac spine (ASIS) avulsion: sartorius, tensor fascia lata, and inguinal ligament.

D. Lesser trochanter avulsion: iliopsoas.

E. Pubic symphysis.

F. Iliac crest avulsion: abdominal musculature; also crest apophysitis is a repetitive overuse traction injury; differentiate per Risser's staging (U.S. system):

    1. Stage 0: no ossification of apophysis.

    2. Stage 1: most anterior one-fourth of apophysis ossified.

    3. Stage 2: most anterior half of apophysis ossified.

    4. Stage 3: most anterior three-fourths of apophysis ossified.

    5. Stage 4: apophysis ossified, but not yet fused to the iliac wing.

    6. Stage 5: completely ossified apophysis fuses to the iliac wing.

G. Greater trochanter avulsion: hip abductors.

Anatomic Considerations

I. Unique blood supply of proximal femur (**Fig. 12.2**)[8,9]:

A. Infants:

    1. Metaphyseal vessels originating from the medial and lateral femoral circumflex arteries[10]:

      a. Transverse femoral physis and supply the proximal epiphysis.

    2. Artery of ligamentum teres.

B. Age older than 2 years[10]:

    1. Cartilaginous physis of the proximal femur is barrier to the femoral head blood flow.

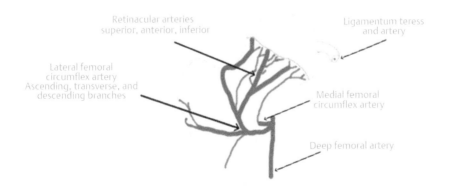

Fig. 12.2 Anterior view of the right proximal femur demonstrating the arterial blood supply.

    2. Main blood supply is via the lateral epiphyseal vessels from the medial femoral circumflex artery:

       a. Posterosuperior and posteroinferior epiphyseal vessels.

       b. Lie on the femoral neck.

       c. Vulnerable to injury with fracture.

  C. Age older than 4 years[11,12]:

    1. Artery of the ligamentum teres diminishes.

    2. Lateral femoral circumflex artery regresses by late childhood.

II. Proximal femur physes[10]:

  A. Proximal femoral epiphysis:

    1. Thirteen percent to 15% of leg length.

    2. Thirty percent length of the femur.

    3. Grows 3 mm per year.

  B. Trochanteric apophysis:

    1. Contributes to femoral neck growth.

    2. Injury can lead to coxa vara or valga.

III. Pelvis ossification[10,13–16]:

  A. Primary ossification centers (triradiate cartilage): endochondral ossification:

    1. Ilium appears on radiographs at 3 weeks.

    2. Ischium appears on radiographs at 16 weeks.

    3. Pubis appears on radiographs at 20 weeks.

    4. Fusion of centers at 12 years in females and at 14 years in males.

  B. Secondary ossification centers of the acetabulum:

    1. Os acetabuli (anterior wall).

    2. Acetabular epiphysis (superior acetabulum).

    3. Secondary ossification center of the ischium (posterior wall).

    4. Appear at 8 years.

    5. Fuse at 17 to 18 years.

  C. Secondary ossification centers of the pelvis:

    1. Iliac crest: appears at 13 years and fuses at 15 to 17 years.

    2. Ischial apophysis: appears at 15 years and fuses at 19 to 25 years.

    3. AIIS: appears at 14 years and fuses at 16 years.

    4. Pubic tubercle.

    5. Angle of pubis.

    6. Ischial spine.

    7. Lateral wing of the sacrum.

Classification

I. Delbet's classification of pediatric proximal femur fractures[17] (**Table 12.1**).

II.   Bucholz's classification of pediatric acetabulum fractures[18] (**Table 12.2**).

III. Letournel's classification of acetabulum fractures[19–23] (**Table 12.3**).

IV.   Torode–Zieg classification of pediatric pelvic ring injuries[24] (**Table 12.4**).

History and Examination

I.   Information from emergency medical transport professionals:
   A. Mechanism of injury.
   B. Level of consciousness.
   C. Initial physical examination.

II. Initial assessment:
   A. Airway.
   B. Breathing.
   C. Circulation.
   D. Disability/neuro status.
   E. Exposure and environment.

III. Symptoms:
   A. Pain.
   B. Inability to bear weight.
   C. Hearing a "pop" during exercise.

IV. Physical examination:
   A. Inspection:
      1. Abnormal lower extremity positioning:
         a. External rotation of one or both extremities.
         b. Leg length shortening.
      2. Skin:
         a. Degloving injury (Morel–Lavallée).
         b. Flank hematoma.
   B. Palpation:
      1. Evaluate for crepitus and tenderness.
      2. Test pelvis stability with gentle lateral compressive or rotational force.
      3. Point tenderness for avulsion injuries.
   C. Neurological examination:
      1. Lower extremity motor examination.
      2. Lower extremity sensory examination.
      3. Rectal examination.
   D. Vascular examination:
      1. Palpate and/or Doppler dorsalis pedis and posterior tibial arteries.

Table 12.1 Delbet's classification of pediatric proximal femur fractures

Type	Description	Incidence (%)	AVN rate (%)
I	Transphyseal separation	8	80
IA	Without dislocation of epiphysis from acetabulum		
IB	With dislocation of epiphysis		
II	Transcervical fracture	40–50	50
III	Cervicotrochanteric (basicervical) fracture	30–35	25
IV	Intertrochanteric fracture	10–20	<10

Abbreviation: AVN, avascular necrosis.

Table 12.2 Bucholz's classification for pediatric acetabulum fractures

Type	Fracture pattern
Shearing	Salter Harris I or II
Crushing/impaction	Salter Harris V

Table 12.3 Letournel's classification system for acetabulum fractures in skeletally mature patients

Type	Notes	Frequency (%)
Elementary		
Posterior wall	Most common	25
Posterior column	Detachment of ischioacetabular segment from innominate bone	3–5
Anterior wall	Rare	1–2
Anterior column	Anterior border of innominate bone displaced form intact ilium	3–5
Transverse	Only elementary fracture to involve both columns	5–19
Associated		
Associated both columns	Acetabulum is completely separate from axial skeleton. "Spur sign" on obturator oblique	23
Transverse and posterior wall	Transverse component may be transtectal, juxtatectal, or infratectal	20
T-shaped	T portion is an inferior vertical fracture	7
Anterior column/wall and posterior hemitransverse	75% will involve anterior column and not wall	7
Posterior column and posterior wall	Only associated fracture that does not involve both columns	3–4

Table 12.4 Torode–Zieg classification for pediatric pelvic ring fractures

Type	Description
I	Avulsion injury
II	Fracture of the iliac wing
III	Fracture of the pelvic ring without segmental instability
IV	Fracture of the pelvic ring with segmental instability

E. Urogenital examination:

1. Scrotal/labial or perineal hematoma.

2. Blood at urethral meatus.

3. Traumatic laceration of perineum.

4. Hematuria.

5. Vaginal/rectal examination for open fracture.

F. Special tests:

1. For low-energy mechanisms, suspicion of avulsion fracture.

2. Resisted activation of muscle group implicated.

Diagnostic Imaging

I. Radiographs:

A. Anteroposterior (AP) of the pelvis (**Fig. 12.3**).

B. AP and cross-table lateral of the affected hip.

C. Pelvic ring injuries:

1. Inlet radiograph:

a. X-ray beam 45 degrees caudad.

2. Outlet radiograph:

a. X-ray beam 45 degrees cephalad.

D. Acetabulum injuries: Judet:

1. Iliac oblique:

a. X-ray beam 45 degrees oblique toward the noninjured side.

2. Obturator oblique:

b. X-ray beam 45 degrees oblique toward the injured side.

E. Plain radiographs will miss about half of the pediatric pelvic fractures.

II. Computed tomography (CT):

A. Routine for evaluation of pelvic ring or acetabulum fractures.

B. Defines comminution, marginal impaction, and rotation.

C. Identifies loose bodies.

D. Three-dimensional reconstructions.

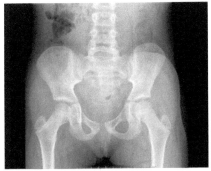

Fig. 12.3 Anteroposterior (AP) radiograph of an 8-year-old skeletally immature girl.

III.   Magnetic resonance imaging (MRI):
    A. Occult fracture.
    B. Stress fracture.
    C. Pathologic fracture.

Differential Diagnosis

I.   Traumatic:
    A. Proximal femur fracture.
    B. Femoral shaft fracture.
    C. Pelvic fracture.
    D. Acetabulum fracture.
    E. Traumatic hip dislocation.
    F. Apophyseal avulsion.
    G. Slipped capital femoral epiphysis.

II. Nontraumatic:
    A. Developmental dysplasia of the hip.
    B. Legg–Calvé–Perthes disease.
    C. Developmental coxa vara.
    D. Stress fracture.
    E. Transient synovitis of the hip.
    F. Septic arthritis of the hip.
    G. Septic arthritis of the knee.
    H. Lyme's disease.
    I. Osteomyelitis.

Treatment

I.   Proximal femur fracture:
    A. Nonoperative[12]:
       1. Indications:
          a. Nondisplaced types IA, II, III, and IV.
          b. Younger than 4 years.
       2. Spica cast in abduction.
       3. Weekly radiographs.
    B. Operative:
       4. Indications[12,25,26]:
          a. Open fracture.
          b. Vessel injury requiring repair.
          c. Concomitant hip dislocation.

d. Significant displacement of fracture.

5. Emergent open reduction and internal fixation and capsulotomy:

a. Type IB.

6. Closed reduction and internal fixation:

a. Types II, III, and IV displaced.

7. Percutaneous pinning:

a. Types II, III, and IV displaced.

8. Open reduction and internal fixation:

a. Type IB.

9. Pediatric dynamic hip screw:

a. Type IV.

II. Acetabulum fracture[3,10]:

A. Nonoperative:

1. Indications:

a. Stable fracture, less than 2 mm displacement.

2. Protected weight bearing to the affected side for 2 to 4 weeks.

3. Physical therapy.

4. Close observation with frequent radiographs to evaluate displacement and premature closure of triradiate cartilage.

B. Operative:

1. Indications:

a. Open fracture.

b. Unstable fracture, greater than 2 mm displacement.

c. Comminuted fracture.

d. Central fracture-dislocation.

e. Joint incongruity.

f. Joint instability.

g. Intra-articular fragments.

2. Open reduction and internal fixation:

a. Physeal sparing when able.

b. Smooth pins across physis if necessary.

c. Removal of pins in 4 to 6 weeks.

III. Pelvic ring fracture[4]:

A. Nonoperative:

1. Indications:

a. Symphysis or SI joint dislocation with minimal displacement:

i. Potential for intact thick periosteal healing.

b. Type I and II injuries with less than 2 cm displacement.

c. Type III injury without segmental instability.

      2. Protected weight bearing for 2 to 4 weeks.

      3. Physical therapy.

  B. Operative:

      1. Indications:

         a. Type I and II injuries with greater than 2 to 3 cm displacement.

         b. Type III injury with displaced acetabulum fracture greater than 2 mm.

         c. Type IV injury with instability and greater than 2 cm pelvic ring displacement.

      2. External fixation followed by definitive open reduction and internal fixation.

      3. Open reduction and internal fixation.

IV. Pelvic avulsion injury[10]:

  A. Nonoperative:

      1. Indications:

         a. Less than 2 cm of displacement.

      2. Protected weight bearing initially with weight bearing as tolerated.

      3. Physical therapy.

  B. Operative:

      1. Indications:

         a. Greater than 2 cm of displacement.

         b. Failure of nonoperative treatment.

      2. Open reduction and internal fixation.

Complications

I. Proximal femur fractures[1,17,27]:

  A. Overall complication rate of 60%.

  B. Avascular necrosis rate of 50%:

      1. Highest (100%) for Delbet type IB[12,28].

      2. Treatment is core decompression or vascularized fibula graft.

  C. Malunion rate of 30%:

      1. Coxa vara:

         a. Most commonly seen with type III.

         b. Treatment:

           i. 0–3 years: nonoperative (will remodel).

           ii. Younger than 6 to 8 years: trochanteric epiphysiodesis.

           iii. Older than 8 years: subtrochanteric/intertrochanteric valgus osteotomy.

      2. Coxa valga:

         i. Most commonly seen with type IV.

  D. Nonunion.

    E. Physeal arrest.

    F. Limb length discrepancy.

    G. Infection.

II. Acetabulum fractures[10]:

    A. Premature closure of triradiate cartilage:

        1. Leads to shallow, dysplastic acetabulum.

        2. Hip subluxation.

        3. Treatment:

            a. Pelvic osteotomy.

    B. Physeal cartilage injury:

        1. Specifically with Bucholz's crushing-type injury.

        2. May lead to shallow acetabulum and hip subluxation.

        3. Leg length discrepancy.

        4. Treatment:

            a. Physeal bar excision.

            b. Pelvic osteotomy.

    C. Post traumatic arthrosis.

    D. Avascular necrosis of the femoral head.

    E. Malunion/nonunion.

    F. Heterotopic ossification.

III. Pelvic ring fractures[4]:

    A. Hemorrhage: rare.

    B. Death: rare:

        1. Most often with accompanying head or visceral injury.

    C. Pelvic asymmetry:

        1. Less than 1 to 2 cm can lead to scoliosis, low back pain, and SI joint pain.

    D. Neurovascular injury.

IV. Pelvis avulsion injury:

    A. Symptomatic nonunion.

    B. Muscle spasm/weakness.

References

1. Canale ST, Bourland WL. Fracture of the neck and intertrochanteric region of the femur in children. J Bone Joint Surg Am 1977;59(4):431–443
2. Flynn JM, Wong KL, Yeh GL, Meyer JS, Davidson RS. Displaced fractures of the hip in children. Management by early operation and immobilisation in a hip spica cast. J Bone Joint Surg Br 2002;84(1):108–112
3. Holden CP, Holman J, Herman MJ. Pediatric pelvic fractures. J Am Acad Orthop Surg 2007;15(3):172–177
4. Banerjee S, Barry MJ, Paterson JM. Paediatric pelvic fractures: 10 years experience in a trauma centre. Injury 2009;40(4):410–413

5. Reina N, Accadbled F, de Gauzy JS. Anterior inferior iliac spine avulsion fracture: a case report in soccer playing adolescent twins. J Pediatr Orthop B 2010;19(2):158–160
6. Rossi F, Dragoni S. Acute avulsion fractures of the pelvis in adolescent competitive athletes: prevalence, location and sports distribution of 203 cases collected. Skeletal Radiol 2001;30(3):127–131
7. Metzmaker JN, Pappas AM. Avulsion fractures of the pelvis. Am J Sports Med 1985;13(5):349–358
8. Chung SM. The arterial supply of the developing proximal end of the human femur. J Bone Joint Surg Am 1976;58(7):961–970
9. Gautier E, Ganz K, Krügel N, Gill T, Ganz R. Anatomy of the medial femoral circumflex artery and its surgical implications. J Bone Joint Surg Br 2000;82(5):679–683
10. Dormans J. Pediatric Orthopaedics. Philadelphia, PA: Elsevier Mosby; 2005
11. Trueta J. The normal vascular anatomy of the human femoral head during growth. J Bone Joint Surg Brit 1957;39-B(2):358–94
12. Boardman MJ, Herman MJ, Buck B, Pizzutillo PD. Hip fractures in children. J Am Acad Orthop Surg 2009;17(3):162–173
13. Ponseti IV. Growth and development of the acetabulum in the normal child. Anatomical, histological, and roentgenographic studies. J Bone Joint Surg Am 1978;60(5):575–585
14. Lindstrom JR, Ponseti IV, Wenger DR. Acetabular development after reduction in congenital dislocation of the hip. J Bone Joint Surg Am 1979;61(1):112–118
15. Scoles PV, Boyd A, Jones PK. Roentgenographic parameters of the normal infant hip. J Pediatr Orthop 1987;7(6):656–663
16. Kahle WK, Coleman SS. The value of the acetabular teardrop figure in assessing pediatric hip disorders. J Pediatr Orthop 1992;12(5):586–591
17. Hughes LO, Beaty JH. Fractures of the head and neck of the femur in children. J Bone Joint Surg Am 1994;76(2):283–292
18. Bucholz RW, Ezaki M, Ogden JA. Injury to the acetabular triradiate physeal cartilage. J Pediatr Orthop 1982;2(3):336
19. Matta JM. Fracture of the acetabulum: accuracy of reduction and clinical results in patients managed operatively within three weeks after the injury. Orthop Trauma Dir 2011;9(2):31–36
20. Moed BR, WillsonCarr SE, Watson JT. Results of operative treatment of fractures of the posterior wall of the acetabulum. J Bone Joint Surg Am 2002;84(5):752–758
21.   Letournel E, Judet R. Fractures of the Acetabulum. Berlin: Springer-Verlag; 1993
22. Borrelli J Jr, Goldfarb C, Catalano L, Evanoff BA. Assessment of articular fragment displacement in acetabular fractures: a comparison of computerized tomography and plain radiographs. J Orthop Trauma 2002;16(7):449–456, discussion 456–457
23. Bucholz R, Court-Brown C, Green D, Heckman J, Rockwood C, Tornetta P. Rockwood and Green's Fractures in Adults. Philadelphia, PA: Wolters Kluwer Health/Lippincott Williams & Wilkins; 2010
24. Torode I, Zieg D. Pelvic fractures in children. J Pediatr Orthop 1985;5(1):76–84
25. Song KS. Displaced fracture of the femoral neck in children: open versus closed reduction. J Bone Joint Surg Br 2010;92(8):1148–1151
26. Hajdu S, Oberleitner G, Schwendenwein E, Ringl H, Vécsei V. Fractures of the head and neck of the femur in children: an outcome study. Int Orthop 2011;35(6):883–888
27. Moon ES, Mehlman CT. Risk factors for avascular necrosis after femoral neck fractures in children: 25 Cincinnati cases and meta-analysis of 360 cases. J Orthop Trauma 2006;20(5):323–329
28. Beaty JH. Fractures of the hip in children. Orthop Clin North Am 2006;37(2):223–232, vii

13 Adult Hip Dysplasia

Luis F. Pulido-Sierra, Carlos J. Meheux

Introduction

I. Common structural hip disorder[1]:
   A. Acetabular deficiency is the primary component in adult hip dysplasia.
   B. Decreased anterior and lateral coverage of the femoral head.
   C. Symptoms are related to level of activity and severity of dysplasia.
   D. Acetabular rim syndrome[2]:
      1. High peak stresses at the superior anterior and lateral rim.
      2. Early failure of the labrum.
      3. Femoral head subluxation.
      4. Early osteoarthritis.
   E. Established cause of hip osteoarthritis[3]:
      1. Tönnis grade:
         a. Grade 0: normal.
         b. Grade 1: mild osteoarthritis.
         c. Grade 2: moderate osteoarthritis.
         d. Grade 3: severe osteoarthritis.
      2. End-stage hip osteoarthritis secondary to hip dysplasia[4]:
         a. Adult hip dysplasia.
         b. Low-grade dislocation.
         c. High-grade dislocation.

II. Epidemiology of adult hip dysplasia:
   A. The prevalence of adult hip dysplasia varies from 2 to 20%.
   B. Multifactorial disease with genetic and environmental risk factors.
   C. Risk factors for adult hip dysplasia:
      1. Residual congenital hip dysplasia:
         a. Female.
         b. Breech presentation.
         c. Oligohydramnios.
         d. Primiparity.
      2. Family history.
      3. First-degree relatives with developmental dysplasia of the hip (DDH):
         a. Twelvefold increase in risk for DDH.
         b. Twenty-seven-fold increase risk for adult hip dysplasia.

    4. Genetics[5,6]:
        a. Multiple susceptibility genes.
        b. Gene CX3CR1 (variants rs3732378 and rs3732379):
            i. 2.25-fold increase risk after adjusting for gender.
            ii. Consistent in different ethnics (Utah and China).
            iii. Affects chondrocyte maturation and bone formation.
        c. GDF5 (growth differentiation factor 5):
            i. CDMP1(cartilage-derived morphogenetic protein-1).
        d. ASP (Asporin).
    5. Higher prevalence in certain ethnicities:
        a. Asians:
            i. Japan.
            ii. China.
        b. Norway.
        c. Italy.
        d. Native Americans.

III. Common cause of osteoarthrosis:
    A. Edge-loading stresses.
    B. Acetabular rim syndrome.
    C. Multiple studies have shown association of dysplasia and osteoarthrosis.
    D. High prevalence (25–50%) of hip dysplasia in patients younger than 50 years who undergo total hip arthroplasty (THA).

Anatomic Considerations

I. Acetabular dysplasia[7–9]:
    A. Classic acetabular dysplasia:
        1. Decreased anterior femoral head coverage.
        2. Decreased lateral femoral head coverage.
        3. Steep upsloping acetabular sourcil.
        4. Lateralized femoral head.
        5. Small acetabular volume.
    B. Acetabular retroversion:
        1. Different acetabular pathology.
        2. Prevalence of acetabular retroversion is one out of six to one out of three symptomatic hips.
        3. Posterior insufficiency and anterior overcoverage.
        4. Cause of anterior femoroacetabular impingement (FAI):
            a. Anterior labral pathology from impingement.
            b. External rotation of the hemipelvis.
            c. Increased anterior coverage.
            d. Decreased posterior coverage.

II. Femoral abnormalities[10-13]:
- A. Femoral neck shaft angle:
  1. Increased neck shaft angle:
     a. More common in adult hip dysplasia (44%).
     b. Coxa valga: neck shaft angle greater than 135 degrees:
        i. Decreased femoral head coverage.
        ii. Decreased femoral lateral offset.
        iii. Decreased abductor moment arm.
        iv. Increased abductor force.
        v. Increased joint contact forces.
  2. Decreased neck shaft angle:
     a. Less common in adult hip dysplasia (4%).
     b. Coxa vara: neck shaft angle less than 120 degrees:
        i. Increased femoral head coverage.
        ii. Increased risk for anterior impingement.
        iii. Increased femoral lateral offset.
        iv. Increased abductor moment arm.
        v. Decreased abductor force.
- B. Femoral version:
  1. Normal femoral version: 5 to 20 degrees.
  2. Large variability in adult hip dysplasia:
     a. Ranges from 0 to 80 degrees of anteversion.
  3. Increased femoral anteversion: greater than 20 degrees:
     a. More common in adult hip dysplasia:
        i. Decreased abductor lever arm.
        ii. Increased abductor force.
        iii. Increased joint contact forces.
  4. Decreased femoral anteversion or retroversion: under 5 degrees:
     a. Less common in hip dysplasia.
     b. Increased risk of anterior impingement.
- C. Femoral head and neck deformity:
  1. Ten percent to 42% prevalence of cam deformity in hip dysplasia.
  2. Elliptical femoral heads.

History and Examination[14]

I. Symptoms present in adult hip dysplasia:
- A. Pain onset:
  1. Insidious (97%).
  2. Acute (1%).
  3. Traumatic (1%).

B. Pain severity:
   1. Severe (26%).
   2. Moderate (51%).
   3. Mild (23%).
C. Pain location:
   1. Groin (72%).
   2. Lateral hip (66%).
   3. Anterior thigh (29%).
   4. Buttock and groin pain (18%).
   5. Isolated buttock pain (0%).
   6. More than one location (63%).
D. Pain quality:
   1. Activity related (87%).
   2. Dull (ache) (78%).
   3. Sharp (72%).
   4. Intermittent (53%).
   5. Constant (42%).
   6. Night pain (59%).
E. Pain duration:
   1. Common delay in diagnosis.
   2. Average 5 years from onset of symptoms to diagnosis.
F. Associated symptoms:
   1. Snapping/popping (67%).
   2. Locking (23%).
   3. Subluxation (22%).
   4. Limping (85%):
      a. Mild limp (54%).
      b. Moderate limp (25%).
      c. Severe limp (6%).
G. Exacerbating factors:
   1. Walking (81%).
   2. Running (80%).
   3. Standing (70%).
   4. Impact (55%).
   5. Pivoting (45%).
   6. Sitting (44%).
   7. Standing from sitting (31%).

   H. Relieving factors:
       1. Rest (75%).
       2. Oral nonsteroidal anti-inflammatory drugs (56%).
       3. Oral narcotics (8%).
II. Physical examination[14]:
   A. Inspection:
       1. Deformity.
       2. Gait:
           a. Limp (85%).
           b. Intoeing.
           c. Negative foot progression angle.
       3. Single leg stance:
           a. Positive Trendelenburg sign (38%).
   B. Range of motion:
       1. Unrestricted.
       2. Internal rotation with hip flexion of 90 degrees:
           a. Limited:
               i. Associated FAI cam morphology.
           b. Excessive:
               i. Increased femoral anteversion:
                   (1) evaluate in prone position.
   C. Strength:
       1. Abductor weakness and abductor fatigue.
   D. Special testing:
       1. Impingement test (flexion, adduction, and internal rotation [FADIR])
       2. Apprehension test (extension, abduction, and external rotation).
       3. Hip adduction and axial load.
       4. Stinchfield's test (resisted hip flexion during straight leg raise).

Diagnostic Imaging

I.   Plain radiographs[15]:
   A. Weight-bearing anteroposterior (AP) pelvis and false profile:
       1. Better acetabular morphology evaluation.
   B. Lateral and Dunn views:
       1. Better femoral head and neck morphology evaluation.
   C. AP pelvis (**Fig. 13.1**):
       1. Technique:
           a. Beam at the center of the pelvis.
           b. Bilateral feet in 15 degrees of internal rotation.
           c. Tube perpendicular to the film.

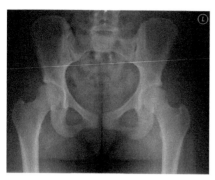

Fig. 13.1 Standing anteroposterior pelvis radiograph showing mild bilateral hip dysplasia.

    d. Tube-to-film distance of 120 cm:

       i. Standing:

         (1) better assessment of the joint space

         (2) functional view:

           (a) spinopelvic.

      ii. Supine:

         (1) underestimation:

           (a) hip joint space

           (b) osteoarthritis.

2. Evaluation:

    a. Joint space.

    b. Degree of osteoarthritis:

       i. Tönnis classification.

    c. Acetabular inclination:

       i. Tönnis angle.

    d. Lateral coverage:

       i. Lateral center edge angle (LCEA) of Wiberg.

    e. Hip congruity.

    f. Cranial subluxation of the femoral head.

       i. Shenton's line.

    g. Femoral head lateralization:

       i. Femoral head relative to lateral teardrop.

      ii. Distance greater than 10 mm.

    h. Acetabular depth:

       i. Protrusio acetabuli:

         (1)medial femoral head crosses the ilioischial line.

      ii. Coxa profunda.

    i. Acetabular version:

       i. Anterior and posterior walls:

(1) acetabular retroversion:

    (a) crossover sign (may be prominent subspine rather than focal retroversion),

    (b) posterior wall sign,

    (c) ischial spine sign.

  j. Femoral head and neck:

    i. Shape: deformities:

      (1) associated cam morphology

      (2) head sphericity.

    ii. Angle:

      (1) coxa vara.

      (2) coxa valga.

D. False profile (**Fig. 13.2**):

  1. Technique:

    a. Standing.

    b. Affected hip against the film.

    c. Pelvis rotated 65 degrees.

    d. Tube-to-film distance of 102 cm.

  2. Evaluation:

    a. Anterior coverage:

      i. Anterior center edge angle (of Lequesne).

    b. Anterior joint space.

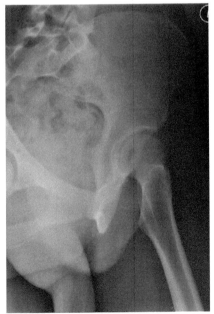

Fig. 13.2 Standing false-profile radiograph illustrating anterior hip dysplasia and mildly incongruent hip joint.

      c. Degree of osteoarthritis.

      d. Anterior inferior iliac spine.

      e. Hip congruity.

  E. Cross-table lateral:

    1. Technique:

      a. Supine.

      b. Neutral extension of the affected hip and 15-degree internal rotation.

      c. Contralateral hip flexion of 90 degrees.

      d. X-ray beam at 45-degree angle to the affected hip.

    2. Evaluation:

      a. Posterior hip joint space.

      b. Degree of osteoarthritis.

      c. Anterior cam.

  F. Frog leg lateral:

    1. Technique:

      a. Supine.

      b. Affected hip abducted 45 degrees and flexed 30 to 40 degrees.

      c. The heel rests on the contralateral medial knee.

      d. Beam at the center of the pelvis.

      e. Tube-to-film distance of 102 cm.

    2. Evaluation:

      a. Femoral head and neck.

      b. Hip reduction with abduction.

  G. Dunn 45 degrees:

    1. Technique:

      a. Supine.

      b. Affected hip abducted 20 degrees, flexed 45 degrees, and neutral rotation.

      c. Beam at the center of the pelvis.

      d. Tube-to-film distance of 102 cm.

    2. Evaluation:

      a. Femoral head and neck.

      b. Sensitive for anterolateral cam detection.

  H. Dunn 90 degrees:

    1. Technique:

      a. As Dunn 45 degrees, but with the hip flexed at 90 degrees.

    2. Evaluation:

      a. Femoral head and neck.

II. Radiographs interpretation:

  A. Degree of osteoarthritis:

1. Tönnis classification:
   a. Grade 0: normal.
   b. Grade 1: mild:
      i. Increased sclerosis.
      ii. Slight joint space narrowing.
   c. Grade 2: moderate:
      i. Small cysts.
      ii. Moderate joint space narrowing.
      iii. Moderate loss of femoral head sphericity.
   d. Grade 3: severe:
      i. Large cysts.
      ii. Severe joint space narrowing.
      iii. Joint space obliteration.
      iv. Severe deformity of the femoral head.
B. Evaluation of acetabular dysplasia[15]:
   1. Tönnis angle (**Fig. 13.3**):
      a. Acetabular roof angle of Tönnis.
      b. Evaluation of acetabular inclination.
      c. Measurement of the angle of Tönnis:
         i. AP pelvis radiograph.

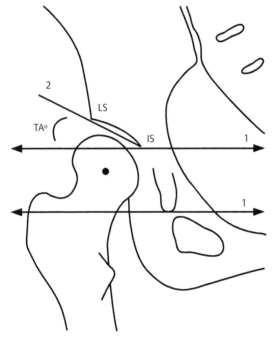

Fig. 13.3 Anteroposterior pelvis radiograph illustration on how to measure the acetabular inclination using the acetabular roof angle of Tönnis. Draw a horizontal inter teardrop line (line 1) to correct the pelvic obliquity. Bring line 1 at the level of the inferior sourcil (IS). Identify the lateral margin of the sclerotic sourcil (LS) and draw line 2 connecting the inferior sourcil with the lateral sourcil. The Tönnis angle (TA) is formed by the intersection of lines 1 and 2.

    ii. Line 1:

      (1) horizontal inter-teardrop line,

      (2) raise line 1 to the inferior sourcil,

      (3) corrects pelvic obliquity.

    iii. Line 2:

      (1) inferior point of the sclerotic sourcil;

      (2) lateral point of acetabular sourcil:

        (a) lateral margin of the sclerotic sourcil;

      (3) connect the lateral and inferior sourcil.

    iv. Angle is formed by the intersection of lines 1 and 2.

  d. Normal angle is 0 to 10 degrees.

  e. Hip dysplasia if angle is greater than 10 degrees.

2. LCEA (**Fig. 13.4**):

  a. Evaluation of the femoral head lateral coverage.

  b. LCEA of Wiberg.

  c. Measurement:

    i. AP pelvis.

    ii. Mark the center of the femoral head.

    iii. Line 1:

      (1) horizontal inter-teardrop line.

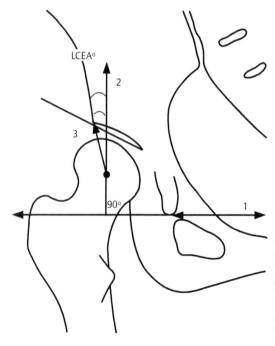

Fig. 13.4 Anteroposterior pelvis illustration on how to measure the acetabular lateral center edge angle (LCEA) of Wiberg. Identify and mark the center of the femoral head. Draw a horizontal inter-teardrop line (line 1) to correct the pelvic obliquity. Draw a vertical line (line 2) perpendicular to the inter-teardrop line and through the center of the femoral head. Draw a line from the center of the femoral head to the lateral margin of the sclerotic sourcil (line 3). The lateral center angle of Wiberg is formed by the intersection of lines 2 and 3.

iv. Line 2:

    (1) vertical line through the center of the femoral head

    (2) perpendicular to line 1 inter-teardrop (90 degrees).

v. Line 3:

    (1) center femoral head.

    (2) lateral margin of the sclerotic sourcil.

vi. Angle formed by the intersection of lines 2 and 3.

d. Normal angle is between 25 and 45 degrees.

e. Hip dysplasia if angle is less than 25 degrees:

  i. Twenty to 25 degrees = borderline dysplasia.

  ii. Less than 20 degrees = dysplasia:

    (1) mild—15 to 20 degrees.

    (2) moderate—5 to 15 degrees.

    (3) severe: less than 5 degrees.

f. Overcoverage if angle is greater than 40 degrees (pincer morphology).

3. Hip joint congruity:

  a. Relationship of the femoral head contour to the acetabulum.

  b. Hip congruity:

    i. The femoral head matches the arc of the acetabulum.

  c. Hip incongruity:

    i. The femoral head does not match the arc of the acetabulum:

      (1) shape of the femoral head,

      (2) shape of the acetabulum,

      (3) severity of acetabular dysplasia,

      (4) prognostic factor in surgical treatment,

      (5) skeletally immature:

        (a) salvage or shelf osteotomy.

4. Anterior center edge angle (**Fig. 13.5**):

  a. Evaluation of the femoral head anterior coverage.

  b. Anterior center edge angle of Lequesne and de Seze.

  c. Affected by the spinopelvic position.

  d. Measurement:

    i. False-profile view.

    ii. Mark the center of the femoral head.

    iii. Line 1:

      (1) vertical line through the center of the head.

    iv. Line 2:

      (1) anterior margin of the sclerotic sourcil.

    v. Angle formed by the intersection of lines 1 and 2.

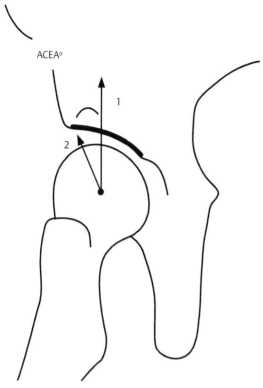

ACEA°

Fig. 13.5 False-profile illustration on how to measure the acetabular anterior center edge angle (ACEA) of Lequesne. Identify and mark the center of the femoral head. Draw a vertical line through the center of the femoral head (line 1). Draw a line from the center of the femoral head to the anterior margin of the sclerotic sourcil (line 2). The ACEA of Lequesne is formed by the intersection of lines 1 and 2.

   e. Normal angle is ≥20 degrees.

    f. Anterior instability or dysplasia if angle is less than 20 degrees.

III. Computed tomography (CT):

  A. Supplementary diagnostic test:

   1. Not routinely performed.

  B. Useful in the evaluation of:

   1. Femoral torsional deformity.

   2. Mild hip dysplasia.

  C. Pelvis with distal femur acquisition:

   1. Femoral version.

   2. Acetabular version.

  D. Three-dimensional reconstructions.

IV. Magnetic resonance imaging (MRI):

  A. Supplementary diagnostic test:

   1. Not routinely performed.

  B. Useful in the evaluation of:

   1. Mechanical hip symptoms.

   2. Associated cam morphology.

C. Hip at 3.0 T.
D. MRI arthrogram:
  1. Better labral evaluation.
E. Biochemical MRI[16]:
  1. Delayed gadolinium-enhanced MRI of the cartilage (DGEMRIC).
  2. Limited access:
    a. Not routinely used in clinical practice.
  3. Measures the glycosaminoglycan content of the cartilage.
  4. Low biochemical index may precede structural cartilage damage.

Treatment

I. Factors to consider:
  A. Age.
  B. Severity of hip dysplasia.
  C. Severity of hip arthritis.
  D. Obesity.
  E. Physical activity.
II. Nonoperative:
  A. Activity modification.
  B. Physical therapy.
    1. Strengthening:
      a. Abductors.
      b. Core.
    2. Increase lumbosacral lordosis:
      a. Improve anterior and lateral acetabular coverage.
  C. Medical treatment:
    1. Oral anti-inflammatory medications.
III. Operative:
  A. Hip arthroscopy:
    1. Does not address hip dysplasia pathomechanism.
    2. High risk of failure due to instability.
    3. Potential role at the time of osteotomy:
      a. Associated cam morphology and labral injury.
    4. Indication in borderline dysplasia (LCEA of 20–25 degrees):
      a. Predominant cam morphology.
      b. Labral injury due to impingement.
  B. Periacetabular osteotomy (PAO):
    1. Ganz's or Bernese's PAO:
      a. Developed by R. Ganz and JW Mast.[17]
      b. Performed since 1982.

2. Forefront of pelvic osteotomies for adult hip dysplasia:
   a. Young patients with closed triradiate cartilage.
3. Advantages:
   a. Realignment hip preservation procedure.
   b. Allows acetabular correction of the main dysplastic features:
      i. Anterior coverage:
         (1) avoid retroversion.
      ii. Lateral coverage.
      iii. Medialization.
   c. Decreased acetabular rim load.
   d. Intact posterior column:
      i. Early ambulation and rehabilitation.
      ii. Stable osteotomy:
         (1) fixation with two to three screws.
   e. Does not alter the shape of the pelvis:
      i. Allows vaginal childbirth delivery.
   f. Single incision.
   g. Abductors intact.
   h. Preserved vascularity of the acetabular fragment.[18]
   i. Access to anterior hip capsule.
   j. Does not compromise results of THA.[19]
   k. Durable and reliable clinical results.
4. Indications:
   a. Symptomatic hip dysplasia.
   b. Mild or no arthritis (Tönnis grades 0 and 1).
5. Surgical technique (**Fig. 13.6**):
   a. Patient supine on radiolucent table.
   b. Check hip range of motion before surgery:
      i. Internal rotation at 90 degrees of flexion.
   c. Modified Smith–Petersen approach:
      i. Incision of 10 to 12 cm:
         (1) **C**-shaped over anterior superior iliac spine (ASIS),
         (2) oblique skin crease distal to ASIS.
   d. Fluoroscopy:
      i. AP and lateral at 60- to 65-degree "supine false profile."
   e. Osteotomies:
      i. Four bone cuts:
         (1) ischial osteotomy,
         (2) superior pubic rami osteotomy,

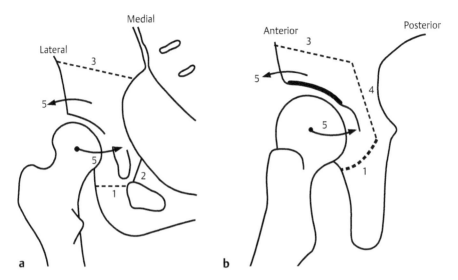

Fig. 13.6 (a) Anteroposterior illustration. **(b)** False-profile illustration. The periacetabular osteotomy consist of four bone cuts: (1) ischial osteotomy, (2) superior pubic rami osteotomy, (3) iliac osteotomy, (4) retroacetabular osteotomy, and (5) mobilization of the acetabular fragment and dysplasia correction of lateral coverage, anterior coverage, and medialization of the acetabular fragment.

        (3) iliac osteotomy,

        (4) retroacetabular osteotomy.

   f. Correction of acetabular dysplasia:

     i. Acetabular fragment mobilization and correction:

        (1) lateral coverage,

        (2) anterior coverage,

        (3) medialization of the fragment.

     ii. Radiographic evaluation of correction:

        (1) goals (**Fig. 13.7**):

           (a) flat sourcil: angle of Tönnis of 0 to 10 degrees;

           (b) lateral coverage: LCEA of 25 to 35 degrees;

           (c) medialization;

           (d) avoid impingement: retroversion and overcoverage.

   g. Check the hip range of motion following correction:

     i. Internal rotation at 90 degrees of flexion.

   h. Fixation of mobile fragment:

     i. Two to three screws:

        (1) 4.0 to 4.5 mm,

        (2) long screws (60–110 mm),

        (3) from stable ilium to mobile fragment.

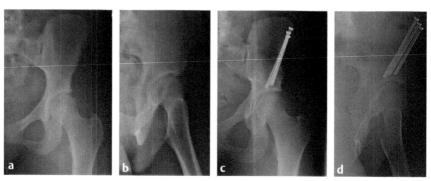

Fig. 13.7 Radiographs of a 16-year-old adolescent girl with symptomatic left hip dysplasia treated successfully with left periacetabular osteotomy (PAO). **(a)** Preoperative anteroposterior (AP) pelvis radiograph with the angle of Tönnis of 20 degrees and lateral center edge angle (LCEA) of 17 degrees. **(b)** Preoperative false profile with an anterior center edge angle (ACEA) of 17 degrees. **(c)** Postoperative AP pelvis radiograph 2 years following PAO with healed osteotomy. Angle of Tönnis of 4 degrees and LCEA of 30 degrees. **(d)** Postoperative false profile following PAO with ACEA of 28 degrees.

    i. Anterior capsular exposure:

        i. Originally described in all cases.

        ii. Controversial.

        iii. Rectus takedown.

        iv. Longer incision.

6. Postoperative care after PAO:

    a. Clinical and radiographic evaluation:

        i. Three weeks:

            (1) wound evaluation.

        ii. Six weeks:

            (1) stable fixation,

            (2) no fractures,

            (3) advance to weight bearing as tolerated (WBAT).

        iii. Twelve weeks:

            (1) healed osteotomy

            (2) advance return to sports and physical therapy.

    b. Rehabilitation:

        i. Protected weight bearing for first 4 to 6 weeks:

            (1) two crutches,

            (2) partial weight bearing of 25 lb for 4 weeks,

            (3) partial weight bearing of 50 lb for the next 2 weeks (weeks 4–6),

            (4) WBAT after 6 weeks:

               (a) satisfactory evaluation.

        ii. Off walking aids at 8 to 10 weeks.

   c. Rehabilitation program:
      i. Twelve weeks: return to low-demand activities.
      ii. Twenty-four weeks: return to higher demand activities.
7. Outcomes:
   a. Level IV evidence:
      i. Retrospective.
      ii. Single center.
      iii. Single institution.
   b. Complications[20]:
      i. Nerve injury[21]:
         (1) sciatic femoral nerve (2%):
            (a) 50% recover;
         (2) lateral femoral cutaneous nerve palsy (5%).
      ii. Superficial and deep surgical site infection (1%).
      iii. Hematoma.
      iv. Blood loss:
         (1) allogenic blood transfusion (20%),[22]
         (2) lower with use of tranexamic acid,
         (3) blood salvage:
            (a) intraoperative autotransfusion
            (b) blood loss of 200 mL to 4 L.[23]
      v. Intra-articular extension:
         (1) fluoroscopy to avoid this complication.
      vi. Disruption of the posterior column:
         (1) fluoroscopy to avoid this complication,
         (2) aggressive early rehabilitation:
            (a) early full weight bearing associated with insufficiency fractures of the ischium.
      vii. Overcorrection of acetabular deformity:
         (1) iatrogenic impingement,
         (2) cause of failure.
      viii. Undercorrection of acetabular deformity:
         (1) residual dysplasia.
      ix. Nonunion of the superior pubic ramus osteotomy.
   c. Survivorship:
      i. All patients:
         (1) 73% at 10 years,
         (2) 60% at 20 years,[24]

        (3) 44% at 30 years[25]:

           (a) 70% of patients at 30 years:

- increase pain,
- hip osteoarthritis,
- conversion THA.

  ii. No preoperative hip arthritis:

    (1) improved survivorship,

    (2) 88% at 10 years,

    (3) 75% at 20 years.[24]

 iii. Poor prognostic factors:

    (1) preoperative:

      (a) hip in congruency,

      (b) obesity,[26]

    (2) postoperative:

      (a) anterior over-correction:

- acetabular retroversion,
- anterior impingement.

    (3) hip osteoarthritis:

- Tönnis grades 2 and 3[24];
- age older than 40 years.[27]

d. Functional outcomes:

  i. Improved functional scores following PAO[28]:

    (1) University of California, Los Angeles (UCLA) function score,

    (2) WOMAC (Western Ontario and McMaster Universities) pain scores,

    (3) Harris' hip scores,

    (4) abductor strength,

    (5) gait improved but not normal.

8. Prospective level II outcomes:

  a. Prospective multicenter cohort study.[29]

  b. ANCHOR (Academic Network of Conservational Hip Outcomes Research).

  c. Four hundred and twenty-three hips and 391 patients.

  d. Early outcomes scores: minimum follow-up of 2 years.

  e. Ninety-three percent satisfied with result.

  f. Improvement in functional outcomes scores:

    i. Harris' hip score.

    ii. UCLA activity score.

   iii. HOOS (Hip disability and Osteoarthritis Outcome Score):

    (1) symptoms,

    (2) pain,

   (3) activities of daily living,

   (4) sports and recreation,

   (5) quality of life.

   iv. SF-12 (12-item Short Form Survey):

   (1) mental

   (2) physical.

g. Reoperations:

   i. THA (0.8%).

   ii. Hip arthroscopy for persistent pain (2%).

C. THA for hip dysplasia:

1. Indications:

   a. Symptomatic hip dysplasia:

      i. Failed nonsurgical treatment.

      ii. Moderate and severe arthritis (Tönnis grades 2 and 3).

2. Classifications:

   a. Hartofilakidis[4]:

      i. Adult hip dysplasia:

         (1) femoral head contained within the acetabulum.

      ii. Low dislocation:

         (1) false acetabulum comes in contact with true acetabulum.

      iii. High dislocation:

         (1) false acetabulum has no connection with true acetabulum.

   b. Crowe and Ranawat[30]:

      i. Ratio between the height of the pelvis and the distance between the inferior border of the teardrop and the union of the neck and head on the medial aspect:

         (1) type I is less than 0.10,

         (2) type II is 0.10 to 0.15,

         (3) type III is 0.15 to 0.20,

         (4) type IV is greater than 0.20.

      ii. Displacement of the head in relation to the true acetabulum:

         (1) type I is less than 50%,

         (2) type II is 50 to 75%,

         (3) type III is 75 to 100%.

3. Anatomic considerations:

   a. Soft tissues:

      i. Abductors shortening.

      ii. Hamstrings shortening.

      iii. Hypertrophic capsule.

b. Acetabulum:
   i. Small.
   ii. High hip center.
   iii. Elongated.
   iv. Shallow.
   v. Superior anterior and lateral deficiency.
   vi. Neoacetabulum.
c. Femur:
   i. Small femoral head.
   ii. Increased anteversion.
   iii. Narrow medullary canal
d. Previous surgery:
   i. Previous incision.
   ii. Deformity.
   iii. Retained hardware
e. Technical tips for THA:
   i. Template:
       (1) small cup size available.
   ii. Acetabulum:
       (1) true hip center of location:
           (a) avoid high hip center;
       (2) improve lateral coverage:
           (a) acetabular medialization: avoid protrusion;
           (b) femoral head autograft;
       (3) screw fixation for better stability.
   iii. Femur:
       (1) uncemented:
           (a) version:
               • Wagner stem,
               • S-ROM stem.
           (b) shortening osteotomy:
               • Wagner stem,
               • S-ROM stem,
               • cylindrical fully coated.
       (2) cemented:
               • version,
               • Charnley trochanteric osteotomy.
   iv. Maximum lengthening of 2 cm:
       (1) avoid nerve-stretching injury,

(2) short femoral neck cut:

(a) avoid trochanteric impingement;

(3) consider shortening femoral osteotomy.

References

1. Engesæter IO, Laborie LB, Lehmann TG, et al. Prevalence of radiographic findings associated with hip dysplasia in a population-based cohort of 2081 19-year-old Norwegians. Bone Joint J 2013;95-B(2):279–285

2. Klaue K, Durnin CW, Ganz R. The acetabular rim syndrome. A clinical presentation of dysplasia of the hip. J Bone Joint Surg Br 1991;73(3):423–429

3. Thomas GE, Palmer AJ, Batra RN, et al. Subclinical deformities of the hip are significant predictors of radiographic osteoarthritis and joint replacement in women. A 20 year longitudinal cohort study. Osteoarthritis Cartilage 2014;22(10):1504–1510

4. Hartofilakidis G, Stamos K, Karachalios T. Treatment of high dislocation of the hip in adults with total hip arthroplasty. Operative technique and long-term clinical results. J Bone Joint Surg Am 1998;80(4):510–517

5. Feldman GJ, Parvizi J, Levenstien M, et al. Developmental dysplasia of the hip: linkage mapping and whole exome sequencing identify a shared variant in CX3CR1 in all affected members of a large multigeneration family. J Bone Miner Res 2013;28(12):2540–2549

6. Li L, Wang X, Zhao Q, et al. CX3CR1 polymorphisms associated with an increased risk of developmental dysplasia of the hip in human. J Orthop Res 2017;35(2):377–380

7. van Bosse H, Wedge JH, Babyn P. How are dysplastic hips different? A three-dimensional CT study. Clin Orthop Relat Res 2015;473(5):1712–1723

8. Sankar WN, Beaulé PE, Clohisy JC, et al. Labral morphologic characteristics in patients with symptomatic acetabular dysplasia. Am J Sports Med 2015;43(9):2152–2156

9. Ganz R, Leunig M. Morphological variations of residual hip dysplasia in the adult. Hip Int 2007;17(Suppl 5):S22–S28

10. Argenson JN, Flecher X, Parratte S, Aubaniac JM. Anatomy of the dysplastic hip and consequences for total hip arthroplasty. Clin Orthop Relat Res 2007;465(465):40–45

11. Fabricant PD, Sankar WN, Seeley MA, et al. Femoral deformity may be more predictive of hip range of motion than severity of acetabular disease in patients with acetabular dysplasia: an analysis of the ANCHOR cohort. J Am Acad Orthop Surg 2016;24(7):465–474

12. Steppacher SD, Tannast M, Werlen S, Siebenrock KA. Femoral morphology differs between deficient and excessive acetabular coverage. Clin Orthop Relat Res 2008;466(4):782–790

13. Anderson LA, Erickson JA, Swann RP, et al. Femoral morphology in patients undergoing periacetabular osteotomy for classic or borderline acetabular dysplasia: are cam deformities common? J Arthroplasty 2016;31(9, Suppl):259–263

14. Nunley RM, Prather H, Hunt D, Schoenecker PL, Clohisy JC. Clinical presentation of symptomatic acetabular dysplasia in skeletally mature patients. J Bone Joint Surg Am 2011;93(Suppl 2):17–21

15. Clohisy JC, Carlisle JC, Beaulé PE, et al. A systematic approach to the plain radiographic evaluation of the young adult hip. J Bone Joint Surg Am 2008;90(Suppl 4):47–66

16. Jessel RH, Zurakowski D, Zilkens C, Burstein D, Gray ML, Kim YJ. Radiographic and patient factors associated with pre-radiographic osteoarthritis in hip dysplasia. J Bone Joint Surg Am 2009;91(5):1120–1129

17. Ganz R, Klaue K, Vinh TS, Mast JW. A new periacetabular osteotomy for the treatment of hip dysplasias. Technique and preliminary results. Clin Orthop Relat Res 1988;(232):26–36

18. Hempfing A, Leunig M, Nötzli HP, Beck M, Ganz R. Acetabular blood flow during Bernese periacetabular osteotomy: an intraoperative study using laser Doppler flowmetry. J Orthop Res 2003;21(6):1145–1150

19. Amanatullah DF, Stryker L, Schoenecker P, et al. Similar clinical outcomes for THAs with and without prior periacetabular osteotomy. Clin Orthop Relat Res 2015;473(2):685–691

20. Thawrani D, Sucato DJ, Podeszwa DA, DeLaRocha A. Complications associated with the Bernese periacetabular osteotomy for hip dysplasia in adolescents. J Bone Joint Surg Am 2010;92(8):1707–1714
21. Sierra RJ, Beaule P, Zaltz I, Millis MB, Clohisy JC, Trousdale RT; ANCHOR group. Prevention of nerve injury after periacetabular osteotomy. Clin Orthop Relat Res 2012;470(8):2209–2219
22. Pulido LF, Babis GC, Trousdale RT. Rate and risk factors for blood transfusion in patients undergoing periacetabular osteotomy. J Surg Orthop Adv 2008;17(3):185–187
23. Lee CB, Kalish LA, Millis MB, Kim YJ. Predictors of blood loss and haematocrit after periacetabular osteotomy. Hip Int 2013;23(Suppl 9):S8–S13
24. Steppacher SD, Tannast M, Ganz R, Siebenrock KA. Mean 20-year followup of Bernese periacetabular osteotomy. Clin Orthop Relat Res 2008;466(7):1633–1644
25. Lerch TD, Steppacher SD, Liechti EF, Tannast M, Siebenrock KA. One-third of hips after periacetabular osteotomy survive 30 years with good clinical results, no progression of arthritis, or conversion to THA. Clin Orthop Relat Res 2017;475(4):1154–1168
26. Novais EN, Potter GD, Clohisy JC, et al. Obesity is a major risk factor for the development of complications after peri-acetabular osteotomy. Bone Joint J 2015;97-B(1):29–34
27. Millis MB, Kain M, Sierra R, et al. Periacetabular osteotomy for acetabular dysplasia in patients older than 40 years: a preliminary study. Clin Orthop Relat Res 2009;467(9):2228–2234
28. Novais EN, Heyworth B, Murray K, Johnson VM, Kim YJ, Millis MB. Physical activity level improves after periacetabular osteotomy for the treatment of symptomatic hip dysplasia. Clin Orthop Relat Res 2013;471(3):981–988
29. Clohisy JC, Ackerman J, Baca G, et al. Patient-reported outcomes of periacetabular osteotomy from the prospective ANCHOR cohort study. J Bone Joint Surg Am 2017;99(1):33–41
30. Crowe JF, Mani VJ, Ranawat CS. Total hip replacement in congenital dislocation and dysplasia of the hip. J Bone Joint Surg Am 1979;61(1):15–23

14 Legg–Calvé–Perthes Disease

Brian D. Lewis, Robert C. Kollmorgen

Introduction

I. Pathophysiology:
    A. Generally accepted that disruption of the vascular supply to the femoral head is the key pathogenic event.[1,2,3]
    B. Pathologic processes affect articular cartilage and the osseous epiphysis and, in some patients, the metaphysis and the physis[4,5]:
        1. Articular cartilage changes observed in deep layer of cartilage.
        2. Cessation of endochondral ossification at the articular cartilage–subchondral bone junction.
        3. Changes in the bony epiphysis include the following:
            a. Necrosis of the marrow space and trabecular bone.
            b. Compression fracture of the trabeculae.
            c. Osteoclastic resorption.
            d. Fibrovascular granulation tissue invasion of the necrotic head.
        4. Physeal changes seen most frequently in the anterior femoral head, areas of cartilage extending below the endochondral ossification line.

II. Pathogenesis of femoral head deformity:
    A. Mechanical: femoral head begins to deform when forces applied are greater than the ability to resist deformation.[4,6]
    B. Healing potential better in younger children: better outcomes in children younger than 6 years at age of onset compared to older than 8 years.[7]

III. Natural history:
    A. Limited by small sample sizes.
    B. Long-term outcomes better in patients with spherical femoral heads.[4]
    C. Degree of femoral head deformity at skeletal maturity is associated with onset of osteoarthritis.[8]

IV. Epidemiology:
    A. Males are five times more likely to be affected.[5,9]
    B. Highest documented incidence in Northern European invidivuals.[9]
    C. Lower incidence among African Americans versus Caucasians.[9]
    D. Multiple studies showing variations within regions of the same country.[9]
    E. Significant variation even found within small areas (variations between children in different social classes within Merseyside, UK).[9–11]
    F. Variation patterns indicate environmental influence on cause of disease.[9,12]

Imaging

I.   Plain radiographs include weight-bearing anteroposterior (AP) and frog leg lateral views of bilateral hips.

II. May be radiographically silent for the first 3 to 6 months.[13]

III. Classifications:

A. Waldenstrom's classification: defines stages, no prognosis[4,14] (**Fig. 14.1**):

1. Initial stage.

2. Fragmentation stage.

3. Reossification stage.

4. Residual stage.

B. Salter–Thompson classification: prognostic based on extent of subchondral fracture (crescent sign)[4,15]:

1. Group A: less than 50% femoral head involvement.

2. Group B: greater than 50% femoral head involvement.

C. Catterall's classification: prognostic based on extent of epiphyseal involvement, recognized during the fragmentation stage[13,16] (**Fig. 14.2**).

1. Group I: 25% involvement—better outcomes.

2. Group II: 50% involvement—better outcomes.

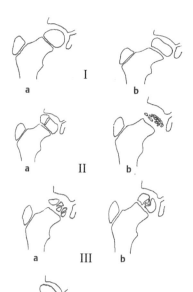

Fig. 14.1 Waldenstrom chronological stages of Perthes: I, sclerosis of epiphysis; II, fragmentation; III, early healing; IV, complete healing. (Source: Femoral Neck Fractures, In: Mullis B, Gaski G, eds. Synopsis of Orthopaedic Trauma Management. New York, NY:. Thieme; 2020.)

3. Group III: 75% involvement—worse outcomes

4. Group IV: 100% involvement—worse outcomes.

5. Simplification into groups I and II and III and IV improves interobserver reliability.[17]

D. Lateral pillar classification: based on the femoral head of the lateral pillar (the lateral 15–30%) radiolucency during fragmentation[18] (**Fig. 14.3**):

1. Group A: normal height.

2. Group B: less than 50% height loss.

3. Group B/C: around 50% height loss.

4. Group C: greater than 50% height loss.

E. Stulberg's classification: applied at skeletal maturity to prognosticate long-term outcome[8]:

1. I: normal hip.

2. II: spherical head with enlargement, short neck, or steep acetabulum.

3. III: nonspherical head, aspherically congruent joint.

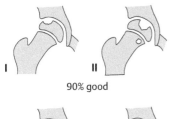
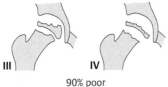

Fig. 14.2 Schematic representation of femoral head involvement in the Catterall classification. (Source: Articular Osteochondroses. In: Bohndorf K, Anderson M, Davies E, et al., eds. Imaging of Bones and Joints: A Concise, Multimodality Approach. Stuttgart, Germany: Thieme; 2016)

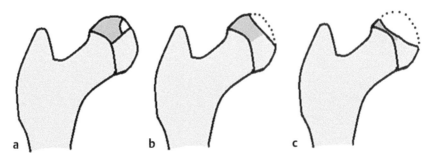

Fig. 14.3 (**a-c**) Schematic representation showing the lateral pillar involvement during the fragmentation phase. (Source: Herregods N, Vanhoenacker FM, Jaremko JL, et al. Update on Pediatric Hip Imaging. Seminars in Musculoskeletal Radiology 2017;21(05):561-581)

    4. IV: flat head, aspherically congruent joint.

    5. V: flat head with incongruent joint.

    6. Simplification proposed: groups I and II with spherical heads have good outcomes, while groups III to V with aspherical heads are much more likely to progress to osteoarthritis.[19]

  F. The problem with all the radiographic/prognostic classification systems is that they cannot be applied until fragmentation, although this may be changing with proposed modifications to the Waldenstrom classification.[20]

    1. In patients requiring treatment, outcomes may be better if initiated prior to fragmentation.

IV. Conway's classification using bone scintigraphy at diagnosis and again 4 to 5 months later: precedes radiographic changes by 3 months[13,21]:

  A. Type A: early and rapid revascularization.

  B. Type B:

    1. Centrally located activity or absence of activity in the epiphysis after 5 months.

    2. Higher risk of a poor prognosis.

  C. Type C: regression from a type A to a type B, very rare.

V. Magnetic resonance imaging (MRI): can provide a good anatomic picture[5,13]:

  A. Flat or round femoral head.

  B. Degree of extrusion of the femoral head.

  C. Extent of necrosis.

  D. Not accurate enough to describe stages of healing.

  E. When progressive subluxation of the femoral head is suspected, MRI can be used instead of arthrography.

  F. Dynamic gadolinium-enhanced subtraction MRI allows early detection of ischemia and revascularization patterns, excellent agreement with bone scintigraphy to determine favorable prognosis or not.

VI. Arthrography: useful to evaluate coverage and mobility under direct visualization prior to treatment for containment.[13]

VII. Ultrasonagraphy[13]:

  A. Likely will show hip effusion.

  B. Nonspecific.

Prognostic Factors

I. Age at onset of symptoms: strong prognostic factor with best prognosis in children younger than 5 years.[22,23]

II. Gender: conflicting results on whether outcomes are worse in girls.[16,22–24]

III. Salter–Thompson size of crescent sign: strong prognostic factor but only present in one-third of plain radiographs.[15]

IV. Epiphyseal involvement (Catterall): strong prognostic factor, only moderate reproducibility.[16]

V.   Lateral pillar involvement: strong prognostic factor, good reproducibility.[18]

VI. Metaphyseal abnormalities (osteoporosis, cysts, widening), poor prognostic indicators.[22]

VII. Altered acetabular contour (bicompartmentalization), poor prognostic factor.[22]

VIII. Catterall's "head-at-risk" signs[16]:

A. Diffuse metaphyseal reaction.

B. Calcification lateral to the epiphysis: questionable.

C. Gage's sign: triangular lucent are on the lateral epiphysis.

D. Horizontal capital femoral epiphysis: questionable.

E. Epiphyseal extrusion.

IX. Femoral epiphyseal extrusion: most important[22]:

A. Loss of containment.

B. Lateral subluxation.

C. Predisposes to femoral head deformation.

D. When more than 20% of the width of the femoral head extrudes, there is high chance of the femoral head becoming deformed.

E. More pronounced in older children and with more epiphyseal involvement.

F. Only modifiable factor.

X.   Long-term factors associated with poor outcomes in adulthood/development of osteoarthritis[8,22]:

A. Femoral head asphericity.

B. Steepness of the acetabular roof.

Early Interventions

I.   Self-limiting disease, but with potential to develop long-term deformities.

II. Early treatments are undertaken in an attempt to prevent long-term femoral head deformities.[25]

III. Extrusion:

A. Important because if more than 20% of the width of the epiphysis extrudes outside the acetabular margin, there is very high risk of irreversible femoral head deformation.[26]

B. Most vulnerable during late fragmentation stage and early reconstitution.

C. Treatment to prevent deformation should be initiated prior to late fragmentation stage: odds ratio is 16.6 times higher to avoid deformation if containment achieved in early fragmentation stage as opposed to later.[27]

IV. Children older than 8 years invariably develop extrusion and should be offered containment; children younger than 8 should be monitored closely for development of extrusion.[5,25–28]

V.   Adequate range of motion must be present prior to containment treatment; can be achieved by traction or casting if needed.[25]

VI.   Options to prevent femoral head deformation[5,29]:
   A.   Prevent/reverse extrusion (containment):
      1.   Femoral approach: proximal varus osteotomy:
         a.   Outcomes equal to acetabular osteotomies.
         b.   May be less suitable in children ≥9 years as remodeling is less reliable.
         c.   Disadvantage: limb shortening, coxa breva, and trochanteric prominence.
         d.   May be combined with acetabular procedure.
      2.   Acetabular approaches:
         a.   Salter osteotomy:
            i.   Osteotomy from sciatic notch to just above AIIS (anterior inferior iliac spine).
            ii.   Increases anterior and lateral coverage.
            iii.   Increases lever arm of the abductor muscles.
         b.   Shelf procedure:
            i.   Extend weight-bearing surface of the acetabulum.
            ii.   Does not change orientation.
         c.   Triple osteotomy:
            i.   May be useful in patients with more severe disease.
            ii.   Provides greater containment.
            iii.   May be used in more advanced cases if hinge abduction can be avoided.
      3.   All surgical approaches may allow weight bearing and resumption of light activities by 8 weeks.
   B.   Bracing/minimize weight bearing is controversial; its use is not supported by the literature[5,29]:
      1.   Petrie casting or bracing including the thigh and leg holding the hip in abduction and internal rotation.
      2.   Must be continued until the end of the fragmentation stage.
      3.   May be 12 to 18 months.
      4.   Community mobility may be challenging.

Interventions after Early Fragmentation

I.   Femoral head deformity and collapse are already present.
II.   Hinge abduction:
   A.   Abnormal pattern of movement where the outer portion of the femoral head impinges on the lateral acetabulum.[30–32]
   B.   Reducible[30]:
      1.   Femoral head will re-center under the acetabulum when the leg is brought into abduction.

2. May still be appropriate for containment procedures, although odds of achieving a spherical head are worse than those done earlier in the disease.

3. May be best in younger children with more remodeling potential.

C. Irreducible (salvage):

1. Radiographic measures do not improve with hip abduction; arthrogram shows medial dye pooling and deformation of the lateral labrum.[30]

2. Femoral valgus osteotomy: useful to realign the femoral head and acetabulum in a best-fitting configuration (restore congruity with weight bearing)[33]:

   a. Useful when joint is congruent in adduction, but incongruent in progressive abduction.

   b. Restores congruent motion in a functional range.

   c. Improves abductor lever arm.

   d. May be combined with an acetabular osteotomy simultaneously or staged.

   e. Femoral head should be in the healing or healed stage.

3. Acetabular augmentation: remove impingement by extending the effective edge of the acetabulum laterally (Chiari or shelf).[30]

4. Articulated hip distraction[34]:

   a. Attempt to neutralize deforming forces on the epiphysis and prevent further femoral head deformation.

   b. Maintained until adequate ossification of the lateral pillar seen (4–5 months).

   c. Studies with small number of patients and short follow-up.

Sequela of Healed Perthes Hip

I. Presents similar to hip pain in other young adults:

A. Groin pain after activities or extended periods of sitting.

B. Instability symptoms during activities such as walking or running.

C. Mechanical symptoms of locking or catching.

II. Coxa magna/impingement (**Fig. 14.4**): may be cam morphology or combined impingement. May be treated in isolation or in combination with other procedures to treat other residual deformities.

III. Coxa breva[35]:

A. Trochanteric abutment.

B. Due to trochanteric overgrowth or as a result of varus osteotomy for containment.

C. Relative femoral neck lengthening/trochanteric advancement[36] (**Fig. 14.5**):

1. Resolves trochanteric impingement.

2. Improves abductor lever arm.

3. Does not improve any existing leg length discrepancy:

   a. Mean 8-year follow-up in 38 patients (39 hips).

   b. All included open osteochondroplasty.

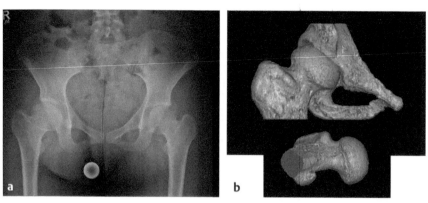

Fig. 14.4 Anteroposterior **(a)** radiograph and **(b)** CT scan of Stulberg type II healed right hip with coxa breva and coxa magna. The patient shows coxa breva on the contralateral hip as well and had a normal gait. This hip is amenable to treatment of impingement alone through either open or arthroscopic methods.

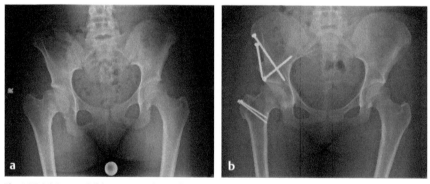

Fig. 14.5 (a) Pre- and **(b)** postoperative radiographs of a patient with a Stulberg type II right hip treated with relative femoral neck lengthening, open femoroplasty, open labral repair, and periacetabular osteotomy for concomitant hip dysplasia.

     c. Four converted to total hip arthroplasty.

     d. Range of motion improved.

     e. Proportion with a limp decreased from 76 to 9%.

     f. Normal abductor strength increased from 17 to 91%.

     g. Ten-percent complications resulting in reoperation.

     h. Forty-percent progression of osteoarthritis.

  D. Correction of coxa breva and leg length discrepancy:

    1. Femoral valgus osteotomy combined with trochanteric advancement (Wagner's osteotomy): useful when joint more congruent in adduction.

    2. Morcher's osteotomy: coxa breva, congruent joint, leg length discrepancy greater than 2 to 3 cm.[37]

IV.   Femoral head deformity:

    A.   Femoral heads with good central portion amenable to open or arthroscopic femoral osteochondroplasty[38]:

        1.   Two-year outcomes on 22 patients treated with hip arthroscopy.

        2.   Mean improvement in Modified Harris Hip Score (mHHS) of 28 points (56.7 to 82).

        3.   No complications.

        4.   No difference in mHHS from Stulberg stages I to IV.

    B.   Femoral head reduction osteotomy, for femoral heads with central deformity or wear[39,40] (**Fig. 14.6**).

V.   Labral tears: may be treated in conjunction with other procedures, either arthroscopic or open techniques.[41]

VI.   Acetabular dysplasia: treatment with periacetabular osteotomy.

VII.   Acetabular retroversion: may be corrected by acetabular rim trimming (open or arthroscopic) or acetabular reorientation.

VIII. Osteochondritis dissecans lesion: amenable to open or arthroscopic treatment.

Development of Osteoarthritis

I.   Related to the shape of the femoral head when healed (Stulberg's classification[8]; **Fig. 14.7**).

II.   Hip resurfacing[42]:

    A.   Good short- to mid-term results.

    B.   May be more technically demanding in these patients given femoral head/neck deformity.

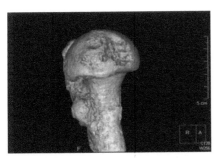

Fig. 14.6 Three-dimensional rendering of a femoral head with a large central defect.

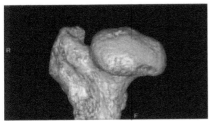

Fig. 14.7 Stulberg type 5 hip with a high likelihood of progression to osteoarthritis.

    C. May be combined with trochanteric advancement to correct trochanteric abutment and improve abductor function.

III. Total hip replacement[43]:

    A. Good outcomes reported; revision rate may be slightly higher than standard cohort.

    B. May be more technically challenging due to previous osteotomy or distorted anatomy:

        1. Rate of fracture is 11% when using standard stems.

        2. Use of reamed/modular or custom stems may decrease intraoperative fracture rate.

    C. May correct leg length discrepancy and trochanteric abutment if present:

        1. Higher rate of sciatic nerve palsy than standard cohort.

        2. All sciatic nerve palsies were in patients with previous hip surgeries.

    D. May be technically more challenging in patients with previous surgery.

References

1. Legg AT. An obscure affection of the hip joint. 1910. Clin Orthop Relat Res 2006;451(451):11–13
2. Calvé J. On a particular form of pseudo-coxalgia associated with a characteristic deformity of the upper end of the femur. 1910. Clin Orthop Relat Res 2006;451(451):14–16
3. Perthes G. The classic: on juvenile arthritis deformans. 1910. Clin Orthop Relat Res 2012;470(9):2349–2368
4. Kim HK, Herring JA. Pathophysiology, classifications, and natural history of Perthes disease. Orthop Clin North Am 2011;42(3):285–295, v
5. Ibrahim T, Little DG. The pathogenesis and treatment of Legg-Calvé-Perthes disease. JBJS Rev 2016;4(7): pii:01874474-201607000-00003
6. Koob TJ, Pringle D, Gedbaw E, Meredith J, Berrios R, Kim HK. Biomechanical properties of bone and cartilage in growing femoral head following ischemic osteonecrosis. J Orthop Res 2007;25(6):750–757
7. Rosenfeld SB, Herring JA, Chao JC. Legg-Calve-Perthes disease: a review of cases with onset before six years of age. J Bone Joint Surg Am 2007;89(12):2712–2722
8. Stulberg SD, Cooperman DR, Wallensten R. The natural history of Legg-Calvé-Perthes disease. J Bone Joint Surg Am 1981;63(7):1095–1108
9. Perry DC, Hall AJ. The epidemiology and etiology of Perthes disease. Orthop Clin North Am 2011;42(3):279–283, v
10. Hall AJ, Barker DJ, Dangerfield PH, Taylor JF. Perthes' disease of the hip in Liverpool. Br Med J (Clin Res Ed) 1983;287(6407):1757–1759
11. Perry DC, Bruce CE, Pope D, Dangerfield P, Platt MJ, Hall AJ. Perthes' disease of the hip: socio-economic inequalities and the urban environment. Arch Dis Child 2012;97(12):1053–1057
12. Bahmanyar S, Montgomery SM, Weiss RJ, Ekbom A. Maternal smoking during pregnancy, other prenatal and perinatal factors, and the risk of Legg-Calvé-Perthes disease. Pediatrics 2008;122(2):e459–e464
13. Dimeglio A, Canavese F. Imaging in Legg-Calvé-Perthes disease. Orthop Clin North Am 2011;42(3):297–302,
14. Waldenstrom H. The classic. The first stages of coxa plana by Henning Waldenström. 1938. Clin Orthop Relat Res 1984;(191):4–7
15. Salter RB, Thompson GH. Legg-Calvé-Perthes disease. The prognostic significance of the subchondral fracture and a two-group classification of the femoral head involvement. J Bone Joint Surg Am 1984;66(4):479–489
16. Catterall A. The natural history of Perthes' disease. J Bone Joint Surg Br 1971;53(1):37–53

17. Wiig O, Terjesen T, Svenningsen S. Inter-observer reliability of radiographic classifications and measurements in the assessment of Perthes' disease. Acta Orthop Scand 2002;73(5):523–530

18. Herring JA, Neustadt JB, Williams JJ, Early JS, Browne RH. The lateral pillar classification of Legg-Calvé-Perthes disease. J Pediatr Orthop 1992;12(2):143–150

19. Neyt JG, Weinstein SL, Spratt KF, et al. Stulberg classification system for evaluation of Legg-Calvé-Perthes disease: intra-rater and inter-rater reliability. J Bone Joint Surg Am 1999;81(9):1209–1216

20. Hyman JE, Trupia EP, Wright ML, et al; International Perthes Study Group Members. Interobserver and intraobserver reliability of the modified Waldenström classification system for staging of Legg-Calvé-Perthes disease. J Bone Joint Surg Am 2015;97(8):643–650

21. Conway JJ. A scintigraphic classification of Legg-Calvé-Perthes disease. Semin Nucl Med 1993;23(4):274–295

22. Joseph B. Prognostic factors and outcome measures in Perthes disease. Orthop Clin North Am 2011;42(3):303–315, v–vi

23. Rampal V, Clément JL, Solla F. Legg-Calvé-Perthes disease: classifications and prognostic factors. Clin Cases Miner Bone Metab 2017;14(1):74–82

24. Wiig O, Terjesen T, Svenningsen S. Prognostic factors and outcome of treatment in Perthes' disease: a prospective study of 368 patients with five-year follow-up. J Bone Joint Surg Br 2008;90(10):1364–1371

25. Joseph B, Price CT. Principles of containment treatment aimed at preventing femoral head deformation in Perthes disease. Orthop Clin North Am 2011;42(3):317–327, vi

26. Joseph B, Varghese G, Mulpuri K, Narasimha Rao K, Nair NS. Natural evolution of Perthes disease: a study of 610 children under 12 years of age at disease onset. J Pediatr Orthop 2003;23(5):590–600

27. Joseph B, Nair NS, Narasimha Rao K, Mulpuri K, Varghese G. Optimal timing for containment surgery for Perthes disease. J Pediatr Orthop 2003;23(5):601–606

28. Nguyen NA, Klein G, Dogbey G, McCourt JB, Mehlman CT. Operative versus nonoperative treatments for Legg-Calvé-Perthes disease: a meta-analysis. J Pediatr Orthop 2012;32(7):697–705

29. Price CT, Thompson GH, Wenger DR. Containment methods for treatment of Legg-Calvé-Perthes disease. Orthop Clin North Am 2011;42(3):329–340, vi

30. Choi IH, Yoo WJ, Cho TJ, Moon HJ. Principles of treatment in late stages of Perthes disease. Orthop Clin North Am 2011;42(3):341–348, vi

31. Grossbard GD. Hip pain during adolescence after Perthes' disease. J Bone Joint Surg Br 1981;63B(4):572–574

32. Quain S, Catterall A. Hinge abduction of the hip. Diagnosis and treatment. J Bone Joint Surg Br 1986;68(1):61–64

33. Yoo WJ, Choi IH, Moon HJ, et al. Valgus femoral osteotomy for noncontainable Perthes hips: prognostic factors of remodeling. J Pediatr Orthop 2013;33(6):650–655

34. Hosny GA, El-Deeb K, Fadel M, Laklouk M. Arthrodiastasis of the hip. J Pediatr Orthop 2011;31(2, Suppl):S229–S234

35. Standard SC. Treatment of coxa brevis. Orthop Clin North Am 2011;42(3):373–387, vii

36. Albers CE, Steppacher SD, Schwab JM, Tannast M, Siebenrock KA. Relative femoral neck lengthening improves pain and hip function in proximal femoral deformities with a high-riding trochanter. Clin Orthop Relat Res 2015;473(4):1378–1387

37. Eidelman M, Keshet D, Nelson S, Bor N. Intermediate to long-term results of femoral neck lengthening (Morscher osteotomy). J Pediatr Orthop 2019;39(4):181–186

38. Freeman CR, Jones K, Byrd JW. Hip arthroscopy for Legg-Calvè-Perthes disease: minimum 2-year follow-up. Arthroscopy 2013;29(4):666–674

39. Siebenrock KA, Anwander H, Zurmühle CA, Tannast M, Slongo T, Steppacher SD. Head reduction osteotomy with additional containment surgery improves sphericity and containment and reduces pain in Legg-Calvé-Perthes disease. Clin Orthop Relat Res 2015;473(4):1274–1283

40. Paley D. The treatment of femoral head deformity and coxa magna by the Ganz femoral head reduction osteotomy. Orthop Clin North Am 2011;42(3):389–399, viii

41. Ross JR, Nepple JJ, Baca G, Schoenecker PL, Clohisy JC. Intraarticular abnormalities in residual Perthes and Perthes-like hip deformities. Clin Orthop Relat Res 2012;470(11):2968–2977
42. Boyd HS, Ulrich SD, Seyler TM, Marulanda GA, Mont MA. Resurfacing for Perthes disease: an alternative to standard hip arthroplasty. Clin Orthop Relat Res 2007;465(465):80–85
43. Hanna SA, Sarraf KM, Ramachandran M, Achan P. Systematic review of the outcome of total hip arthroplasty in patients with sequelae of Legg-Calvé-Perthes disease. Arch Orthop Trauma Surg 2017;137(8):1149–1154

15 Slipped Capital Femoral Epiphysis

Robert C. Kollmorgen, Brian D. Lewis

Introduction

I. Slipped Capital Femoral Epiphysis

  A. Etiology:

    1. Most common hip disorder affecting adolescents:

      a. 1.5:1 male-to-female ratio:

        i. Unstable slips: 1:1 male-to-female ratio.

      b. Strong association with socioeconomic level and obesity.

      c. Bilateral 20 to 80%:

        i. Second slipped capital femoral epiphysis (SCFE) usually occurs within the first year after index slip.

      d. Racial variability:

        i. Increased incidence in African Americans, Native Americans, Hispanics, and Polynesians.

      e. Age of onset:

        i. Boys: 12.7 to 13.5 years.

        ii. Girls: 11.2 to 12.1 years.

      f. Incidence:

        i. 4.8/100,000 (0–16 years of age).

  B. Pathogenesis:

    1. Multifactorial and unknown:

      a. Slippage secondary to collagen disturbance around the pubescent growth spurt: at hypertrophic zone of physis.

      b. Metabolic, endocrine, and mechanical postulates for cause of SCFE:

        i. Metabolic:

          (1) Serum leptin levels:

            (a) Elevated in obese patients.

            (b) According to Halverson et al, regardless of body mass index (BMI), leptin greater than 4.9 increases the odds ratio of SCFE.

        ii. Endocrine disorders.

        iii. Mechanical factors:

          (1) Obesity:

            (a) Eighty percent of SCFE patients.

            (b) May be due to increased loads on physis, morphology, and endocrine disorders in obese patients.

(2) Morphology:

(a) Relative femoral retroversion.

(b) Acetabular retroversion.

(c) More vertically orientated physis.

C. Histopathology and pathomorphology:

1. Proximal capital physiolysis.

2. Damage occurs at the zone of provisional calcification (hypertrophic).

3. Deformity:

a. Anterior translation, external rotation of the femoral neck (metaphysis).

b. Posterior, inferior displacement of femoral head (epiphysis).

c. Variable posterior tilt of the femoral epiphysis.

d. Varus, extension, and external rotation deformity of the femoral neck.

e. Rare "valgus slip":

i. Anterior, medial neck translation.

ii. Posterior, valgus inclination of the femoral head.

D. Natural history:

1. Directly related to degree of slip and durations of treatment:

a. According to Loder et al's retrospective study of 328 "stable" SCFE:

i. Older children had more severe slip (age):

(1) Mild: 12.3 years.

(2) Moderate: 13 years.

(3) Severe: 13.8 years.

ii. Duration of symptoms (months):

(1) Mild: 3.5.

(2) Moderate: 7.7.

(3) Severe: 8.8.

iii. Regression analysis:

(1) Stable SCFE:

(a) Two times more likely for moderate or severe slip if older than 12.5 years.

(b) If duration longer than 2 months, 4.1 times more likely for moderate or severe slip.

1. Femoroacetabular impingement (FAI) after SCFE:

a. Remodeling occurs at head–neck junction:

i. Variable degrees.

ii. Cam morphology occurs.

iii. Regardless of remodeling, damage to anterior chondrolabral junction.

b. Multiple studies report chondrolabral injury even after mild slips.

c. Thirty-one percent painful hips in the first decade after pinning.

d. Hundred percent decreased head–neck offset = 100% cam morphology:

    i. Less physically demanding lifestyle after remodeling may improve symptoms.

    ii. Recommended to closely monitor SCFE patients in adulthood for FAI syndrome.

    iii. Leads to anterior chondrolabral injury:

        (1) Severity of damage depends on:

            (a) Duration of slip.

            (b) Deformity severity.

            (c) Activity level.

        (2) Damage occurs early:

            (a) Basheer et al reviewed 18 patients at mean 29-month follow-up: significant correlation between outcome scores and time to arthroscopy following SCFE; recommend early FAI treatment after painful presentation.

            (b) Leunig et al found damage in 13 consecutive adolescent SCFE hips with FAI chondrolabral damage when the metaphysis extends beyond the epiphysis.

    iv. FAI syndrome may be risk factor for osteoarthritis.

2. Avascular necrosis of the femoral head:

    a. Devastating and can lead to osteoarthritis.

    b. Associated with physeal stability.

    c. Unstable slips are at 9.4 times greater risk.

3. Osteoarthritis:

    d. SCFE deformity role in osteoarthritis:

        i. Castañeda et al:

            (1) One hundred and twenty one stable slips treated with pinning at 20-year follow-up.

            (2) Hundred percent had signs of osteoarthritis.

II. Classification System

  A. Southwick's classification system:

    1. Based on head (epiphyseal)–shaft (diaphyseal) angle (**Fig. 15.1**).

    2. Preslip (widening of the physis; no displacement).

    3. Mild: less than 30 degrees, up to one-third displacement.

    4. Moderate: 30 to 60 degrees, one-third to one-half displacement.

    5. Severe: greater than 60 degrees; greater than one-half displacement.

  B. Loder's classification system: weight-bearing status:

    1. Unstable:

        a. Severe pain.

        b. Unable to bear weight with crutches:

            i. Fourteen of 30 (47%) unstable hips developed avascular necrosis (AVN).

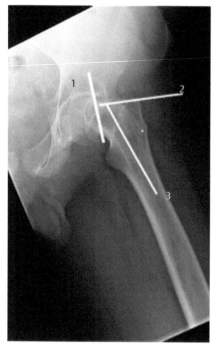

Fig. 15.1 Frog-leg lateral left hip radiograph of a 9.7-year-old boy who presented with 3 weeks of vague left knee pain, after which he fell and was unable to bear weight. Southwick's angle is formed by tracing an epiphyseal line (1), a line perpendicular to the epiphyseal line (2), and a line parallel to the center of the femoral shaft (3). The *asterisk* represents the angle to be measured. Image is classified as a severe slip greater than 60 degrees.

2. Stable:
   a. Can bear weight with or without crutches:
      i. Zero percent of stable slips developed AVN.
   C. Duration:
      1. Acute: symptoms less than 3 weeks.
      2. Chronic: symptoms greater than 3 weeks.
      3. Acute-on-chronic: acute exacerbation of symptoms in the setting of a chronic slip.
   D. Prognosis:
      1. Mild: good prognosis.
      2. Moderate and severe have increased chance of developing arthritis.

III. Physeal stability:
   A. Standard is based on inability to bear weight:
      1. Ziebarth et al questioned this:
         a. Retrospective analysis of 82 patients:
            i. Complete physeal disruption observed in 28/82 hips (34%) at surgery.
            ii. Acute versus chronic classification: 82% sensitive and 44% specific.
            iii. Stable versus unstable classification: 39% sensitive and 76% specific.
            iv. Calls into question current SCFE classification systems and there are more unstable hips than expected based on ability to weight bear.

Anatomical Considerations

I.   Proximal femoral Physis
   A.   Zone of provisional calcification (in hypertrophic zone) is damaged.
   B.   Proximal femur responsible for 3 mm of growth per year.

II. Blood supply:
   A.   Deep branch of the medial femoral circumflex artery:
      1.   Most important blood supply to the femoral head/epiphysis.
      2.   Lesser contributions from lateral femoral circumflex artery, artery of ligamentum teres.

History and Physical Examination

I.   History
   A.   Symptoms:
      1.   Vague pain:
         a.   Groin, hip, and knee pain.
         b.   May be severe enough to prevent ambulation.
      2.   Limp:
         a.   Children presenting with knee pain have a longer diagnostic delay than those with hip pain.
   B.   Past medical history: evaluate for endocrinopathy:
      1.   Strong association with SCFE.
   C.   Obesity:
      1.   Increased awareness in all preadolescent patients with pain.

II. Physical Examination
   A.   No pathognomonic finding for SCFE.
   B.   Gait:
      1.   Antalgic gait.
   C.   Seated or supine:
      1.   Limited flexion and internal rotation (most frequent finding).

Diagnostic Testing

I.   Imaging
   A.   Radiographs:
      1.   Anteroposterior (AP) pelvis and frog-leg lateral (**Fig. 15.2**):
         a.   Orthogonal radiographs: gold standard for diagnosis:
            i.   Southwick's angle (SA):
               (1) Also known as the slip angle, epiphyseal–diaphyseal angle,
               (2) Measured on frog-leg lateral.

        (3) Angle between a line connecting the corners of the femoral epiphysis and a line perpendicular to the longitudinal axis of the femoral shaft.

        (4) Difference is taken between affected and normal side.

        (5) When there is bilateral involvement, 12 degrees are subtracted from the angle measured.

    b. Lateral view head–neck index (LVHNI):

      i. Developed to measure residual head–neck deformity.

      ii. Forty-five-degree flexion/45-degree abduction/30-degree external rotation view.

      iii. Threshold of 9%:

        (1) Index greater than 9% is 89% sensitive and 82% specific for detecting pistol grip deformity.

B. Ultrasound:

    1. Can detect effusion of initial slip and quantify degree of slip.

    2. Reliable for moderate and severe SCFE detection.

    3. Radiographs best served to follow remodeling over time.

C. CT scan:

    1. Limited utility.

    2. May be useful in cases of chronic slips where fusion of physis or fracture is in question (**Fig. 15.3**).

D. MRI:

    1. Can show abnormalities in "preslip" time frame.

Differential Diagnosis

I. Early Diagnosis

    A. Foundation of better outcomes:

    B. Delay is common due to:

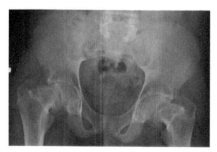

Fig. 15.2 Anteroposterior radiograph of the pelvis of a 16-year-old adolescent boy with acute-on-chronic bilateral slipped capital femoral epiphysis.

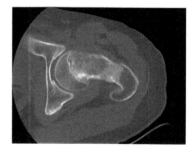

Fig. 15.3 Axial hip CT of chronic slipped capital femoral epiphysis in a 16-year-old adolescent boy.

    1. Lack of awareness.

    2. Vagueness of pain complaints not localizing to the hip.

    3. Obesity alone can be the cause of lower extremity pain.

II. Differential

  A. Legg–Calvé–Perthes disease.

  B. Avascular necrosis.

  C. Infection.

  D. FAI.

  E. Dysplasia.

Nonsurgical Management

I. Indicated only in a completely asymptomatic patient

  A. Controversy exists regarding prophylactic pinning.

  B. Monitor closely:

    1. No established criteria for follow-up.

    2. The authors recommend follow-up every 3 to 6 months if pain free.

Surgical Management: Acute

I. Stable

  A. Commonly managed with in situ fixation.

  B. Goal is to stabilize femoral head and reducing risk of chondrolysis and AVN.

  C. Bilateral (prophylactic) pinning:

    1. Controversial.

    2. Relative indications:

      a. Young age at diagnosis.

      b. Unstable SCFE.

      c. Endocrine disorders.

      d. Unreliable patient.

  D. Percutaneous single-screw fixation:

    1. Recommended screw placement (**Fig. 15.4**):

      a. Center of epiphysis.

      b. Perpendicular to physis.

      c. No consensus on elective screw removal:

        i. Surgeon preference based on practice experience:

          (1) Less than 10 years' practice: 16% remove screws.

          (2) ≥10 years' practice: 7% remove screws.

          (3) Our current recommendation is for screw removal: secondary FAI is a concern.

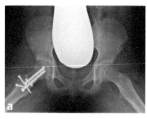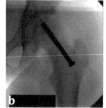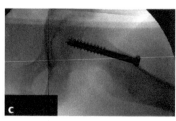

Fig. 15.4 Frog-leg lateral radiograph (**a**) of an 11-year-old girl who presented with 4 weeks of left hip pain after modified Dunn's procedure on the right side. The patient was unable to bear weight on the left side. Left side demonstrating mild slipped capital femoral epiphysis. Anteroposterior (**b**) and frog-leg lateral (**c**) radiograph demonstrating single screw placement.

      2. Techniques described with oblique screw placement to allow for femoral neck osteoplasty.

II. Unstable

    A. Urgent gentle reduction with internal fixation.

    B. Initial open reduction with internal fixation.

    C. Modified Dunn's osteotomy.

III. Osteotomies

    A. Several osteotomies described to improve dysfunction and malposition of the femoral head:

        1. Southwick's osteotomy through the lesser trochanter.

        2. Imhauser's intertrochanteric femoral osteotomy:

           a. Goal is to decrease impingement.

           b. Combines an intertrochanteric osteotomy with epiphysiodesis.

        3. Dunn's osteotomy:

           a. Subcapital osteotomy.

        4. Modified Dunn's osteotomy (**Fig. 15.5**):

           a. Combines surgical dislocation greater trochanteric osteotomy (SDO) with Dunn's osteotomy:

              i. Allows for anatomic reduction.

           b. Goal is to preserve blood supply, decrease risk of AVN, and increase offset:

              i. Procedure:

                  (1) Standard SDO.

                  (2) Femoral head separated from neck through the physis.

                  (3) Femoral neck callus removed without excessive shortening.

                  (4) Remaining physis removed with curet.

                  (5) Head reduced, provisionally fixed with threaded pin through the fovea.

                  (6) A second pin is placed distal to proximal.

                  (7) Pins cut and trochanteric fragment fixed.

IV.   Vascularized Free Fibula Graft

    A. Hip preservation option for AVN from SCFE.

Surgical Management: Chronic

I.   Goal is to preserve native hip if possible

    A. If open physis and greater than 2 mm of joint space:

        1. Osteotomy for realignment and containment (**Fig. 15.6**).

    B. FAI following SCFE management:

        1. SDO or hip arthroscopy are options to correct FAI:

            a. Arthroscopic treatment of FAI at short-term follow-up shows significant improvement in all patient-reported outcomes.

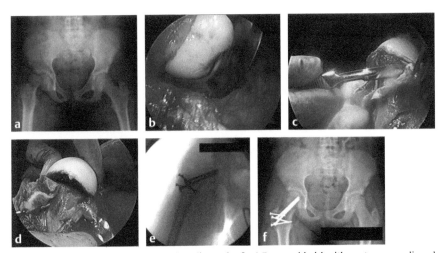

Fig. 15.5 (a) Anteroposterior (AP) pelvis radiograph of a 9.7-year-old girl with acute severe slipped capital femoral epiphysis after a fall. **(b)** Operative photograph of surgical hip dislocation, with **(c)** subperiosteal flaps created to protect the blood supply to the femoral head. **(d)** Head is reduced. **(e)** Fluoroscopic image illustrating head reduction, fixation of epiphysis, and trochanteric osteotomy. **(f)** Postoperative AP pelvis radiograph showing healed epiphysis and trochanter.

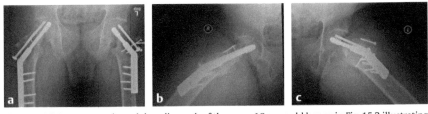

Fig. 15.6 (a) Anteroposterior pelvis radiograph of the same 16-year-old boy as in Fig. 15.2 illustrating bilateral healed modified Dunn's osteotomies and subtrochanteric osteotomies at 2-year follow-up (18 years of age). Right **(b)** and left **(c)** Dunn's 45-degree plain radiographs. Patient was ambulating without assistive device and had 0/10 pain.

C. Osteoarthritis secondary to SCFE:

1. Total hip arthroplasty (THA):

a. Reliable option for pain relief and shows improved patient-reported outcomes.

b. Reported higher revision rate with cementless prosthesis as compared with non-SCFE cohort at 11 years' follow-up (19–50%).

c. We recommend a ceramic femoral head bearing on highly cross-linked acetabular bearing surface for this young population to decrease wear rate over time.

Outcomes

I. In Situ Pinning

A. Leads to decreased head–neck offset.

B. Long-term follow-up studies have shown evidence of remodeling.

C. Internal rotation deficit occurs, but not clinically relevant:

1. Mean follow-up of 19.6 years.

2. Seventy-two percent obese.

3. No association between initial slip angle and outcome.

4. Male sex and lower BMI predicted better long-term scores.

D. Patients with severe slips have significantly worse long-term outcomes (18-year follow-up):

1. Severe SCFE: 75% developed arthritis.

2. Moderate SCFE: 11% developed arthritis.

3. Mild SCFE: 1% developed arthritis.

II. Osteotomies

A. Imhauser's versus modified Dunn's osteotomy for moderate to severe stable SCFE:

1. Higher rate of AVN in modified Dunn's osteotomy (29 vs. 0%).

2. Similar complication rate (33% Imhauser vs. 36% modified Dunn).

3. Similar reoperation rate (33% Imhauser vs. 21% modified Dunn).

III. Vascularized Free Fibular Graft

A. Hip preservation option for AVN after SCFE:

1. At short-term follow-up, 8% converted to THA and 2% to hip fusion.

2. Significant patient-reported outcome improvements in those without re-operation.

IV. Femoroacetabular impingement after Slipped Capital Femoral Epiphysis

1. Systematic review of the efficacy of surgical management of FAI following SCFE comparing arthroscopy, surgical dislocation, open osteotomy (150-level IV studies with 266 hips):

a. Treatment groups:

       i. Arthroscopic osteochondroplasty.

      ii. Surgical hip dislocation.

     iii. Traditional open osteotomy.

   b. Major complication rate lowest after arthroscopy (1.6%), followed by osteotomy (6.7%) and surgical dislocation (11%).

   b. Alpha angle significantly improved after arthroscopy (32 degrees) and surgical dislocation (41 degrees), but not after osteotomy (6 degrees).

Future Directions

I.   Early detection and increasing awareness among musculoskeletal care providers.

II.   Obesity epidemic in the United States correlated to SCFE.

III.   Long-term studies on postsurgical FAI correction to alter natural history of arthritis are needed.

Acknowledgments

The authors thank Dr Steven A. Olson and Dr Robert Lark for providing images for this chapter.

Suggested Readings

Alves C, Steele M, Narayanan U, Howard A, Alman B, Wright JG. Open reduction and internal fixation of unstable slipped capital femoral epiphysis by means of surgical dislocation does not decrease the rate of avascular necrosis: a preliminary study. J Child Orthop 2012;6(4):277–283

Aronsson DD, Loder RT, Breur GJ, Weinstein SL. Slipped capital femoral epiphysis: current concepts. J Am Acad Orthop Surg 2006;14(12):666–679

Basheer SZ, Cooper AP, Maheshwari R, Balakumar B, Madan S. Arthroscopic treatment of femoroacetabular impingement following slipped capital femoral epiphysis. Bone Joint J 2016;98-B(1):21–27

Bertrand T, Urbaniak JR, Lark RK. Vascularized fibular grafts for avascular necrosis after slipped capital femoral epiphysis: is hip preservation possible? Clin Orthop Relat Res 2013;471(7):2206–2211

Carney BT, Weinstein SL, Noble J. Long-term follow-up of slipped capital femoral epiphysis. J Bone Joint Surg Am 1991;73(5):667–674

Castañeda P, Ponce C, Villareal G, Vidal C. The natural history of osteoarthritis after a slipped capital femoral epiphysis/the pistol grip deformity. J Pediatr Orthop 2013;33(Suppl 1):S76–S82

Castriota-Scanderbeg A, Orsi E. Slipped capital femoral epiphysis: ultrasonographic findings. Skeletal Radiol 1993;22(3):191–193

Chahla J, Lapradre RF, Mardones R, Huard J, Phillippon MJ, Mei-Dan O, Garirido CP. Biological therapies for cartilage lesions in the hip: a new horizon. Orthopedics 2016;39(4):e715–e723

de Poorter JJ, Beunder TJ, Gareb B, et al. Long-term outcomes of slipped capital femoral epiphysis treated with in situ pinning. J Child Orthop 2016;10(5):371–379

Davis RL II, Samora WP III, Persinger F, Klingele KE. Treatment of unstable versus stable slipped capital femoral epiphysis using the modified Dunn procedure. J Pediatr Orthop 2017

Dodds MK, McCormack D, Mulhall KJ. Femoroacetabular impingement after slipped capital femoral epiphysis: does slip severity predict clinical symptoms? J Pediatr Orthop 2009;29(6):535–539

Dunn DM. The treatment of adolescent slipping of the upper femoral epiphysis. J Bone Joint Surg Br 1964;46:621–629

Escott BG, De La Rocha A, Jo CH, Sucato DJ, Karol LA. Patient-reported health outcomes after in situ percutaneous fixation for slipped capital femoral epiphysis: an average twenty-year follow-up study. J Bone Joint Surg Am 2015;97(23):1929–1934

Ganz R, Parvizi J, Beck M, Leunig M, Nötzli H, Siebenrock KA. Femoroacetabular impingement: a cause for osteoarthritis of the hip. Clin Orthop Relat Res 2003;(417):112–120

Gourineni P. Oblique in situ screw fixation of stable slipped capital femoral epiphysis. J Pediatr Orthop 2013;33(2):135–138

Halverson SJ, Warhoover T, Mencio GA, Lovejoy SA, Martus JE, Schoenecker JG. Leptin elevation as a risk factor for slipped capital femoral epiphysis independent of obesity status. J Bone Joint Surg Am 2017;99(10):865–872

Leunig M, Casillas MM, Hamlet M, et al. Slipped capital femoral epiphysis: early mechanical damage to the acetabular cartilage by a prominent femoral metaphysis. Acta Orthop Scand 2000;71(4):370–375

Loder RT, Richards BS, Shapiro PS, Reznick LR, Aronson DD. Acute slipped capital femoral epiphysis: the importance of physeal stability. J Bone Joint Surg Am 1993;75(8):1134–1140

Loder RT, Starnes T, Dikos G, Aronsson DD. Demographic predictors of severity of stable slipped capital femoral epiphyses. J Bone Joint Surg Am 2006;88(1):97–105

Makhni EC, Stone AV, Ukwuani GC, et al. A critical review: management and surgical options for articular defects in the hip. Clin Sports Med 2017;36(3):573–586

Morlock MM, Bishop N, Huber G. Biomechanics of Hip Arthroplasty. In: Knahr K, eds. Tribology in Total Hip Arthroplasty. Berlin: Springer; 2011

Millis MB. SCFE: clinical aspects, diagnosis, and classification. J Child Orthop 2017;11(2):93–98

Murgier J, Chiron P, Cavaignac E, Espié A, Bayle-Iniguez X, Lepage B. The lateral view headneck index (LVHNI): a diagnostic tool for the sequelae of slipped capital femoral epiphysis. Orthop Traumatol Surg Res 2013;99 (5):501–508

Novais EN, Millis MB. Slipped capital femoral epiphysis: prevalence, pathogenesis, and natural history. Clin Orthop Relat Res 2012;470(12):3432–3438

Oduwole KO, de Sa D, Kay J, et al. Surgical treatment of femoroacetabular impingement following slipped capital femoral epiphysis: a systematic review. Bone Joint Res 2017;6(8):472–480

Perry DC, Metcalfe D, Costa ML, Van Staa T. A nationwide cohort study of slipped femoral epiphysis. Arch Dis Child 2017;102(12):1132–1136

Schoof B, Citak M, O'Loughlin PF, et al. Eleven year results of total hip arthroplasty in patients with secondary osteoarthritis due to slipped capital femoral epiphysis. Open Orthop J 2013;7:158–162

Sikora-Klak J, Bomar JD, Paik CN, Wenger DR, Upasani V. Comparison of surgical outcomes between a triplane proximal femoral osteotomy and the modified Dunn procedure for stable, moderate to severe slipped capital femoral epiphysis. J Pediatr Orthop 2019;39(7):338–346

Southwick WO. Osteotomy through the lesser trochanter for slipped capital femoral epiphysis. J Bone Joint Surg Am 1967;49(5):807–835

Terjesen T. Ultrasonography for diagnosis of slipped capital femoral epiphysis. Comparison with radiography in 9 cases. Acta Orthop Scand 1992;63(6):653–657

Thawrani DP, Feldman DS, Sala DA. Current practice in the management of slipped capital femoral epiphysis. J Pediatr Orthop 2016;36(3):e27–e37

Witbreuk MM, Bolkenbaas M, Mullender MG, Sierevelt IN, Besselaar PP. The results of downgrading moderate and severe slipped capital femoral epiphysis by an early Imhauser femur osteotomy. J Child Orthop 2009;3(5):405–410

Wylie JD, Beckmann JT, Maak TG, Aoki SK. Arthroscopic treatment of mild to moderate deformity after slipped capital femoral epiphysis: intra-operative findings and functional outcomes. Arthroscopy 2015;31(2):247–253

Ziebarth K, Domayer S, Slongo T, Kim YJ, Ganz R. Clinical stability of slipped capital femoral epiphysis does not correlate with intraoperative stability. Clin Orthop Relat Res 2012;470(8):2274–227

Ziebarth K, Zilkens C, Spencer S, Leunig M, Ganz R, Kim Y-J. Capital realignment for moderate and severe SCFE using a modified Dunn procedure. Clin Orthop Relat Res 2009;467(3):704–716

16 Femoroacetabular Impingement

Joshua D. Harris

Introduction

I. Femoroacetabular impingement (FAI) refers to hip joint pathomorphology.

  A. FAI does not necessarily imply symptoms of pain or dysfunction.

    1. First defined by Professor Reinhold Ganz and colleagues as abnormal contact that may arise as a result of either of the following[1]:

      a. Abnormal morphological features.

      b. Subjecting the hip to excessive supraphysiological motion.

    2. Definition expanded by (American Academy of Orthopaedic Surgeons (AAOS)[2]:

      a. Abnormal morphology of femur and/or acetabulum.

      b. Abnormal contact between femur and acetabulum.

      c. Especially vigorous supraphysiological motion that results in such abnormal contact and collision.

      d. Repetitive motion resulting in the continuous insult.

      e. Presence of soft-tissue damage.

  B. Presence of symptoms = FAI syndrome (Warwick Agreement):

    1. Defined by Warwick Agreement International Consensus Statement (**Fig. 16.1**).[3]

    2. Motion-related clinical disorder of the hip with a triad of:

      a. Symptoms.

      b. Clinical signs.

      c. Imaging findings.

    3. Represents symptomatic premature contact between proximal femur and acetabulum.

  C. No role for prophylactic surgery in asymptomatic FAI.[4]

II. Two main types of FAI pathomorphology:

  A. Cam:

    1. Proximal femoral asphericity:

      a. Loss of head–neck junction offset.

  B. Pincer:

    1. Acetabular overcoverage:

      a. Retroversion:

        i. Focal loss of cranial acetabular anteversion.

        ii. Global retroversion.

      b. General overcoverage (protrusio acetabula).

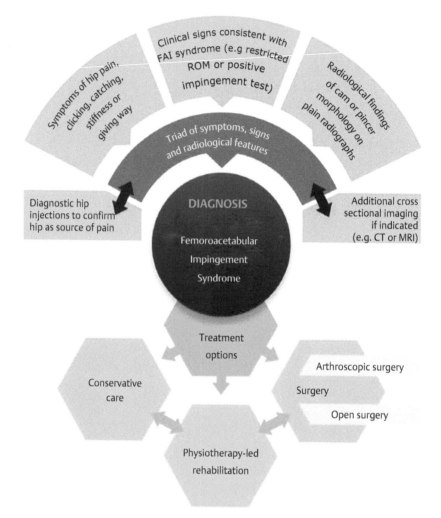

Fig. 16.1 Warwick Agreement diagnosis of femoroacetabular impingement syndrome including the triad of clinical symptoms, signs, and imaging findings. Management involves a triad of nonsurgical observation and education, physical therapy, or surgery. (Reproduced with permission of BMJ Publishing Group Ltd.)

    C. Combined cam and pincer:

        1. More common than either cam or pincer in isolation.

III. Prevalence of FAI morphology:

    A. Common in asymptomatic individuals.

    B. Cam:

        1. Ranges from 29[5] to 37[6] to 76%.[7]

        2. 2.4 times more common in athletes than nonathletes.[6]

        3. Participation in competitive sports as young adult associated with increased prevalence of FAI pathomorphology (odds ratio 1.49).[7]

C. Pincer:

    1. Ranges from 28[7] to 57[5] to 67%.[6]

D. Mixed cam and pincer.

IV. Common cause of labral injury:

A. Plain radiograph- and CT-based studies have shown high prevalence of FAI structural abnormalities in patients with labral tears (>90%).[8–11]

B. Cam leads to primarily delamination articular surface chondrolabral junction injury.

C. Pincer leads to primarily labral pinching, crushing, tearing injury.

V. Common cause of osteoarthrosis:

A. Dynamic, motion-related femoral abutment against acetabular rim leads to joint damage in nondysplastic hips.[1,12]

B. Multiple large-scale, population-based, longitudinal or cross-sectional investigations have shown significant association of FAI and osteoarthrosis:

    1. Cohort Hip and Cohort Knee (CHECK).[13]

    2. Chingford.[14]

    3. Rotterdam.[15]

    4. Sumiswald.[16]

    5. Genetics of Osteoarthritis and Lifestyle (GOAL) (Nottingham).[17]

    6. Copenhagen.[18]

    7. Korean Longitudinal Study on Health and Aging (KLoSHA).[19]

Anatomic Considerations

I. The "layer" concept of hip pain generators:

A. Layer I: osteochondral (femur, acetabulum/pelvis).

B. Layer II: static soft tissue (labrum, capsule).

C. Layer III: dynamic soft tissue (muscles, tendons).

D. Layer IV: neurokinetic, neuromechanical (nerves, vessels).

II. The hip is a multiaxial, diarthrodial synovial, deep, highly congruent joint:

A. Convex femur.

B. Concave acetabulum.

III. Shape largely believed as spherical ("ball-and-socket"). This is not exactly true.

A. Actually, shape is elongated in neck axis, "egg-shaped," or conchoidal:[20]

    1. Femoral head forms two-thirds of a sphere.[21]

    2. Acetabulum has slightly smaller diameter than the femoral head[22]:

        a. Covers approximately 170 degrees of femoral head.[23]

        b. Globally covers 40 ± 2%.[24]

B. Primarily a rotational joint, with minimal rolling or gliding (translation).

C. Greater degrees of incongruity (such as those observed in FAI) may increase the translational (shearing stress) motion of the joint, leading to articular cartilage injury, and eventual joint degeneration (osteoarthrosis).

IV. Extra-articular femoral and pelvic anatomy plays significant role in FAI syndrome:

A. Femur:

1. Neck–shaft angle:

a. Decreased (coxa vara): increases femoral offset (and abductor moment arm) and femoral head coverage.

b. Increased (coxa valga): decreases femoral offset (and abductor moment arm) and increases abductor force and joint contact forces.

2. Version:

a. Increased (excessive anteversion): decreases abductor lever arm and increases abductor force and joint contact forces.

b. Decreased (relative retroversion): increases impingement risk due to insufficient head–neck offset during flexion and rotation.

B. Pelvis:

1. Spinopelvic parameters:

a. Normal sagittal balance: C7 plumb line from center of C7 to posterosuperior corner of S1 superior end plate:

i. Also known as sagittal vertical axis (SVA).

b. Negative sagittal balance: axis falls posterior to sacrum:

i. In patients with lumbar hyperlordosis.

c. Positive sagittal balance: axis falls anterior to sacrum:

i. In patients with hip flexion contracture or flat back.

d. Pelvic incidence (PI; fixed, position independent):

i. Sacral slope (SS; positional).

ii. Pelvic tilt (PT; positional).

iii. PI = SS + PT:

(1) Mean normal PI is 53 ± 7 degrees in men and 49 ± 7 degrees in women.[25]

(2) In general, PI = lumbar lordosis + 9 degrees.

e. Normal sagittal balance aligns forces behind lumbar spine and femoral heads:

i. When standing, the pelvis tilts anteriorly, PT decreases, and SS increases, but PI remains constant.

ii. When supine, lumbar lordosis increases, PT decreases (more than standing), and SS increases (more than standing).

iii. When sitting, lumbar lordosis decreases, PT increases, and SS decreases.

iv. With hip flexion contracture, the body tilts forward, and lumbar lordosis must increase to maintain sagittal balance.

v. Increased PI associated with increased lumbar lordosis, forcing posterior PT to maintain sagittal balance: reduces anterior impingement.

      vi. Decreased PI associated with decreased lumbar lordosis, forcing anterior PT to maintain sagittal balance: increases anterior impingement:[26]

        (1) May cause "dynamic" pincer FAI.[27,28]

        (2) Essentially, patients with decreased PI cannot posteriorly tilt the pelvis more to open the anterior acetabulum, increasing impingement.

    f. T1 pelvic angle (position independent):

      i. The angle formed by the line formed from the femoral head axis to the centroid of T1 and the line from the femoral head axis to the middle of the S1 superior end plate.[29]

      ii. Sum of T1 spinopelvic inclination and PT.

      iii. Does not change with PT.

History and Examination

I.   History:

   A. A thorough history and physical examination, without any imaging, may diagnose an intra-articular hip problem (FAI syndrome, dysplasia, and arthritis) in majority of cases.

   B. Warwick Agreement: primary symptom of FAI syndrome is motion- or position-related pain in the hip or groin. Pain may also be felt in the back, buttock, or thigh. Patients may also complain clicking, catching, locking, stiffness, restricted range of motion, or giving way.[3]

   C. Pain onset:

    1. Acute.

    2. Chronic.

    3. Acute on chronic.

   D. Pain location:

    1. Typically deep groin, rather than superficial.

    2. "C" sign (**Fig. 16.2a**).

    3. "Between the fingers" sign (**Fig. 16.2b**).

    4. Anterior most common location (groin), followed by lateral, posterolateral, and posterior.

   E. Pain duration:

    1. May go undiagnosed for significant duration, frequently mistaken for other cause of groin pain (gastrointestinal, genitourinary, obstetric, gynecologic, pelvic floor disorder, neurovascular, extra-articular impingement, and other musculoskeletal pains).

    2. Patients have a mean duration of symptoms 32.0 months prior to diagnosis of labral tear and FAI, see a mean of 4.0 health care providers, mean of 3.4 diagnostic imaging tests, attempted mean of 3.1 treatments prior to diagnosis, and mean amount spent prior to diagnosis of $2,456.97.[30]

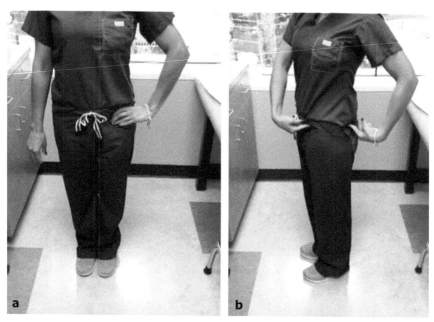

Fig. 16.2 (a) The "C" sign, with the patient making the letter "C" with the hand and reaching around the hip, indicative of intra-articular source of hip pain. **(b)** The "between the fingers" sign, with the patient pointing with two fingers in the front and back of the hip, indicative of intra-articular source of hip pain.

F. Exacerbating factors:

　　1. Deep flexion, rotational maneuvers.

　　2. Sports: six categories[31]:

　　　　a. Cutting.

　　　　b. Flexibility.

　　　　c. Contact.

　　　　d. Impingement.

　　　　e. Asymmetric/overhead.

　　　　f. Endurance.

　　3. Sitting typically affects patients more than standing.

G. Relieving factors:

　　1. Rest, activity modification, oral medications (nonsteroidal anti-inflammatory).

H. Associated symptoms:

　　1. Low back or sacroiliac (SI) joint pain ("hip-spine syndrome").

　　2. Coughing, sneezing (athletic pubalgia, core muscle injury, sports hernia).

　　3. Stiffness, loss of hip motion.

　　4. Weakness.

5. Snapping:

    a. Deep, audible: usually iliopsoas.

    b. Deep, palpable: iliopsoas, labral tear.

    c. Superficial, lateral, visible: usually iliotibial band.

6. Difficulty sleeping.

II. Physical examination:

  A. Inspection:

    1. No deformity, no cutaneous abnormalities.

    2. Gait, single leg stance, single leg squat.

  B. Palpation:

    1. All bony and soft-tissue landmarks.

    2. Typically no peritrochanteric, proximal hamstring, adductor, inguinal, pubis, rectus abdominis, deep gluteal space, SI tenderness.

  C. Motion:

    1. Always remember to assess contralateral limb for symmetry.

    2. Typically, a loss of motion: usually hip flexion, internal rotation in 90 degrees of flexion, total arc sum of rotational motion (internal and external).

  D. Strength:

    1. Typically not limited, unless by pain.

  E. Special testing:

    1. FADIR (flexion, adduction, and internal rotation): most sensitive test for FAI syndrome, but poorly specific.

    2. Impingement maneuvers: assure that an affirmative response to pain during the maneuver reproduces the patient's symptoms prompting the evaluation:

      a. Anterior: taking hip from flexed, abducted, and externally rotated position to a position of FADIR:

        i. Note clockface arc perception and localization of pain (typically 12 o'clock to 3 o'clock position).

      b. Subspine: straight hip flexion in sagittal plane.

      c. Lateral: straight hip abduction in coronal plane, with permissive limb external rotation:

        i. Once end of abduction is reached, internal rotation to a gentle stop indicates trochanteric–pelvic impingement.

      d. Posterior: extension, external rotation causing pain:

        i. Differentiate from apprehension, fear: indicative of anterior hip instability, microinstability.

    3. FABER (flexion, abduction, and external rotation): assess for asymmetry in distance of lateral knee to table (vs. contralateral hip)—inquire with patient if pain is deep in the hip (anterior groin) versus SI joint.

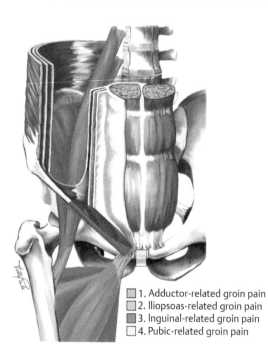

☐ 1. Adductor-related groin pain
☐ 2. Iliopsoas-related groin pain
■ 3. Inguinal-related groin pain
☐ 4. Pubic-related groin pain

Fig. 16.3 Four defined clinical entities for groin pain: (1) adductor related, (2) iliopsoas related, (3) inguinal related, and (4) pubic related. (Reproduced with permission of BMJ Publishing Group Ltd.)

III.   The Doha agreement resolved the problem of heterogeneity in terminology and definitions in groin pain in athletes.[32]

A.   Defined clinical entities for groin pain (**Fig. 16.3**):

1.   Adductor related.

2.   Pubic related.

3.   Iliopsoas related.

4.   Inguinal related.

B.   Hip-related groin pain.

C.   Other causes of groin pain in athletes.

Diagnostic Imaging

I.   Plain radiographs:

A.   At a minimum, two orthogonal views necessary:

1.   Anteroposterior (AP) pelvis (standing; **Fig. 16.4a**):

a.   Detects lateral/posterolateral cam, lateral acetabular coverage, and joint space (**Fig. 16.4b**).

b.   Crossover sign: focal retroversion (loss of cranial acetabular anteversion) pincer morphology (**Fig. 16.4c**):

i.   Fifty percent of positive crossover signs due to prominent antero-inferior iliac spine (AIIS) in the presence of anteverted acetabulum.

c.   Prominent ischial spine sign and posterior wall sign: global acetabular retroversion pincer morphology.

    d. General overcoverage pincer morphology:

       i. Protrusio acetabula.

      ii. Lateral center edge angle greater than 40 degrees.

     iii. Coxa profunda poorly sensitive for pincer.

2. Lateral view(s):

    a. Dunn 45-degree view: most sensitive for typical anterolateral cam detection (**Fig. 16.4d**).

    b. Dunn 90-degree view: detects more anterior cam.

    c. False profile: detects AIIS type, anterior center edge angle (greater than 40-degree anterior pincer FAI), anterior joint space, cam, and posterior joint congruity.

    d. Frog leg: detects more anterior cam.

    e. Cross-table: detects more anterior cam.

3. Spinopelvic views:

    a. EOS:

       i. AP (**Fig. 16.4e**):

         (1) Measurement of any coronal plane spinopelvic deformity or lower extremity mechanical axis malalignment.

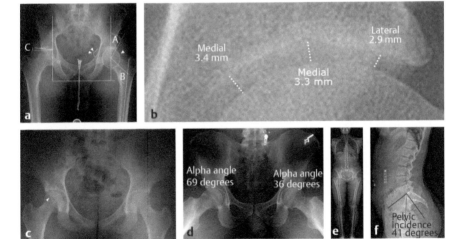

Fig. 16.4 (a) Standing anteroposterior (AP) pelvis view. Angle A is the lateral center edge angle, angle B is the neck-shaft angle, and angle C is the Tönnis angle. The two vertical lines are perpendicular to the most inferior aspect of the ischial tuberosities to account for any coronal plane pelvic tilt (alternatively, the teardrops may be used). Single arrowhead indicates a far lateral cam and double arrowhead indicates a prominent ischial spine sign. **(b)** Standing AP pelvis view with increased magnification at joint space at medial, middle, and lateral sourcil. **(c)** Standing AP pelvis view illustrating a positive crossover sign with the anterior wall (black dotted line) crossing over the posterior wall (white dotted line). **(d)** Dunn 45-degree lateral radiograph with α angle measurements on bilateral hips; right hip with symptomatic femoroacetabular impingement syndrome (α angle 69 degrees); left hip 6 weeks following arthroscopic hip preservation surgery, cam osteoplasty (α angle 36 degrees). **(e)** AP full-body EOS radiograph illustrating lower extremity mechanical axis measurement, between the medial and lateral tibial spines bilaterally. It also permits leg length discrepancy analysis, coronal plane spinal deformity (scoliosis). **(f)** Lateral full-body EOS radiograph illustrating measurement of pelvic incidence at 41 degrees.

ii. Lateral (**Fig. 16.4f**):

(1)Measurement of SS, PT, PI, and T1 pelvic angle.

II. MRI (magnetic resonance imaging):

A. Minimum of 1.5-T magnet strength; preferred magnet strength is 3.0 T.

B. Hip versus pelvis MRI:

   1. Hip: increased resolution; greater detail for ipsilateral hip.

   2. Pelvis: permits assessment of bilateral hips, at expense of decreased dedicated detailed hip resolution:

      a. Intrapelvic disorders (gynecologic, genitourinary, gastrointestinal, oncologic, and pelvic floor).

      b. Adductor, iliopsoas, inguinal canal, rectus abdominis, pubis, pubic symphysis, proximal hamstring, SI joint, ischiofemoral space, L5–S1 disk, and possible L4–L5 disk.

C. Nonarthrogram:

   1. Permits assessment of effusion.

   2. Less expensive than arthrogram.

   3. Easier scheduling for patient.

   4. No pain from an injection. However, misses possible diagnostic component of injection.

D. Arthrogram:

   1. Better assessment of capsular integrity.

   2. Better assessment of capsular volume.

   3. Increased sensitivity of labral tear detection.

E. Series: combination of T1, proton density, and T2 weighting:

   1. Axial (**Fig. 16.5a**).

   2. Sagittal.

   3. Coronal.

   4. Axial oblique: original description of α angle measurement.[33]

   5. Sagittal oblique.

   6. Radial: best 360-degree circumferential cam, labral assessment (**Fig. 16.5b**):

      a. Can measure omega angle, where α angle exceeds considered normal threshold (45 degrees) and begins to be abnormal and where it returns to normal.[34]

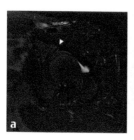 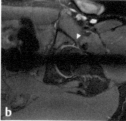

Fig. 16.5 (a) Axial T2-weighted magnetic resonance image illustrating an acetabular labral tear (*white arrowhead*). **(b)** Radial magnetic resonance image illustrating an acetabular labral tear (*white arrowhead*).

F. Helps rule out stress fracture, soft tissue, or osseous mass.

G. Assessment of subchondral edema, paralabral cyst (acetabular, femoral impingement; synovial herniation pit), capsular thickness, synovial disorders (synovial chondromatosis), and loose bodies.

H. Three-dimensional (3D) reconstructions improving with advanced MR technologies.

I. Advanced MRI primarily research application, not everyday clinical care:

1. dGEMRIC (delayed gadolinium-enhanced MRI of cartilage).

2. T2 mapping.

3. T2*.

4. Na imaging.

5. T1 rho.

III. Computed Tomography (CT):

A. Best evaluation for osseous anatomy, including complex deformities.

B. Several low-dose protocols exist to reduce radiation exposure.

C. Pelvis with distal femur acquisition:

1. Acetabular version:

a. Cranial (1–3 o'clock position).

b. Central.

c. Caudal.

2. Femoral version.

D. 3D reconstructions commonplace at most facilities:

1. Various proprietary and public hardware and software programs exist to independently manipulate femur and acetabulum/pelvis to evaluate FAI (**Fig. 16.6**).

2. Permits 3D printing of femur, pelvis to manipulate hip joint for illustration of motion, impingement.

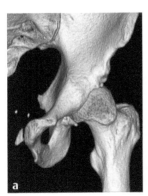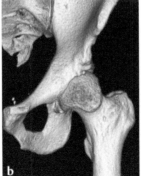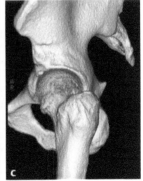

Fig. 16.6 (a–c) Computed tomography three-dimensional reconstructions of left hip with complex anterior osseous deformity, osteochondroma, creating a cam effect impingement.

Table 16.1 Differential diagnosis of patients with intra-articular hip pain and possible FAI syndrome

Intra-articular	Extra-articular
• FAI syndrome	• Peritrochanteric pain syndrome
• Labral tear	• Trochanteric bursitis
• Dysplasia	• Gluteal tendinopathy
• Osteoarthritis	• Deep gluteal space syndrome
• Hip instability, microinstability	• Ischiofemoral impingement
• Iliopsoas impingement	• Proximal hamstring syndrome
• AIIS subspine impingement	• Trochanteric-pelvic impingement
• Inflammatory arthritis	• Athletic pubalgia
• Avascular necrosis	• Muscle strain
• Pigmented villonodular synovitis	• Nerve or vessel injury
• Synovial chondromatosis	• Lumbosacral spine pathology
• Fracture, stress fracture	• Sacroiliac joint pathology
	• Nonmusculoskeletal (obstetric, gynecologic, gastrointestinal, genitourinary)

Abbreviations: AIIS, anteroinferior iliac spine; FAI, femoroacetabular impingement.

Differential Diagnosis

Imaging-guided (ultrasound, fluoroscopy), intra-articular diagnostic (and therapeutic) injection beneficial in establishing presence or absence of joint (FAI syndrome, labrum) as source of symptoms (**Table 16.1**).

Treatment

I.   Nonoperative:

   A. Education, rest, activity modification, and avoidance of provocative maneuvers.

   B. Physical therapy:

      1. Improves hip strength, motion, stability, neuromuscular control, and movement patterns.

      2. Very little evidence on success of physical therapy, as it does not alter hip morphology or heal labral injury.[35]

      3. Only one evidence-based nonsurgical physical therapy program currently exists; contains four core components.[35]

      4. Core 1: patient assessment—formalizes individualization, personalization, and customization of therapy program.

      5. Core 2: patient education and advice—identify, receive advice on, and avoid provocative (deep flexion, rotation) activities (behavior modification) and encourage posterior PT.

      6. Core 3: help with pain relief—oral nonsteroidal anti-inflammatory medications for 2 to 4 weeks; commencement and commitment to an exercise program.

7. Core 4: exercise-based hip program—begins with muscle control and stability (pelvis, hip, abdominals, and gluteals) and progresses to strengthening and stretching:

   a. Primary muscles: gluteus maximus, abdominals, abductors, and short external rotators.

8. Key avoidance: vigorous stretching (no painful hard end stretches).

9. Requires minimum of 12 weeks (minimum of six visits with therapist).

C. Medical (oral anti-inflammatory; intra-articular anti-inflammatory).

D. Education, observation.

II. Operative:

A. Surgical goal: perfect correction of FAI morphology, labral preservation:

   1. Labral repair significantly better outcomes than debridement:

      a. No significant difference in looped versus pierced labral base refixation technique.[36,37]

   2. Cam correction: improve femoral head–neck offset, improve α angle (<45 degrees) on all views (**Fig. 16.7a**).

   3. Pincer correction: convert offending retroverted acetabulum to anteverted—use lateral center edge angle, anterior center edge angle, and femoral head extrusion index (**Fig. 16.7b**):

      a. Change in lateral center edge angle = 1.8 + (0.64 × rim reduction in millimeters).[38]

      b. One-millimeter resection = 2.4-degree lateral center edge reduction.

      c. Five-millimeter resection = 5.0-degree lateral center edge reduction.

B. Open: includes surgical hip dislocation, mini-open anterior approach.

C. Arthroscopic:

   1. General anesthesia; complete muscle relaxation permits easier distraction and fewer traction-related complications (perineum, nerve).

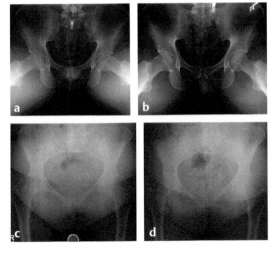

Fig. 16.7 Dunn 45-degree (**a**) preoperative and (**b**) 6 weeks postoperative lateral radiographs illustrating left hip cam correction using hip arthroscopy, labral repair. Radiographically, significant reduction in α angle, increased head–neck offset, and resection of head–neck junction sclerosis are observed. (**c, d**) Standing anteroposterior preoperative and 6 weeks postoperative radiographs illustrating far lateral and posterior pincer correction using hip arthroscopy, labral repair. Radiographically, significant reduction in lateral center-edge angle and posterior/lateral coverage are observed.

2. Multiple available portals: most techniques utilize:
    a. Anterolateral (**Fig. 16.8a**).
    b. Modified mid-anterior.
    c. Accessory portal(s): distal anterolateral.
    d. Posterolateral.

3. Seventy-degree arthroscope more commonly used than 30-degree arthroscope.

4. Central compartment—in traction—requires variable degree of interportal capsulotomy:
    a. Acetabular rim treatment: rim resection.
    b. AIIS decompression.
    c. Labral treatment (**Fig. 16.8b–d**): repair, debride, reconstruction.
    d. Articular cartilage management: debridement and marrow stimulation (microfracture, drilling).
    e. Ligamentum teres (debridement, reconstruction).
    f. Iliopsoas (tenotomy).

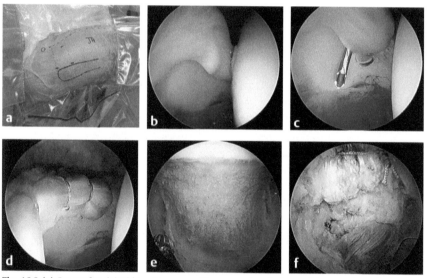

Fig. 16.8 (a) Set-up for right hip arthroscopy. Three-portal technique with anterolateral, modified mid-anterior, and distal anterolateral accessory portal. (**b**) Right hip arthroscopy, anterolateral viewing portal, instrumenting via modified mid-anterior portal. Labral tear is visualized in a 16-year-old adolescent girl with cam femoroacetabular impingement. (**c**) Right hip arthroscopy, anterolateral viewing portal, passing suture around labrum at chondrolabral junction via modified mid-anterior portal (same patient as in Fig. 16.8b). (**d**) Right hip arthroscopy, anterolateral viewing portal, completed labral repair with five suture anchors and looped technique (same patient as in Fig. 16.8b). (**e**) Right hip arthroscopy, modified mid-anterior viewing portal, comprehensive cam correction from 12:00 to 6:00, visualized via "T" capsulotomy. (**f**) Right hip arthroscopy, anterolateral viewing portal, completed capsular closure with three sutures in the "T" capsulotomy and three additional sutures in the interportal capsulotomy.

5. Peripheral compartment—no traction—can be visualized with either an interportal or "T" capsulotomy:

a. Comprehensive cam correction (**Fig. 16.8e**).

b. Dynamic arthroscopic and/or fluoroscopic examination to confirm head–neck offset correction, retention of labral suction seal.

c. With lateral and posterolateral cam resection, avoid lateral ascending vessel iatrogenic injury (lateral synovial fold).

6. Capsular closure: repair/plication is controversial:

a. Growing evidence demonstrates better outcomes with repair[39,40] (**Fig. 16.8f**).

b. If the capsulotomy is left open, the hip is susceptible to instability (microinstability to dislocation).[41-44]

Outcomes

I. Generally excellent short- and mid-term improvements in multiple patient-reported outcome measures[45]:

A. Utilized and recommended outcome scores:

1. iHOT-12 (International Hip Outcome Tool), iHOT-33.

2. HAGOS (The Copenhagen Hip and Groin Outcome Score).

3. HOOS (Hip Dysfunction and Osteoarthritis Outcome Score).

4. HOS (Hip Outcome Score), ADL (Activities of Daily Living), and SSS (Sport-Specific subscale).

5. mHHS (Modified Harris Hip Score).

6. General health (SF-12 [12-item Short-Form Survey], SF-36, Patient-Reported Outcomes Measurement Information System (PROMIS); EQ-5D = EuroQol 5 Dimensions

7. Activity (UCLA [University of California, Los Angeles], Marx, Tegner).

II. No long-term investigations yet define natural history of FAI syndrome and progression to osteoarthrosis and the role treatment may have on altering that progression:

A. Without treatment (surgical or nonsurgical).

B. With treatment (surgical or nonsurgical).

III. Most common reason for failure of FAI surgery: incomplete correction of FAI morphology, leaving residual FAI.

IV. Complication rate[46,47]:

A. Major: 0.45 to 0.58%.

B. Minor: 7.5 to 7.9%.

C. Reoperation: 6.3%.

D. Conversion to total hip arthroplasty: 2.9%.

V. Although most early FAI literature was retrospective, small case series without comparator groups, now there are several ongoing prospective, well-designed, high-quality randomized and nonrandomized international investigations:

A. Feasibility of Arthroscopic Surgery for Hip Impingement compared with Non-operative Care (FASHIoN) (UK): arthroscopic treatment of FAI/labrum versus nonsurgical treatment (physical therapy).

B. FASHIoN (Australia): arthroscopic treatment of FAI/labrum versus nonsurgical treatment (physical therapy).

C. Femoroacetabular Impingement Trial (FAIT) (UK): arthroscopic treatment of FAI/labrum versus nonsurgical treatment (physical therapy).

D. Femoroacetabular Impingement Randomized Controlled Trial (FIRST) (Canada and Finland): arthroscopic treatment of FAI/labrum versus washout sham.

E. HIPARTI (HIP ARThroscopy International) (Australia and Norway): arthroscopic treatment of FAI/labrum versus diagnostic arthroscopy.

F. U.S. MHS (US Military Health System) (United States): arthroscopic treatment of FAI/labrum versus nonsurgical treatment (physical therapy).

References

1. Ganz R, Parvizi J, Beck M, Leunig M, Nötzli H, Siebenrock KA. Femoroacetabular impingement: a cause for osteoarthritis of the hip. Clin Orthop Relat Res 2003;(417):112–120
2. Sankar WN, Nevitt M, Parvizi J, Felson DT, Agricola R, Leunig M. Femoroacetabular impingement: defining the condition and its role in the pathophysiology of osteoarthritis. J Am Acad Orthop Surg 2013;21(Suppl 1):S7–S15
3. Griffin DR, Dickenson EJ, O'Donnell J, et al. The Warwick agreement on femoroacetabular impingement syndrome (FAI syndrome): an international consensus statement. Br J Sports Med 2016;50(19):1169–1176
4. Collins JA, Ward JP, Youm T. Is prophylactic surgery for femoroacetabular impingement indicated? A systematic review. Am J Sports Med 2014;42(12):3009–3015
5. Nardo L, Parimi N, Liu F, et al; Osteoporotic Fractures in Men (MrOS) Research Group. Femoroacetabular impingement: prevalent and often asymptomatic in older men—the osteoporotic fractures in men study. Clin Orthop Relat Res 2015;473(8):2578–2586
6. Frank JM, Harris JD, Erickson BJ, et al. Prevalence of femoroacetabular impingement imaging findings in asymptomatic volunteers: a systematic review. Arthroscopy 2015;31(6):1199–1204
7. Anderson LA, Anderson MB, Kapron A, et al. The 2015 Frank Stinchfield Award: radiographic abnormalities common in senior athletes with well-functioning hips but not associated with osteoarthritis. Clin Orthop Relat Res 2016;474(2):342–352
8. Dolan MM, Heyworth BE, Bedi A, Duke G, Kelly BT. CT reveals a high incidence of osseous abnormalities in hips with labral tears. Clin Orthop Relat Res 2011;469(3):831–838
9. Peelle MW, Della Rocca GJ, Maloney WJ, Curry MC, Clohisy JC. Acetabular and femoral radiographic abnormalities associated with labral tears. Clin Orthop Relat Res 2005;441(441):327–333
10. Guevara CJ, Pietrobon R, Carothers JT, Olson SA, Vail TP. Comprehensive morphologic evaluation of the hip in patients with symptomatic labral tear. Clin Orthop Relat Res 2006;453(453):277–285
11. Wenger DE, Kendell KR, Miner MR, Trousdale RT. Acetabular labral tears rarely occur in the absence of bony abnormalities. Clin Orthop Relat Res 2004;(426):145–150
12. Ganz R, Leunig M, Leunig-Ganz K, Harris WH. The etiology of osteoarthritis of the hip: an integrated mechanical concept. Clin Orthop Relat Res 2008;466(2):264–272
13. Agricola R, Heijboer MP, Bierma-Zeinstra SM, Verhaar JA, Weinans H, Waarsing JH. Cam impingement causes osteoarthritis of the hip: a nationwide prospective cohort study (CHECK). Ann Rheum Dis 2013;72(6):918–923

14. Nicholls AS, Kiran A, Pollard TC, et al. The association between hip morphology parameters and nineteen-year risk of end-stage osteoarthritis of the hip: a nested case-control study. Arthritis Rheum 2011;63(11):3392–3400

15. Saberi Hosnijeh F, Zuiderwijk ME, Versteeg M, et al. Cam deformity and acetabular dysplasia as risk factors for hip osteoarthritis. Arthritis Rheumatol 2017;69(1):86–93

16. Reichenbach S, Leunig M, Werlen S, et al. Association between cam-type deformities and magnetic resonance imaging-detected structural hip damage: a cross-sectional study in young men. Arthritis Rheum 2011;63(12):4023–4030

17. Doherty M, Courtney P, Doherty S, et al. Nonspherical femoral head shape (pistol grip deformity), neck shaft angle, and risk of hip osteoarthritis: a case-control study. Arthritis Rheum 2008;58(10):3172–3182

18. Gosvig KK, Jacobsen S, Sonne-Holm S, Palm H, Troelsen A. Prevalence of malformations of the hip joint and their relationship to sex, groin pain, and risk of osteoarthritis: a population-based survey. J Bone Joint Surg Am 2010;92(5):1162–1169

19. Chung CY, Park MS, Lee KM, et al. Hip osteoarthritis and risk factors in elderly Korean population. Osteoarthritis Cartilage 2010;18(3):312–316

20. Menschik F. The hip joint as a conchoid shape. J Biomech 1997;30(9):971–973

21. Kelly BT, Williams RJ III, Philippon MJ. Hip arthroscopy: current indications, treatment options, and management issues. Am J Sports Med 2003;31(6):1020–1037

22. Konrath GA, Hamel AJ, Olson SA, Bay B, Sharkey NA. The role of the acetabular labrum and the transverse acetabular ligament in load transmission in the hip. J Bone Joint Surg Am 1998;80(12):1781–1788

23. Bharam S. Labral tears, extra-articular injuries, and hip arthroscopy in the athlete. Clin Sports Med 2006;25(2):279–292, ix

24. Larson CM, Moreau-Gaudry A, Kelly BT, et al. Are normal hips being labeled as pathologic? A CT-based method for defining normal acetabular coverage. Clin Orthop Relat Res 2015;473(4):1247–1254

25. Legaye J, Duval-Beaupère G, Hecquet J, Marty C. Pelvic incidence: a fundamental pelvic parameter for three-dimensional regulation of spinal sagittal curves. Eur Spine J 1998;7(2):99–103

26. Yoshimoto H, Sato S, Masuda T, et al. Spinopelvic alignment in patients with osteoarthrosis of the hip: a radiographic comparison to patients with low back pain. Spine 2005;30(14):1650–1657

27. Gebhart JJ, Streit JJ, Bedi A, Bush-Joseph CA, Nho SJ, Salata MJ. Correlation of pelvic incidence with cam and pincer lesions. Am J Sports Med 2014;42(11):2649–2653

28. Hellman MD, Haughom BD, Brown NM, Fillingham YA, Philippon MJ, Nho SJ. Femoroacetabular impingement and pelvic incidence: radiographic comparison to an asymptomatic control. Arthroscopy 2017;33(3):545–550

29. Protopsaltis T, Schwab F, Bronsard N, et al; International Spine Study Group. TheT1 pelvic angle, a novel radiographic measure of global sagittal deformity, accounts for both spinal inclination and pelvic tilt and correlates with health-related quality of life. J Bone Joint Surg Am 2014;96(19):1631–1640

30. Kahlenberg CA, Han B, Patel RM, Deshmane PP, Terry MA. Time and cost of diagnosis for symptomatic femoroacetabular impingement. Orthop J Sports Med 2014;2(3):2325967114523916

31. Nawabi DH, Bedi A, Tibor LM, Magennis E, Kelly BT. The demographic characteristics of high-level and recreational athletes undergoing hip arthroscopy for femoroacetabular impingement: a sports-specific analysis. Arthroscopy 2014;30(3):398–405

32. Weir A, Brukner P, Delahunt E, et al. Doha agreement meeting on terminology and definitions in groin pain in athletes. Br J Sports Med 2015;49(12):768–774

33. Nötzli HP, Wyss TF, Stoecklin CH, Schmid MR, Treiber K, Hodler J. The contour of the femoral head-neck junction as a predictor for the risk of anterior impingement. J Bone Joint Surg Br 2002;84(4):556–560

34. Rego PR, Mascarenhas V, Oliveira FS, et al. Morphologic and angular planning for cam resection in femoro-acetabular impingement: value of the omega angle. Int Orthop 2016;40(10):2011–2017
35. Wall PD, Dickenson EJ, Robinson D, et al. Personalised Hip Therapy: development of a non-operative protocol to treat femoroacetabular impingement syndrome in the FASHIoN randomised controlled trial. Br J Sports Med 2016;50(19):1217–1223
36. Sawyer GA, Briggs KK, Dornan GJ, Ommen ND, Philippon MJ. Clinical outcomes after arthroscopic hip labral repair using looped versus pierced suture techniques. Am J Sports Med 2015;43(7):1683–1688
37. Jackson TJ, Hammarstedt JE, Vemula SP, Domb BG. Acetabular labral base repair versus circumferential suture repair: a matched-paired comparison of clinical outcomes. Arthroscopy 2015;31(9):1716–1721
38. Philippon MJ, Wolff AB, Briggs KK, Zehms CT, Kuppersmith DA. Acetabular rim reduction for the treatment of femoroacetabular impingement correlates with preoperative and postoperative center-edge angle. Arthroscopy 2010;26(6):757–761
39. Frank RM, Lee S, Bush-Joseph CA, Kelly BT, Salata MJ, Nho SJ. Improved outcomes after hip arthroscopic surgery in patients undergoing T-capsulotomy with complete repair versus partial repair for femoroacetabular impingement: a comparative matched-pair analysis. Am J Sports Med 2014;42(11):2634–2642
40. Weber AE, Kuhns BD, Cvetanovich GL, et al. Does the hip capsule remain closed after hip arthroscopy with routine capsular closure for femoroacetabular impingement? A magnetic resonance imaging analysis in symptomatic postoperative patients. Arthroscopy 2017;33(1):108–115
41. Bayne CO, Stanley R, Simon P, et al. Effect of capsulotomy on hip stability–a consideration during hip arthroscopy. Am J Orthop 2014;43(4):160–165
42. Abrams GD, Hart MA, Takami K, et al. Biomechanical evaluation of capsulotomy, capsulectomy, and capsular repair on hip rotation. Arthroscopy 2015;31(8):1511–1517
43. Harris JD, Gerrie BJ, Lintner DM, Varner KE, McCulloch PC. Microinstability of the hip and the splits radiograph. Orthopedics 2016;39(1):e169–e175
44. Duplantier NL, McCulloch PC, Nho SJ, Mather RC III, Lewis BD, Harris JD. Hip dislocation or subluxation after hip arthroscopy: a systematic review. Arthroscopy 2016;32(7):1428–1434
45. Nwachukwu BU, Rebolledo BJ, McCormick F, Rosas S, Harris JD, Kelly BT. Arthroscopic versus open treatment of femoroacetabular impingement: a systematic review of medium- to long-term outcomes. Am J Sports Med 2016;44(4):1062–1068
46. Harris JD, McCormick FM, Abrams GD, et al. Complications and reoperations during and after hip arthroscopy: a systematic review of 92 studies and more than 6,000 patients. Arthroscopy 2013;29(3):589–595
47. Weber AE, Harris JD, Nho SJ. Complications in hip arthroscopy: a systematic review and strategies for prevention. Sports Med Arthrosc Rev 2015;23(4):187–193

17 Extra-Articular Impingement

Joshua D. Harris

Introduction

I. Femoroacetabular impingement (FAI) syndrome has been defined, via the Warwick Agreement International Consensus statement, as a motion-related clinical disorder of the hip with a triad of[1]:

   A. Symptoms.

   B. Clinical signs.

   C. Imaging findings.

II. FAI syndrome represents symptomatic premature contact between the proximal femur and the acetabulum.

III. Similarly, extra-articular impingement refers to other osseous or soft-tissue sources of abnormal contact, with symptoms, clinical signs, and imaging findings consistent with the two impinging structures around the hip.

IV. Several different sources of extra-articular impingement have been described:

   A. Subspine (anteroinferior iliac spine [AIIS]) impingement.

   B. Ischiofemoral impingement.

   C. Iliopsoas impingement.

   D. Trochanteric–pelvic impingement.

Anatomic Considerations

I. Subspine impingement:

   A. Contact between AIIS and distal anterior femoral neck (or anterior edge of the greater trochanter).

   B. AIIS is origin for direct head of rectus femoris and iliocapsularis[2]:

      1. Composed of two facets, divided by horizontal AIIS ridge (**Fig. 17.1**)[3]:

         a. Superior: occupied entirely by direct head rectus femoris (teardrop-shaped attachment, tapered proximally).

         b. Inferior: occupied by iliocapsularis origin (iliocapsularis lies immediately superficial, and adherent, to anteromedial iliofemoral ligament).[4]

II. Ischiofemoral impingement:

   A. Contact between the lesser trochanter and the ischium[5] in the ischiofemoral interval (narrowest distance between the apex of the medial cortex of the lesser trochanter and the lateral cortex of the ischial tuberosity)[6]:

      1. Lesser trochanter is insertion of the iliopsoas tendon (**Fig. 17.2**).

      2. Ischium is origin of the hamstring (superolateral semimembranosus and central–inferomedial conjoint tendon semitendinosus and biceps femoris long head).

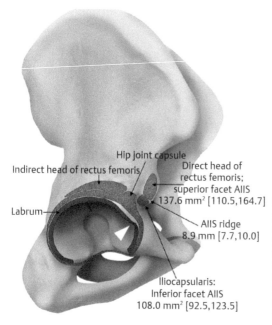

Hip joint capsule
Indirect head of rectus femoris
Direct head of rectus femoris; superior facet AIIS
137.6 mm² [110.5,164.7]
Labrum
AIIS ridge
8.9 mm [7.7,10.0]
Iliocapsularis: Inferior facet AIIS
108.0 mm² [92.5,123.5]

Fig. 17.1 Right hip illustrating AIIS morphology, with superior facet occupied by direct head rectus femoris, separated from the inferior facet, occupied by iliocapsularis, by the AIIS ridge. *White arrowhead* represents 3:00 o'clock position, indicated by the most superior aspect of the psoas "U." (Reproduced with permission of Wolters Kluwer Health, Inc.)

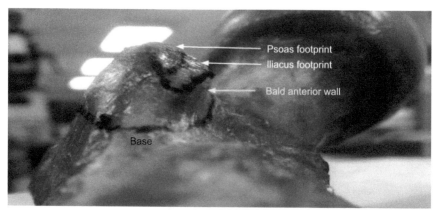

Psoas footprint
Iliacus footprint
Bald anterior wall
Base

Fig. 17.2 Left hip, view from distal, posterior. The bald anterior wall can be observed clearly on this dissection as well as its relationship with the tendinous footprint and lesser trochanteric height. The mean ratio between the bald anterior wall and the lesser trochanteric height is ~38%. (Reproduced with permission of Oxford University Press.)

3. Up to 84% of cadaveric specimens may demonstrate ischiofemoral impingement in 10-degree extension, 10-degree adduction, and 29-degree external rotation.[5]

B. Leads to compression of the quadratus femoris and the sciatic nerve (**Fig. 17.3**).

C. May also occur between the posterior edge of the greater trochanter and the lateral ischium in extreme hip external rotation.[7]

D. Deep gluteal space borders[8]:

1. Posterior: gluteus maximus.

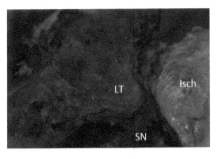

Fig. 17.3 Posteroinferior view of left hip. Entrapment of the sciatic nerve (SN) between the ischium (Isch) and the lesser trochanter (LT) in the ischiofemoral impingement test position—10-degree extension, then 10-degrees adduction, and then maximal external rotation. (Reproduced with permission of Springer.)

2. Anterior: posterior column of the acetabulum, posterior hip capsule, proximal posterior femur.

3. Lateral: linea aspera and gluteal tuberosity.

4. Medial: sacrotuberous ligament, falciform fascia.

5. Superior: inferior margin of the sciatic notch.

6. Inferior: proximal origin of the hamstring at ischial tuberosity.

7. Contains sciatic nerve, piriformis, blood vessel containing fibrous bands, gluteal muscles, hamstring tendons, gemelli–obturator internus complex:

   a. Sciatic nerve excursion 28 mm during hip flexion.[9]

III. Iliopsoas impingement:

A. Contact between iliopsoas and anterior hip (3 o'clock position on acetabular clockface with 3 o'clock denoting the superior margin of the psoas-u) with compression on the labrum.[3,10]

B. Iliopsoas tendon is a confluence of the psoas and iliacus muscles:

   1. Psoas major muscle originates from transverse processes and bodies of T12–L5 and their intervertebral disks.

   2. Iliacus muscle originates from the iliac fossa, overlying the anterior sacroiliac joint, and the lateral sacrum.

   3. Iliopsoas is composed of 40% tendon and 60% muscle at the level of the labrum.[11,12]

C. Iliopsoas tendon may be multibanded (single tendon, bifid, trifid)[13]:

   1. Single banded: 28.3%.

   2. Double banded: 64.2%.

   3. Triple banded: 7.5%.

D. Iliopsoas tendon is an anterior stabilizer from 0 to 15 degrees of hip flexion[14]:

   1. As the iliopsoas crosses the superior pubic ramus (at an angle of 35–45 degrees), the relative anterior position increases its leverage for hip flexion (**Fig. 17.4**):

      a. As the hip flexes, the iliopsoas loses contact with the femoral head at approximately 14 degrees (7–19 degrees) and loses contact with the iliopectineal eminence at 54 degrees (42–67 degrees).[14]

      b. Increased lesser trochanteric retroversion (further posterior relative position of the lesser trochanter) observed in patients with symptomatic iliopsoas impingement.[15]

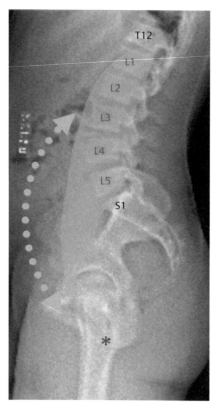

Fig. 17.4 Lateral plain radiograph of the spinopelvic association with the psoas major (*blue*) illustrated. Iliopsoas contraction (or contracture) leads to anterior pelvic tilt as the pelvis rotates anteriorly (*dotted line*) over an axis of rotation between the femoral heads.

E. Iliopsoas contraction (or contracture) causes anterior pelvic tilt.

F. Psoas tunnel is the groove in which the iliopsoas tendon passes, medial to the AIIS and iliopectineal eminence[16]:

1. For suture anchor placement during labral repair between 2 and 4 o'clock positions, there is concern for perforation through the anteromedial cortex of the acetabular dome: the psoas tunnel.[16,17]

IV. Trochanteric–pelvic impingement:

A. Contact between the greater trochanter and ilium with the hip abducted and extended:

1. Repetitive impingement will cause both compressive and tensile injuries to the abductor (gluteus medius, minimus) insertion.

2. Repetitive impingement will cause a levering effect with greater femoral head translation (vs. rotation).

B. Abductor (gluteus medius and minimus) tension is decreased.

History and Examination

I. Subspine impingement:

A. Four diagnostic criteria[18]:

1. Anterior hip pain aggravated by hip flexion, kicking, and sprinting.

2. Positive subspine impingement test (straight sagittal plane flexion, with limited terminal hip flexion motion)[19] and tender AIIS:

    a. Greater degrees of flexion loss with increasing AIIS type[19]:

        i. Type I: 120 ± 12 degrees.

        ii. Type II: 107 ± 10 degrees.

        iii. Type III: 93 ± 20 degrees.

    b. Greater degrees of internal rotation loss at 90 degrees of hip flexion with increasing AIIS type[19]:

        i. Type I: 21 ± 10 degrees.

        ii. Type II: 11 ± 9 degrees.

        iii. Type III: 8 ± 9 degrees.

3. Negative response to intra-articular injection.

4. Prominent AIIS (type II or III) on radiographs and/or CT.

B. Frequently observed in one of five possible clinical scenarios:

1. Old rectus femoris avulsion/AIIS avulsion as adolescent.[18,20,21]

2. Hypermobile dancers.[20,22–24]

3. Acetabular retroversion.[20,25]

4. Post-periacetabular osteotomy (post-PAO) overcorrection.

5. Valgus neck, anteverted femur.[26]

II. Ischiofemoral impingement:

A. Patients typically complain of chronic, insidious onset, atraumatic, deep posterior buttock pain (100%), especially with sitting (88%), with radiation distally, with or without sciatica[27]:

1. Shortened stride during gait is frequently observed (avoidance of hip extension).

2. If Trendelenburg gait with abductor weakness, there is relative limb adduction in extension, exacerbating pain due to lesser trochanter impingement on the lateral ischium.

3. Patients may have a variety of relevant past orthopaedic history issues:

    a. Ischial tuberosity avulsion.

    b. Medialized total hip replacement (or low offset).

    c. Previous peritrochanteric hip fracture.

    d. Prior valgus proximal femoral osteotomy.

    e. Legg–Calvé–Perthes disease.

4. Patients tend to be older than cam and pincer FAI syndrome patients (~47 years of age), greater female distribution (~82%), with a long duration of symptoms (~30 months).[27]

B. Physical examination should assess for tenderness of the ischiofemoral space and the presence/absence of Tinel's sign of the sciatic nerve:

1. Ischiofemoral impingement test involves hip extension, adduction, and maximal external rotation: reproduction of the symptoms accounting for the chief complaint of pain's location is a positive test.

2. Long-stride walking test: pain reproduction and forced stride shortening due to pain when attempting to take long strides.

3. The active piriformis (sensitivity 0.78; specificity 0.80; positive likelihood ratio 3.9; diagnostic odds ratio 14.4) and seated piriformis stretch test (sensitivity 0.52; specificity 0.90; positive likelihood ratio 5.22; diagnostic odds ratio 9.8) combined (sensitivity 0.91; specificity 0.80; positive likelihood ratio 4.57; diagnostic odds ratio 42.0) are the optimal tests to identify sciatic nerve entrapment in deep gluteal space.[28]

C. Diagnostic injection (ultrasound or CT guided) into ischiofemoral space with local anesthetic with or without steroid is useful adjunct in accurate diagnosis of ischiofemoral impingement.[29]

III. Iliopsoas impingement:

A. Patients typically complain of deep anterior hip or groin pain (with a "C" sign or "between the fingers" sign), with focal iliopsoas tenderness (body habitus permitting), sitting pain, and infrequently with internal snapping:

1. Audible "pop" is usually iliopsoas.

2. Visible lateral "pop" (patient will report "my hip is dislocating") is usually iliotibial band.

B. Patients tend to be athletic, younger, greater female distribution.

C. Physical examination reveals a similar examination to that of FAI syndrome with positive anterior impingement maneuver:

1. Positive Stinchfield, positive hip extension pain, positive Ludloff, positive iliopsoas test,[30] positive FABER (flexion, abduction, and external rotation).

IV. Trochanteric–pelvic impingement:

A. Patients typically are bimodally distributed:

1. Young hypermobile female patients who frequently perform high-flexibility sports (ballet, gymnastics, rhythmic gymnastics, figure skating, yoga, cheerleading).[31,32]

2. Older female patients with chronic lateral peritrochanteric pain.

B. Pain is located deep anterior, lateral, and posterior with provocative activities, including excessive abduction (in variable degrees of rotation determining the location of impingement).

C. A limp (with Trendelenburg gait and/or sign) is frequently present.

D. Physical examination should scrutinize range of motion, especially the amount of abduction (in several different degrees of internal/external rotation), and abductor muscle strength (manual muscle testing, hand-held dynamometry)[33]:

1. Typically less abduction in internal rotation (vs. external).[32]

2. Pain within 30 seconds of single leg stance is highly specific (100%, positive likelihood ratio ~12) of gluteal tendinopathy.[34]

3. No pain on palpation of greater trochanter highly sensitively (80%) rules out gluteal tendinopathy.[34]

E. Beighton score should be assessed for joint hypermobility syndrome, as it has been shown to significantly influence hip motion.[35]

Diagnostic Imaging

I. Subspine impingement:

    A. Plain radiographs:

        1. False profile is useful for evaluation of AIIS morphology.

        2. Anteroposterior (AP) pelvis may illustrate prominent AIIS (crossover sign):

            a. Caution: only 50% of subjects with a positive crossover sign actually have a retroverted acetabulum on CT (the other 50% have a type II or III AIIS).[25]

    B. CT scan is optimal imaging modality for visualization of AIIS morphology.

    C. Three types of AIIS morphology[19]:

        1. Type I: smooth section of the ilium (without bony prominences) between the most caudal aspect of the AIIS and the most cranial aspect of the acetabular rim.

        2. Type II: AIIS sits at the level of the acetabular rim, appearing as "rooflike" prominence over the anterior hip (at the level of the sourcil on the AP radiograph).

        3. Type III: AIIS extends distally to the anterosuperior rim (extends distal to the sourcil on the AP radiograph; **Fig. 17.5**).

II. Ischiofemoral impingement:

    A. Definitions (Torriani's classification[36,37]; **Fig. 17.6**):

        1. Ischiofemoral space: smallest distance between the lateral cortex of the ischial tuberosity and the medial cortex of the lesser trochanter:

            a. Greater than 17 mm is normal.

        2. Quadratus femoris space: smallest space for passage of the quadratus femoris muscle defined by the superolateral surface of the hamstring tendons and the posteromedial surface of the iliopsoas tendon or the lesser trochanter:

            a. Greater than 8 mm is normal.

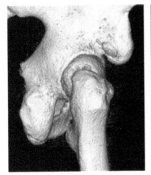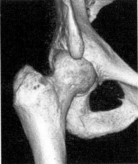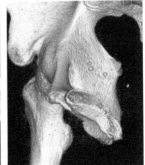

Fig. 17.5 Three-dimensional CT scans of right hip of a 40-year-old man with type III AIIS, extending below the level of the anterosuperior acetabular rim. *Left* is a lateral to medial view, center is an anterior to posterior view, and *right* is a medial to lateral view.

B. FNVLTV (femoral neck version lesser trochanteric version) angle is a measure of the angle between the femoral neck version and the lesser trochanter (**Fig. 17.7**):

1. FNVLTV angle is significantly increased in patients with symptomatic ischiofemoral impingement.

2. Femoral neck version is significantly increased in patients with symptomatic ischiofemoral impingement.

C. Statics measurements from axial MRI significantly overestimate ischiofemoral space (distance) in comparison to dynamic measurements from dual fluoroscopy during walking, hip adduction, extension, and external rotation.[38]

D. Static measurements:

1. Plain radiographs: AP pelvis may illustrate a narrowed ischiofemoral space, decreased femoral offset, coxa valga (neck–shaft angle >135 degrees[39]):

   a. Important to rule out other more common diagnoses (e.g., osteoarthritis, FAI syndrome, hamstring tendon pathology).

2. CT: best bony evaluation for ischiofemoral space.

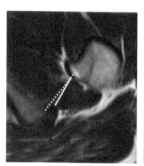 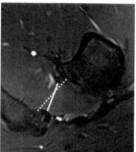 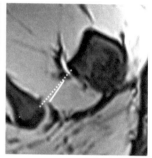

Fig. 17.6 Axial MRI zoomed in on the left hip of a 40-year-old man with posterior hip pain with T1-weighted (*left*), T2-weighted (*middle*), and volumetric interpolated breath-hold sequence examination (VIBE; *right*) sequences demarcating ischiofemoral space measurements (*dotted lines*) and quadratus femoris space measurements (*solid lines*).

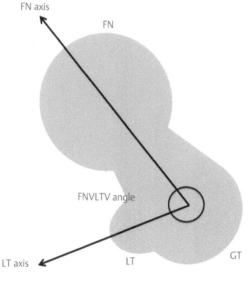

Fig. 17.7 The angle between the femoral neck version and the lesser trochanter (FNVLTV angle) was calculated through the following formula: FNVLTV angle = FNV + LTV. (FN, femoral neck; FNV, femoral neck version; GT, greater trochanter; LT, lesser trochanter; LTV, lesser trochanteric version.) (Reproduced with permission of Elsevier.)

3. MRI:
   a. Quadratus femoris edema (Torriani's classification)[36]:
      i. Grade 1: mild.
      ii. Grade 2: moderate.
      iii. Grade 3: severe.
4. No significant difference in ischiofemoral space dimensions exist using static ultrasound versus MRI in healthy volunteers.[40]

E. Dynamic measurements:
   1. Dual fluoroscopy[38]:
      a. Ischiofemoral space decreases during hip external rotation (minimum), adduction, and extension.
   2. Ultrasound:
      a. Ischiofemoral space increases maximally in abduction and internal rotation (mean 5.2 cm) and decreases maximally in adduction and external rotation (3.1 cm) in healthy volunteers.[6]
   3. Full range-of-motion (FROM) MRI:
      a. In zero degrees of hip flexion, external rotation up to 60 degrees may yield greater trochanteric impingement on the lateral ischium, with compression of the quadratus femoris between—distinguish from lesser trochanter versus ischium ischiofemoral impingement and greater trochanteric tip versus pelvis trochanteric-pelvic impingement.

F. Patients with symptomatic ischiofemoral impingement demonstrate significantly smaller ischiofemoral space and quadratus femoris space in comparison to controls (14.9 vs. 26.0 mm and 9.6 vs. 16.0 mm, respectively).[41]

III. Iliopsoas impingement:
   A. MRI (with arthrography) should be scrutinized for[42]:
      1. Increased signal intensity between iliopsoas and capsule at the 3 o'clock position,
      2. Edema within the iliopsoas tendon or adjacent capsule.
      3. Labral tear at the 3 o'clock position.
      4. Irregularity of the deep margin of the iliopsoas tendon.
      5. Dimensions of iliopsoas tendon.
      6. Location of iliopsoas tendon as it passes over the labrum.

IV. Trochanteric–pelvic impingement:
   A. Plain radiographs should be scrutinized for:
      1. Neck–shaft angle (coxa vara defined as angle <120 degrees or trochanteric tip >7 mm above the head center[39]).
      2. Femoral offset (distance from the center of the femoral head rotation to a line bisecting the center of the long axis of the femur).
      3. Trochanteric height (also known as center–trochanteric distance) relative to the femoral head center).
      4. "Splits" radiograph may demonstrate impingement above the superior rim at approximately 12 o'clock position with the limb maximally internally

rotated, while permissive external rotation may demonstrate impingement behind the posterior rim at approximately 9 o'clock position (**Fig. 17.8**)[32]:

   a. This may cause a levering of the femoral head out of the acetabulum (translation) with loss of the suction seal and a vacuum sign in approximately 36% of patients.[31]

Differential Diagnosis

I. Selective diagnostic injections are useful in differentiating both the source and magnitude of pain around the hip (**Table 17.1**):

   A. Intra-articular:

      1. Ultrasound, fluoroscopic, or landmark guided.[43]

   B. Extra-articular:

      1. Trochanteric bursa.[44]

      2. Ischiofemoral space.[45]

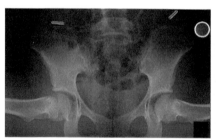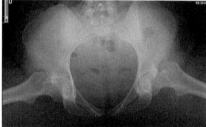

Fig. 17.8 Trochanteric–pelvic impingement observed in a 22-year-old woman ballet dancer with bilateral deep anterior and posterior groin pain. Splits radiograph with the limb permissively externally rotated (*left radiograph*) demonstrates bilateral vacuum signs with hip subluxation as a result of lateral and inferior femoral head translation due to trochanteric levering effect behind the posterior acetabular rim (trochanteric–pelvic impingement). Splits radiograph with the limb forcefully internally rotated (*right radiograph*) demonstrates trochanteric–pelvic impingement over the superior acetabular rim. (Reproduced with permission of SLACK Inc.)

Treatment

I. Nonoperative:

   A. Education, observation, rest, activity modification, and avoidance of provocative maneuvers:

      1. AIIS subspine impingement: avoidance of deep straight hip flexion.

      2. Iliopsoas impingement: avoidance of frequent active hip flexion.

      3. Ischiofemoral impingement: avoidance of extension, adduction, and external rotation.

      4. Trochanteric–pelvic impingement: avoidance of excessive abduction and avoidance of limp with walking and standing.

Table 17.1 Differential diagnosis of patients with hip pain and extra-articular impingement

Intra-articular	Extra-articular
• FAI syndrome, labral tear	• AIIS subspine impingement
• Cam and/or pincer morphology	• Ischiofemoral impingement
• Osteoarthrosis	• Iliopsoas impingement
• Chondral defect	• Trochanteric–pelvic impingement
• Dysplasia	• Peritrochanteric pain syndrome
• Femoral head avascular necrosis	• Trochanteric bursitis
• Hip instability, microinstability	• Gluteal tendinopathy
• Inflammatory arthritis	• Snapping iliotibial band (external coxa saltans)
• Pigmented villonodular synovitis	• Proximal hamstring tendinopathy
• Synovial chondromatosis	• Athletic pubalgia
• Fracture, stress fracture	• Muscle strain
	• Lumbosacral spine pathology
	• Sacroiliac joint pathology
	• Nonmusculoskeletal (neurovascular, obstetric, gynecologic, gastrointestinal, genitourinary)

Abbreviations: AIIS, anteroinferior iliac spine; FAI, femoroacetabular impingement.

    B. Physical therapy:

        1. Improves core, pelvis, hip strength, motion, stability, neuromuscular control, and movement patterns.

    C. Medical:

        1. Oral and injectable nonnarcotic medications.

II.   Operative:

    A. AIIS subspine impingement:

        1. Arthroscopic subspine decompression (**Fig. 17.9**):

            a. Pearls: preoperative imaging (plain radiograph, CT) to fully characterize the location and size of the subspine inferior facet.

            b. Pitfalls:

               i. Capsular management is critical, as larger and more proximal decompression necessarily violates the acetabular side of the interportal capsulotomy.

              ii. Avoidance of direct head rectus femoris release (superior facet of AIIS).

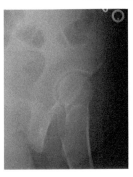 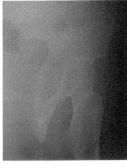

Fig. 17.9 Preoperative (*left*) and 6-week postoperative (*right*) false-profile radiographs of a 17-year-old adolescent ballerina with subspine impingement. At 1 year following surgery, she had returned to elite dance with complete symptom resolution.

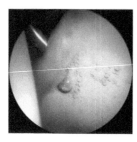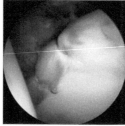

Fig. 17.10 Intraoperative images (viewing anterolateral portal, 70-degree arthroscope) of revision left hip arthroscopy in a 16-year-old female dancer with iliopsoas impingement, a 3 o'clock labral tear (*left*) and looped suture repair (*right*).

B. Iliopsoas impingement:

    1. Arthroscopic labral repair (3 o'clock position; **Fig. 17.10**) and treatment of iliopsoas:

        a. Pearls: thorough subspine assessment and decompression to reduce iliopsoas excursion angle.[46]

        b. Pitfalls: iliopsoas tenotomy has significant risk of hip flexor decrease in size (up to 25%), loss of strength (up to 20% with irreversible atrophy), and pain.[47]

C. Ischiofemoral impingement:

    1. Open or arthroscopic ischiofemoral decompression via lesser trochanter resection:

        a. Pearls: preoperative angiogram or 3D CT angiogram to define medial femoral circumflex artery course near the lesser trochanter.

        b. Pitfalls: iatrogenic sciatic nerve injury:

            i. Monopolar radiofrequency use for 2, 5, and 10 seconds of continuous activation at 10-, 5-, and 3-mm distance from the sciatic nerve is safe during endoscopy with maximum temperature of 28°C well below minimal reported temperature necessary to cause nerve changes (40–45°C).[48]

           ii. Normal nerve appearance upon endoscopic inspection demonstrates presence of blood flow and epineural fat (**Fig. 17.11**). Abnormal sciatic nerve appearance demonstrates a white shoestring appearance without epineural fat.

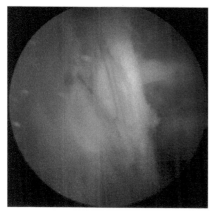

Fig. 17.11 Deep gluteal space endoscopic image of normal sciatic nerve with blood flow and epineural fat in a 48-year-old woman with deep gluteal space syndrome.

Table 17.2 Selected case series outcomes of endoscopic surgical treatment of extra-articular impingement

	Author(s)	Year	No. of patients (hips)	Mean age (y)	Gender: female (%)	Mean follow-up (y)	Outcomes
AIIS subspine	Nawabi et al[150]	2017	26 (34)	19.2 ± 4.1	46	3.0	• 34 soccer hips vs. 87 nonkicking hips • Soccer hips: 16% type I; 52% type II; 32% type III • Significant improvement mHHS, HOS-ADL, HOS-SSS, iHOT-33
	Hapa et al[20]	2013	150 (163)	27.8 (14–52)	50	0.9	• Significant improvement mHHS, SF-12, pain VAS • No rectus femoris avulsions; no hip flexion deficits
	Hetsroni et al[18]	2012	10 (10)	24.9 ± 9.6	0	1.2	• Hip flexion significantly improved from 99 ± 7 to 117 ± 8 degrees • mHHS significantly improved
	Amar et al[51]	2016	21 (21)	37.3 ± 3.6	38	0	• Preoperatively, patients had pain with SLR, FADIR, femoral stretch test • All had labral tear at level of AIIS (17/21 had "wave" sign at same spot)
Iliopsoas	Nelson and Keene al[52]	2014	30 (30)	35 (15–57)	80	2.0	• All had iliopsoas tenotomy (24/30 labral debridement; 3/30 labral repair) • 23/30 patients had significant improvements in mHHS (3 had recurrent snapping, 2 trochanteric bursitis, and 1 AVN, 1 OA)
	Cascio et al[53]	2013	22 (26)	19 (12–25)	95	Minimum 0.5	• 24/26 labral repair; 2/26 labral debridement • Significant improvements in HHS
	Domb et al[10]	2011	25 (25)	25.1 (15–37)	92	1.8	• All had iliopsoas tenotomy; 23/25 labral debridement; 2/25 labral repair • Significant improvements in HHS, HOS-ADL, HOS-SSS

(Continued)

Table 17.2 (*Continued*) Selected case series outcomes of endoscopic surgical treatment of extra-articular impingement

	Author(s)	Year	No. of patients (hips)	Mean age (y)	Gender: female (%)	Mean follow-up (y)	Outcomes
Ischiofemoral	Wilson and Keene[29]	2016	7 (7)	46 (15–66)	86	1.7	• Significant improvement in mHHS • No hip flexion weakness at 12-mo follow-up in any patient
	Hatem et al[54]	2015	5 (5)	33.9 (16–59)	60	2.3	• Significant improvements in mHHS, pain VAS; no hip flexion weakness • Mean return to sport at 4.4 mo post-op (60% at same level)
Trochanteric-pelvic	None						

Abbreviations: AIIS, anteroinferior iliac spine; AVN, avascular necrosis; FADIR, flexion, adduction, and internal rotation; HOS-ADL, Hip Outcome Score—Activities of Daily Living subscore; HOS-SSS, Hip Outcome Score—Sport-Specific Subscore; iHOT-33, International Hip Outcome Tool-33; mHHS, modified Harris Hip Score; OA, osteoarthritis ; SLR, straight leg raise; VAS, visual analog scale.

    D. Trochanteric–pelvic impingement:

       1. Open trochanteric osteotomy:

          a. Open lateral approach with greater trochanteric distalization ("relative neck lengthening").

          b. Goal is to place tip of trochanter level to the center of the femoral head.

Outcomes

I.   Evidence via a large systematic review suggests high rates of success with arthroscopic treatment of subspine and iliopsoas impingement (**Table 17.2**)[49]:

    A. Successful endoscopic management of ischiofemoral impingement.

    B. For both ischiofemoral and trochanteric–pelvic impingement, open surgical treatment has provided anecdotal patient symptom improvement without formal patient-reported outcome score utilization.

II.   No long-term investigations define natural history of extra-articular impingement and the role nonsurgical and surgical treatments may have on that natural history.

References

1. Griffin DR, Dickenson EJ, O'Donnell J, et al. The Warwick Agreement on femoroacetabular impingement syndrome (FAI syndrome): an international consensus statement. Br J Sports Med 2016;50(19):1169–1176

2. Ryan JM, Harris JD, Graham WC, Virk SS, Ellis TJ. Origin of the direct and reflected head of the rectus femoris: an anatomic study. Arthroscopy 2014;30(7):796–802

3. Philippon MJ, Michalski MP, Campbell KJ, et al. An anatomical study of the acetabulum with clinical applications to hip arthroscopy. J Bone Joint Surg Am 2014;96(20):1673–1682

4. Walters BL, Cooper JH, Rodriguez JA. New findings in hip capsular anatomy: dimensions of capsular thickness and pericapsular contributions. Arthroscopy 2014;30(10):1235–1245

5. Kivlan BR, Martin RL, Martin HD. Ischiofemoral impingement: defining the lesser trochanter-ischial space. Knee Surg Sports Traumatol Arthrosc 2017;25(1):72–76

6. Finnoff JT, Bond JR, Collins MS, et al. Variability of the ischiofemoral space relative to femur position: an ultrasound study. PM R 2015;7(9):930–937, quiz 87

7. Singer A, Clifford P, Tresley J, Jose J, Subhawong T. Ischiofemoral impingement and the utility of full-range-of-motion magnetic resonance imaging in its detection. Am J Orthop 2014;43(12):548–551

8. Martin HD, Reddy M, Gómez-Hoyos J. Deep gluteal syndrome. J Hip Preserv Surg 2015;2(2):99–107

9. Coppieters MW, Alshami AM, Babri AS, Souvlis T, Kippers V, Hodges PW. Strain and excursion of the sciatic, tibial, and plantar nerves during a modified straight leg raising test. J Orthop Res 2006;24(9):1883–1889

10. Domb BG, Shindle MK, McArthur B, Voos JE, Magennis EM, Kelly BT. Iliopsoas impingement: a newly identified cause of labral pathology in the hip. HSS J 2011;7(2):145–150

11. Blomberg JR, Zellner BS, Keene JS. Cross-sectional analysis of iliopsoas muscle-tendon units at the sites of arthroscopic tenotomies: an anatomic study. Am J Sports Med 2011;39(Suppl):58S–63S

12. Alpert JM, Kozanek M, Li G, Kelly BT, Asnis PD. Cross-sectional analysis of the iliopsoas tendon and its relationship to the acetabular labrum: an anatomic study. Am J Sports Med 2009;37(8):1594–1598

13. Philippon MJ, Devitt BM, Campbell KJ, et al. Anatomic variance of the iliopsoas tendon. Am J Sports Med 2014;42(4):807–811

14. Yoshio M, Murakami G, Sato T, Sato S, Noriyasu S. The function of the psoas major muscle: passive kinetics and morphological studies using donated cadavers. J Orthop Sci 2002;7(2):199–207

15. Gómez-Hoyos J, Schröder R, Reddy M, Palmer IJ, Khoury A, Martin HD. Is there a relationship between psoas impingement and increased trochanteric retroversion? J Hip Preserv Surg 2015;2(2):164–169

16. Degen RM, O'Sullivan E, Sink EL, Kelly BT. Psoas tunnel perforation-an unreported complication of hip arthroscopy. J Hip Preserv Surg 2015;2(3):272–279

17. Degen RM, Poultsides L, Mayer SW, et al. Safety of hip anchor insertion from the midanterior and distal anterolateral portals with a straight drill guide: a cadaveric study. Am J Sports Med 2017;45(3):627–635

18. Hetsroni I, Larson CM, Dela Torre K, Zbeda RM, Magennis E, Kelly BT. Anterior inferior iliac spine deformity as an extra-articular source for hip impingement: a series of 10 patients treated with arthroscopic decompression. Arthroscopy 2012;28(11):1644–1653

19. Hetsroni I, Poultsides L, Bedi A, Larson CM, Kelly BT. Anterior inferior iliac spine morphology correlates with hip range of motion: a classification system and dynamic model. Clin Orthop Relat Res 2013;471(8):2497–2503

20. Hapa O, Bedi A, Gursan O, et al. Anatomic footprint of the direct head of the rectus femoris origin: cadaveric study and clinical series of hips after arthroscopic anterior inferior iliac spine/subspine decompression. Arthroscopy 2013;29(12):1932–1940

21. Matsuda DK, Calipusan CP. Adolescent femoroacetabular impingement from malunion of the anteroinferior iliac spine apophysis treated with arthroscopic spinoplasty. Orthopedics 2012;35(3):e460–e463

22. Weber AE, Bedi A, Tibor LM, Zaltz I, Larson CM. The hyperflexible hip: managing hip pain in the dancer and gymnast. Sports Health 2015;7(4):346–358

23. Audenaert EA, Peeters I, Vigneron L, Baelde N, Pattyn C. Hip morphological characteristics and range of internal rotation in femoroacetabular impingement. Am J Sports Med 2012;40(6):1329–1336

24. Larson CM, Kelly BT, Stone RM. Making a case for anterior inferior iliac spine/subspine hip impingement: three representative case reports and proposed concept. Arthroscopy 2011;27(12):1732–1737

25. Zaltz I, Kelly BT, Hetsroni I, Bedi A. The crossover sign overestimates acetabular retroversion. Clin Orthop Relat Res 2013;471(8):2463–2470

26. Siebenrock KA, Steppacher SD, Haefeli PC, Schwab JM, Tannast M. Valgus hip with high antetorsion causes pain through posterior extraarticular FAI. Clin Orthop Relat Res 2013;471(12):3774–3780

27. Gómez-Hoyos J, Martin RL, Schröder R, Palmer IJ, Martin HD. Accuracy of 2 clinical tests for ischiofemoral impingement in patients with posterior hip pain and endoscopically confirmed diagnosis. Arthroscopy 2016;32(7):1279–1284

28. Martin HD, Kivlan BR, Palmer IJ, Martin RL. Diagnostic accuracy of clinical tests for sciatic nerve entrapment in the gluteal region. Knee Surg Sports Traumatol Arthrosc 2014;22(4):882–888

29. Wilson MD, Keene JS. Treatment of ischiofemoral impingement: results of diagnostic injections and arthroscopic resection of the lesser trochanter. J Hip Preserv Surg 2016;3(2):146–153

30. Laible C, Swanson D, Garofolo G, Rose DJ. Iliopsoas syndrome in dancers. Orthop J Sports Med 2013;1(3):2325967113500638

31. Mitchell RJ, Gerrie BJ, McCulloch PC, et al. Radiographic evidence of hip microinstability in elite ballet. Arthroscopy 2016;32(6):1038–1044.e1

32. Harris JD, Gerrie BJ, Lintner DM, Varner KE, McCulloch PC. Microinstability of the hip and the splits radiograph. Orthopedics 2016;39(1):e169–e175

33. Allison K, Vicenzino B, Wrigley TV, Grimaldi A, Hodges PW, Bennell KL. Hip abductor muscle weakness in individuals with gluteal tendinopathy. Med Sci Sports Exerc 2016;48(3):346–352

34. Grimaldi A, Mellor R, Nicolson P, Hodges P, Bennell K, Vicenzino B. Utility of clinical tests to diagnose MRI-confirmed gluteal tendinopathy in patients presenting with lateral hip pain. Br J Sports Med 2017;51(6):519–524

35. Naal FD, Hatzung G, Müller A, Impellizzeri F, Leunig M. Validation of a self-reported Beighton score to assess hypermobility in patients with femoroacetabular impingement. Int Orthop 2014;38(11):2245–2250

36. Torriani M, Souto SC, Thomas BJ, Ouellette H, Bredella MA. Ischiofemoral impingement syndrome: an entity with hip pain and abnormalities of the quadratus femoris muscle. AJR Am J Roentgenol 2009;193(1):186–190

37. Gómez-Hoyos J, Schröder R, Reddy M, Palmer IJ, Martin HD. Femoral neck anteversion and lesser trochanteric retroversion in patients with ischiofemoral impingement: a case-control magnetic resonance imaging study. Arthroscopy 2016;32(1):13–18

38. Atkins PR, Fiorentino NM, Aoki SK, Peters CL, Maak TG, Anderson AE. In vivo measurements of the ischiofemoral space in recreationally active participants during dynamic activities: a high-speed dual fluoroscopy study. Am J Sports Med 2017;45(12):2901–2910

39. Reikerås O, Høiseth A, Reigstad A, Fönstelien E. Femoral neck angles: a specimen study with special regard to bilateral differences. Acta Orthop Scand 1982;53(5):775–779

40. Finnoff JT, Johnson AC, Hollman JH. Can ultrasound accurately assess ischiofemoral space dimensions? A validation study. PM R 2017;9(4):392–397

41. Singer AD, Subhawong TK, Jose J, Tresley J, Clifford PD. Ischiofemoral impingement syndrome: a meta-analysis. Skeletal Radiol 2015;44(6):831–837

42. Blankenbaker DG, Tuite MJ, Keene JS, del Rio AM. Labral injuries due to iliopsoas impingement: can they be diagnosed on MR arthrography? AJR Am J Roentgenol 2012;199(4):894–900

43. Hoeber S, Aly AR, Ashworth N, Rajasekaran S. Ultrasound-guided hip joint injections are more accurate than landmark-guided injections: a systematic review and meta-analysis. Br J Sports Med 2016;50(7):392–396

44. Mu A, Peng P, Agur A. Landmark-guided and ultrasound-guided approaches for trochanteric bursa injection: a cadaveric study. Anesth Analg 2017;124(3):966–971

45. Volokhina Y, Dang D. Using proximal hamstring tendons as a landmark for ultrasound- and CT-guided injections of ischiofemoral impingement. Radiol Case Rep 2015;8(1):789

46. Smith KM, Gerrie BJ, McCulloch PC, et al. Arthroscopic hip preservation surgery practice patterns: an international survey. J Hip Preserv Surg 2016;4(1):18–29

47. Brandenburg JB, Kapron AL, Wylie JD, et al. The functional and structural outcomes of arthroscopic iliopsoas release. Am J Sports Med 2016;44(5):1286–1291

48. Martin HD, Palmer IJ, Hatem M. Monopolar radiofrequency use in deep gluteal space endoscopy: sciatic nerve safety and fluid temperature. Arthroscopy 2014;30(1):60–64

49. de Sa D, Alradwan H, Cargnelli S, et al. Extra-articular hip impingement: a systematic review examining operative treatment of psoas, subspine, ischiofemoral, and greater trochanteric/pelvic impingement. Arthroscopy 2014;30(8):1026–1041

50. Nawabi DH, Degen RM, Fields KG, Wentzel CS, Adeoye O, Kelly BT. Anterior inferior iliac spine morphology and outcomes of hip arthroscopy in soccer athletes: a comparison to nonkicking athletes. Arthroscopy 2017;33(4):758–765

51. Amar E, Warschawski Y, Sharfman ZT, Martin HD, Safran MR, Rath E. Pathological findings in patients with low anterior inferior iliac spine impingement. Surg Radiol Anat 2016;38(5):569–575

52. Nelson IR, Keene JS. Results of labral-level arthroscopic iliopsoas tenotomies for the treatment of labral impingement. Arthroscopy 2014;30(6):688–694

53. Cascio BM, King D, Yen YM. Psoas impingement causing labrum tear: a series from three tertiary hip arthroscopy centers. J La State Med Soc 2013;165(2):88–93

54. Hatem MA, Palmer IJ, Martin HD. Diagnosis and 2-year outcomes of endoscopic treatment for ischiofemoral impingement. Arthroscopy 2015;31(2):239–246

55. Gómez-Hoyos J, Schröder R, Palmer IJ, Reddy M, Khoury A, Martin HD. Iliopsoas tendon insertion footprint with surgical implications in lesser trochanterplasty for treating ischiofemoral impingement: an anatomic study. J Hip Preserv Surg 2015;2(4):385–391

18 Soft-Tissue Hip Injuries
Joshua D. Harris

Introduction

I. Soft-tissue injuries are very common athletic and nonathletic injuries.

II. Layered concept of hip pain generators:
  A. Layer I: osteochondral.
  B. Layer II: inert soft tissue—static stability.
  C. Layer III: contractile soft tissue—dynamic stability.
  D. Layer IV: neuromechanical—kinetic and kinematic chain.

III. Soft-tissue structural hierarchy: layer III:
  A. Skeletal muscle:
    1. Muscle bundle:
      a. Surrounded by epimysium.
      b. Contains multiple fascicles.
    2. Muscle fascicle:
      a. Surrounded by perimysium.
      b. Contains multiple fibers (cells).
    3. Muscle fiber:
      a. Surrounded by endomysium.
      b. Contains multiple myofibrils.
    4. Myofibrils:
      a. Surrounded by sarcolemma.
      b. Contains multiple myofilaments.
      c. Sectioned into sarcomeres:
        i. Z-line forms each end of a sarcomere.
        ii. H-zone contains only myosin; bisected by M-line.
        iii. I-band contains only actin; bisected by Z-line.
        iv. A-band is the length of the myosin myofilaments.
    5. Myofilaments:
      a. Thick: myosin.
      b. Thin: actin.
    6. Muscle types:
      a. Type I: slow twitch; red fibers; oxidative:
        i. Aerobic metabolism; fatigue resistant.
        ii. More mitochondria and myoglobin than type II fibers.

   iii. Endurance, posture, balance.

   iv. Low power, low strength.

  b. Type IIa: fast twitch; red fibers; oxidative and glycolytic:

   i. Anaerobic metabolism (up to 30 minutes).

   ii. Medium power, medium strength.

  c. Type IIb: fast twitch; white fibers; glycolytic:

   i. Anaerobic metabolism (up to 1 minute); fatigue prone.

   ii. Sprinting, heavy weightlifting.

   iii. High power, high strength.

 7. Muscle contraction types:

  a. Isometric: muscle length remains the same during contraction:

   i. Static strength.

   ii. Plank or bridge exercise.

  b. Isotonic: muscle tension remains the same during contraction:

   i. Dynamic strength.

   ii. Hamstring curl exercise.

   iii. Concentric: muscle shortens during contraction.

   iv. Eccentric: muscle lengthens during contraction:

    (1) Greatest strengthening potential.

    (2) Greatest injury risk.

  c. Isokinetic: muscles contract and joints move at constant velocity:

   i. Dynamic strength.

   ii. Requires special equipment.

B. Tendon:

 1. Tendon:

  a. Two types:

   i. Paratenon covered:

    (1) Better vascular supply than sheathed tendon.

    (2) Majority of tendons around hip and pelvis.

   ii. Sheathed.

  b. Surrounded by epitenon.

  c. Contains multiple fascicles.

 2. Tendon fascicle:

  a. Surrounded by endotenon.

  b. Contains multiple fibers.

 3. Tendon fiber:

  a. Surrounded by endotenon.

  b. Contains multiple fibrils:

   i. Contains multiple microfibrils.

4. Osseous attachment:
   a. Tendon.
   b. Fibrocartilage.
   c. Mineralized fibrocartilage.
   d. Bone.

C. Injury location:
   1. Most frequently at musculotendinous junction.
   2. Second most frequently at tendon–bone junction.

Anatomic Considerations

I. Muscle groups:
   A. Biarticular (cross two joints):
      1. Cross hip and knee.
      2. Hamstring.
      3. Quadriceps.
   B. Uniarticular (cross one joint):
      1. Adductors.
      2. Abductors.

II. Anterior (**Figs. 18.1** and **18.2**):
   A. Iliopsoas.
   B. Rectus femoris.
   C. Sartorius.
   D. Rectus abdominis.
   E. External oblique, internal oblique, transversus abdominis.

III. Posterior (**Figs. 18.3** and **18.4**):
   A. Gluteus maximus.
   B. Hamstring.
   C. Piriformis.
   D. Short external rotators.

IV. Medial (**Fig. 18.5**):
   A. Adductor longus.
   B. Adductor brevis.
   C. Adductor magnus.
   D. Gracilis.
   E. Pectineus.

V. Lateral (**Fig. 18.3**):
   A. Gluteus medius.
   B. Gluteus minimus.
   C. Tensor fascia lata.

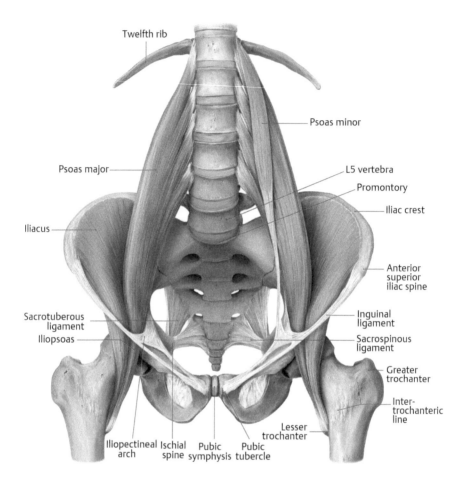

Fig. 18.1 Anterior view of the pelvis: the iliacus and the psoas major unite to form the iliopsoas tendon immediately anterior to the hip joint and insert onto the lesser trochanter. (Source: Schuenke M, Schulte E, Schumacher U. Thieme Atlas of Anatomy. General Anatomy and Musculoskeletal System. 2nd edition, ©2014, Thieme Publishers, New York. Illustrations by Voll M and Wesker K.)

VI.   Pelvic floor:

    A. Levator ani (pubococcygeus, puborectalis, iliococcygeus).

    B. Transversus perineum.

    C. Obturator internus.

VII. Muscle action (**Table 18.1**).

VIII. Sagittal pelvic balance:

    A. Anterior pelvic tilt:

        1. Tight iliopsoas.

        2. Tight rectus femoris/quadriceps.

        3. Tight hip adductors.

        4. Weak gluteus maximus.

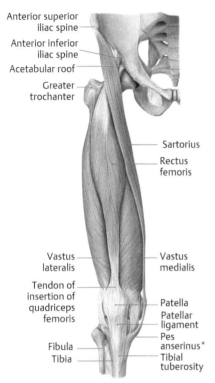

Fig. 18.2 Anterior view of the right hemipelvis and thigh, illustrating the quadriceps and sartorius. The rectus femoris crosses both the hip and knee joints, acting as a hip flexor and a knee extensor. (Source: Schuenke M, Schulte E, Schumacher U. Thieme Atlas of Anatomy. General Anatomy and Musculoskeletal System. 2nd edition, ©2014, Thieme Publishers, New York. Illustrations by Voll M and Wesker K.)

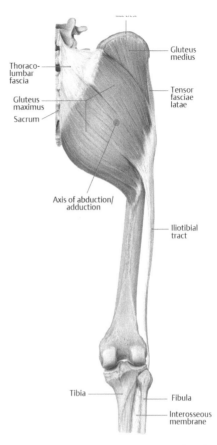

Fig. 18.3 Posterior view of the right hemipelvis. The gluteus maximus is the primary hip extensor, uniting with the tensor fascia lata laterally to form the iliotibial tract. (Source: Schuenke M, Schulte E, Schumacher U. Thieme Atlas of Anatomy. General Anatomy and Musculoskeletal System. 2nd edition, ©2014, Thieme Publishers, New York. Illustrations by Voll M and Wesker K.)

  5. Weak hamstring.
  6. Weak rectus abdominis.
  7. Increased lumbar lordosis:
      a. Exacerbated by tight psoas major.
B. Posterior pelvic tilt.
  1. Tight hamstring.
  2. Weak iliopsoas.
  3. Rectus abdominis activation.
  4. Gluteus maximus activation.
  5. Decreased lumbar lordosis.

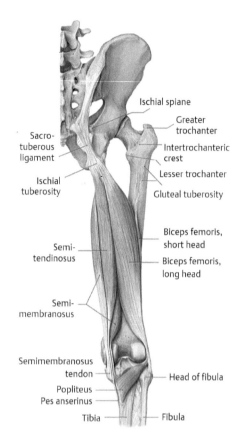

Fig. 18.4 Posterior view of the right hemipelvis and thigh, illustrating the hamstring muscle group. (Source: Schuenke M, Schulte E, Schumacher U. Thieme Atlas of Anatomy. General Anatomy and Musculoskeletal System. 2nd edition, ©2014, Thieme Publishers, New York. Illustrations by Voll M and Wesker K.)

Classification

I.   Acute:

    A. Traumatic mechanism.

    B. Eccentric contraction more common mechanism than concentric contraction.

II.   Chronic:

    A. Overuse mechanism.

    B. Tendinosis.

III. Strain:

    A. Mechanism frequently noncontact.

    B. Commonly in muscle(s) that are biarticular, at musculotendinous junction.

    C. Grade 1: mild injury:

        1. Minimal loss of strength and motion.

        2. MRI may show little to no edema in muscle.

    D. Grade 2: moderate injury:

        1. More extensive damage—partial muscle fiber disruption.

        2. MRI may show edema, partial fiber tear, without retraction.

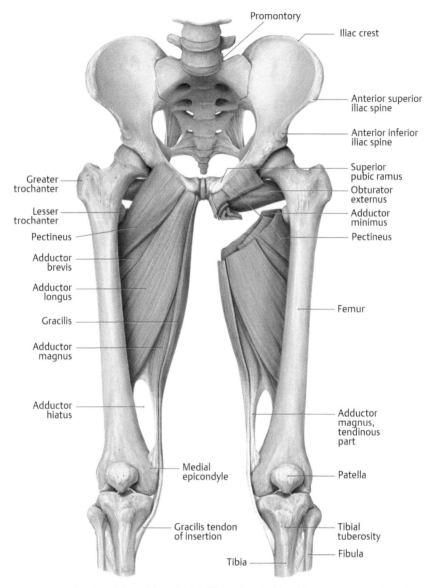

Fig. 18.5   Anterior view of the pelvis and thigh, illustrating the hip adductors. (Source: Schuenke M, Schulte E, Schumacher U. Thieme Atlas of Anatomy. General Anatomy and Musculoskeletal System. 2nd edition, ©2014, Thieme Publishers, New York. Illustrations by Voll M and Wesker K.)

    E.   Grade 3: severe injury:

        1.   Complete tear of muscle or tendon.

        2.   MRI may show complete tear, with retraction.

IV.   Contusion:

    A.   Mechanism: direct contact.

    B.   Quadriceps.

Table 18.1   Muscle actions relative to the hip in the anatomic position

Flexion	Extension	Abduction	Adduction	External rotation	Internal rotation
Iliopsoas	Gluteus maximus	Gluteus medius	Adductor longus	Piriformis	None
Sartorius				Superior gemellus	
Tensor fascia lata	Semimembranosus	Gluteus minimus	Adductor brevis		
	Semitendinosus			Obturator internus	
Rectus femoris	Biceps femoris	Tensor fascia lata	Adductor magnus		
	Adductor magnus			Inferior gemellus	
Adductor longus			Gracilis	Quadratus femoris	
Pectineus			Pectineus		
				Obturator externus	
				Gluteus maximus	

      C. Hamstring.

      D. Lateral hip—Morel–Lavallée lesion.

V.   Muscle quality:

      E. Goutallier/Fuchs classification:

         1. Grade 0: normal muscle.

         2. Grade 1: fatty streaks.

         3. Grade 2: fatty infiltration, more muscle than fat.

         4. Grade 3: equal amounts muscle and fat.

         5. Grade 4: more fat than muscle.

History and Examination

I.   A detailed history and physical examination is required.

II.   History alone may be able to accurately diagnose most soft-tissue hip injuries.

III.   Mechanism of injury:

      A. Contact versus noncontact.

      B. Sport or activity of causation.

      C. Feeling of a "pop" or "tear" or "rip."

      D. Pain with coughing, sneezing, Valsalva, abdominal crunch.

IV.   Location of pain:

      A. Deep anterior, groin, "C" sign: iliopsoas, core muscle injury.

      B. Medial, groin: adductor, core muscle injury.

      C. Lateral: abductor.

      D. Posterior: proximal hamstring.

V.   Location of deformity or bruising:

      A. Medial: adductor tear (**Fig. 18.6**).

      B. Posterior: proximal hamstring tear (**Fig. 18.7**).

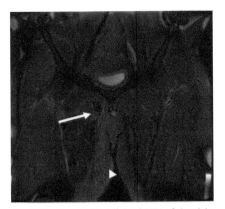

Fig. 18.6 Coronal T2-weighted MRI of the right hip adductor tear with intratendon hemorrhage 8 days following injury (*arrow*), with significant subcutaneous swelling and ecchymosis (*arrowhead*).

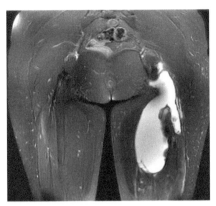

Fig. 18.7 Coronal T2-weighted MRI of the left proximal hamstring complete three-tendon tear with significant distal retraction and surrounding hematoma.

VI. Presence or absence of snapping:

    A. Internal coxa saltans: iliopsoas:

        1. Can "hear" the snap.

    B. External coxa saltans: iliotibial band:

        1. Can "see" the snap laterally.

    C. Intra-articular coxa saltans: labral tear:

        1. Can "feel," but not hear or see the snap.

VII. Physical examination.

VIII. Appearance:

    A. Ecchymosis, deformity, atrophy.

IX. Tenderness:

    A. Bony prominences, muscles, tendons.

X. Motion:

    A. Spine, hip, knee (bilateral).

XI. Strength:

    A. All muscle groups, assess for symmetry.

XII. Special testing:

    A. Impingement: anterior, subspine, lateral, posterior.

    B. Instability:

        1. Anterior: iliofemoral ligament:

            a. External rotation recoil, dial, apprehension.

        2. Posterior: posterior acetabular wall, labrum, capsule:

            a. Flexion, adduction, posterior load and shift.

    C. Snapping iliopsoas: flexed, external rotation to extension, internal rotation.

    D. Snapping iliotibial band: Ober's test, lateral decubitus bicycle test.

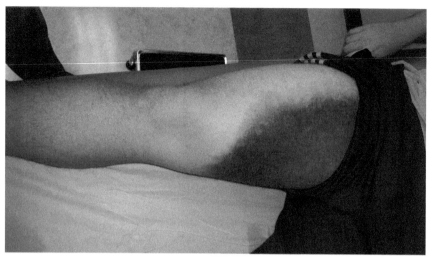

Fig. 18.8 Supine clinical photograph of the same patient as in **Fig. 18.6** with large amount of swelling and ecchymosis 8 days following a right adductor injury sustained while kicking during a soccer match.

Diagnostic Imaging

I.   Plain radiographs:

    A. In acute situation, helpful to evaluate for osseous avulsion:

        1. Lesser trochanter: iliopsoas tendon.

        2. Ischial tuberosity: proximal hamstring.

        3. Anterosuperior iliac spine: tensor fascia lata, sartorius.

        4. Anteroinferior iliac spine: rectus femoris.

    B. In chronic injuries, helpful to evaluate for bony pathomorphology:

        1. Femoroacetabular impingement.

        2. Osteoarthritis.

        3. Stress fracture.

II. MRI:

    A. Contrast (intravenous, intra-articular) unnecessary.

    B. Helpful to diagnose injury location, severity (**Figs. 18.8** and **18.9**).

    C. Assess atrophy, fatty degeneration of muscle.

III. Ultrasound:

    A. Dynamic examination capabilities, user dependent.

    B. Helpful to evaluate tendon/muscle tear, snapping, hematoma.

    C. Helpful to facilitate accurate injection (joint, tendon sheath).

Differential Diagnosis

I.   Diagnostic intra-articular injection useful to quantify pain contribution from joint (**Table 18.2**).

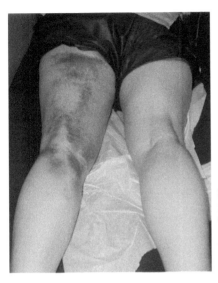

Fig. 18.9 Prone clinical photograph of the same patient as in **Fig. 18.7** with large amount of swelling and ecchymosis 3 weeks following a left proximal hamstring complete three-tendon tear. The patient additionally complained of left foot paresthesias secondary to sciatic nerve compression from the hematoma.

Treatment

I.   Nonoperative:

   A. Generally indicated for most hip soft-tissue injuries.

   B. Rest.

   C. Activity modification:

      1. Avoid provocative painful activity(ies).

      2. Immobilization generally not recommended.

   D. Oral anti-inflammatory medications:

      1. Avoidance of fluoroquinolone antibiotics (tendon compromise).

   E. Ice cryotherapy for soft-tissue swelling, ecchymosis.

   F. Physical therapy:

      1. Proper pelvic posture:

         a. Gluteus maximus activation.

         b. Hamstring strengthening and stretching.

         c. Abductor strengthening, avoidance of Trendelenburg:

            i. Especially if dysplasia (abductor fatigue).

         d. Iliopsoas stretching.

         e. Rectus femoris stretching.

         f. Quadriceps strengthening.

         g. Rectus abdominis strengthening.

         h. Transversus abdominis activation.

      2. Improve muscular strength for objective weakness.

Table 18.2 Differential diagnosis of soft tissue hip injuries

Pathology	Differential
Soft tissue: acute	Muscle strain (iliopsoas, rectus femoris, adductor, hamstring, rectus abdominis)
	Muscle/tendon tear (proximal hamstring, adductor, rectus femoris, iliopsoas)
Soft tissue: chronic	Anterior enthesopathy (iliopsoas, rectus femoris)
	Iliopsoas impingement (iliopsoas-induced labral tear)
	Medial enthesopathy (adductor/rectus abdominis tendinopathy: core muscle injury, "athletic pubalgia," osteitis pubis)
	Lateral enthesopathy (peritrochanteric pain, gluteus medius/minimus tendinopathy/tear)
	Posterior enthesopathy (proximal hamstring syndrome, "piriformis syndrome," deep gluteal space syndrome)
	Hip microinstability (generalized ligamentous laxity, capsular insufficiency, ligamentum teres injury, labral insufficiency)
Bony: acute	Fracture (proximal femur, acetabulum, pelvis)
	Dislocation (hip)
Bony: chronic	Femoroacetabular impingement (cam, pincer) with labral injury
	Extra-articular impingement (subspine, ischiofemoral, trochanteric–pelvic, pectineofoveal)
	Stress fracture (femoral neck, pubis, iliac crest, iliac wing, sacrum, proximal femoral shaft)
Nonhip causes	Obstetric: gynecologic system
	Ovarian cyst
	Pregnancy
	Uterine fibroid
	Malignant/benign tumor
	Infection
	Gastrointestinal
	Hernia (direct, indirect, femoral)
	Appendicitis
	Diverticulitis
	Inflammatory bowel disease
	Genitourinary
	Nephrolithiasis
	Infection
	Nervous system
	Meralgia paresthetica (lateral femoral cutaneous)
	Neuralgia (iliohypogastric, ilioinguinal, genitofemoral, pudendal, obturator, femoral)
	Vascular
	Claudication
	Musculoskeletal
	Lumbosacral spine
	Sacroiliac joint

3. Improve motion for objective loss of motion in the absence of osseous impingement.

4. Modalities as needed:

   a. Active release therapy.

   b. Dry needling, acupuncture.

   c. Ultrasound.

   d. Neuromuscular electrical stimulation.

II. Operative:

A. Tendon tear:

   1. Proximal hamstring:

      a. Indications: two or three tendon tears with ≥2 cm of retraction, with or without sciatic nerve involvement.

      b. Acute repair (less than 4 weeks from injury date) with transverse incision in gluteal crease, anatomic suture anchor repair to ischial tuberosity.

      c. Chronic repair (>4 weeks from injury date) with possible longitudinal (or "**L**"-shaped) incision (depends on magnitude of retraction, necessary mobilization, possible sciatic neurolysis), assessment of primary repair tension, utilization of Achilles bone block allograft if unable to primarily repair without significant tension.

   2. Gluteus medius/minimus:

      a. Indications: failure of nonsurgical treatment for partial tear.

      b. Endoscopic or open suture anchor repair.

      c. Gluteus maximus rotation and advancement in chronic retracted irreparable tear.

   3. Adductor origin:

      a. Indications: no absolute indications.

      b. Suture anchor repair to pubis.

      c. In combination with rectus abdominis (core muscle injury), multiple techniques exist:

         i. Debridement of devitalized tissue.

         ii. Repair of torn tendon(s).

         iii. Decortication, marrow stimulation for tendon–bone healing.

         iv. Decompression of contracted, swollen compartments.

         v. Neurolysis (genitofemoral, ilioinguinal, iliohypogastric).

B. Postoperative management:

   1. Avoidance of tension on repaired musculotendinous unit:

      a. Proximal hamstring:

         i. Knee brace (locked in relative flexion).

         ii. Hip brace (locked in relative extension).

  iii. Rolling walker (permits mobilization, knee flexed, hip extended).

  iv. Avoid passive hip flexion and knee extension.

  v. Avoid active knee flexion and hip extension.

  vi. Progressive return to activities after 3 months.

 b. Abductor:

  i. Hip brace (avoid passive abduction).

  ii. Partial weight bearing for 6 to 8 weeks.

  iii. Avoid Trendelenburg gait.

  iv. Progressive return to activities after 3 months.

 c. Core muscle injury:

  i. Address other concomitant surgically treated (if any) pathology (femoroacetabular impingement, labral injury).

  ii. Avoid passive hip abduction.

  iii. Avoid active adductor/rectus abdominis.

  iv. Ensure optimal pelvic tilt.

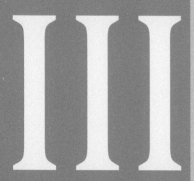

Section III

19 Hip Osteoarthritis

Brian M. Culp, Brett R. Levine

Etiology of Hip Osteoarthritis

I. Primary "idiopathic" hip osteoarthritis (OA):

   A. Historically described as "wear and tear" or overuse.

   B. Common age-related changes, although routine use over time does not account for all aspects of the pathology.

   C. Genetic predisposition[1]:

      1. More common in females.

      2. Possible link to Collagen IX gene (Col9A) phenotype.

II. Secondary OA:

   A. Post slipped capital femoral epiphysis.

   B. Dysplasia of the hip: shallow acetabular socket resulting in edge loading and increased articular contact forces.

   C. Sequela of Legg–Calvé–Perthes disease with resulting femoral head irregularities (the square peg in a round hole):

      1. Development often depends on containment of the femoral head and congruency of the ultimate joint through adolescence and adulthood.

   D. Posttraumatic arthritis: prior damage to chondrocytes, labrum, or osseous structures.

   E. Septic arthritis: infection and inflammatory response resulting in articular damage.

III. Femoroacetabular impingement (FAI):

   A. Cam impingement: prominent bone present at the femoral head–neck junction leading to cartilage damage with hip motion.

   B. Pincer impingement: excessively deep socket or retroversion leading to bony impingement.

   C. Combination FAI frequently demonstrates features of both aspects of the impingement spectrum:

      1. Ganz and several others have suggested that subtle changes in hip anatomy, such as that seen in FAI, lead to abnormal contact forces and progressive changes of the osteochondral and labrocapsular structures.

      2. This concept proposes that idiopathic OA is unrecognized or subtle forms of these secondary diagnoses.

IV. Differential diagnosis: other conditions leading to hip degeneration:

   A. Avascular necrosis of the femur:

      1. Vascular compromise to the femoral head resulting in subchondral osteonecrosis and collapse, cartilage damage, and deterioration.

    2. Risk factors include trauma, corticosteroid use, alcohol abuse, hematologic conditions, irradiation, and cytotoxic insults.

B. Inflammatory arthritis: constellation of conditions leading to joint destruction in the setting of varying degrees of inflammation:

    1. Rheumatoid arthritis: polyarthropathy with characteristic stigma including prolonged morning stiffness and morphology changes to hands/feet.

    2. Systemic lupus erythematosus: "lupus":

        a. Systemic inflammatory condition that affects multiple body parts including skin, brain, kidney, heart, lungs, and joints. Malar rash is a common facial finding.

    3. Ankylosing spondylitis:

        a. Hallmark stiffness at multiple body parts most notably in the sacroiliac joints and spine.

C. Referred back pain:

    1. Often presents as pain in the buttocks and follows a radiating pattern below the level of the knee.

    2. This can present with back pain, or neurologic changes of motor or sensory or both.

    3. A corticosteroid injection into the hip can be useful to distinguish hip versus referred spinal pathology.

Basic Science

I. Macroscopic changes:

A. Loss of articular cartilage leading to increased contact forces and high coefficient of friction.

B. Results in eburnation of bone, activation of ossification centers, osteophyte formation, and labral degeneration.

C. Coxarthrosis—"hip joint inflammation"—misnomer as inflammatory process is not always a major factor:

    1. Loss of proteoglycan content within articular cartilage.[2]

II. Microscopic changes:

A. Loss of proteoglycan bonds to hyaluronic acid:

    1. Increased type VI collagen replaces normal type II collagen.

B. Increased keratin sulfate–decreased chondroitin sulfate composition of glycosaminoglycans.

C. INCREASED water content up to 90%.

D. Elevated proteolytic enzymes[3]:

    1. Metalloproteinases present in joint fluid.

    2. Cathepsins B and D overexpression.

E. Nitric oxide synthase pathway activation.

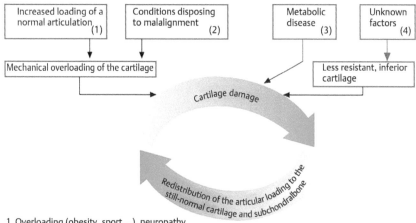

1 Overloading (obesity, sport,...), neuropathy
2 Joint dysplasias, abnormal alignment of neighboring joints, post-traumatic, postinflammatory, damage of the subchondral bone (e.g., ischemia)
3 Crystal deposition disease
4 Genetic dispositons?

Fig. 19.1 Osteoarthritis pathway. (Source: Introduction and Synopsis. In: Bohndorf K, Imhof H, Pope T, eds. Musculoskeletal Imaging. A Concise Multimodality Approach. Stuttgart: Thieme; 2001.)

    F. Inflammatory cytokines upregulated:
        1. Interleukin 1-beta (IL-1β)
        2. Tumor necrosis factor α (TNF-α).
    G. Upregulation of growth factors:
        1. Fibroblast growth factor-2 (FGF-2) decreases aggrecanase activity and upreglulates metalloproteinases.
        2. Transforming growth factor B1 (TFG-B1).
    H. The end result is articular cartilage changes and chondrocyte apoptosis (**Fig. 19.1**).

Patient History

I. Pain quality:
    A. Most frequently patients present with deep groin pain—progressively worsening with the severity of the disease.
    B. "C sign" can represent a deep and difficult-to-localize pain: vague pain described by cupping hand around the lateral hip in a "**C**" shape to describe the location.
    C. Buttocks, thigh, or knee pain may also be present but may represent other pathologies such as lumbar pathology, trochanteric bursitis, or vascular compromise.
    D. Worsened by increased activity or trauma:
        1. Tends to be worse with prolonged inactivity and then attempted motion.
        2. Too much of any one activity is difficult (standing too long, sitting too long, etc.).

II.   Character of symptoms:

    A. The patient may note leg length differences as the disease pattern progresses.

    B. Motion restriction:

        1. Forward flexion through pelvis—hip contracture.

        2. Poor rotational motion is common—particularly internal rotation:

            a. Difficulty donning socks or shoes.

            b. Hard time getting into/out of low chairs or toilet, stair climbing, getting in and out of cars.

    C. Notable feeling with weather and barometric pressure changes.

    D. Symptoms present in the morning or the first few steps after sitting for too long:

        1. Additional symptoms such as:

            a. Radiating pain into the knee.

            b. Throbbing while at rest.

            c. Prolonged stiffness in the morning may suggest inflammatory arthritis or avascular necrosis.

            d. Night pain should trigger thoughts of tumor or infection.

Physical Examination

Clinical evaluation of the hip should take a systematic approach. This requires in-depth knowledge of the local anatomy, as well as a variety of techniques to localize the cause. These specialized examination techniques, when combined with a good clinical history, can allow accurate diagnosis.[4]

I.   Gait pattern changes and limping:

The patient's gait should be observed without the use of a walking aid if the patient can manage. This may reveal specific patterns of disease as follows:

    A. Antalgic gait: shortened stance phase on affected leg to minimize joint reactive forces on painful joint.

    B. Trendelenburg gait: consequence of abductor weakness manifesting as leaning (shifting body weight) over the weak side to prevent the need of pelvic support by the affected gluteal muscles.

    C. Positive foot progression angle: foot externally rotated (suggests external rotation contracture).

    D. Requirement of an assistive device to maintain balance or minimize pain (best when used in the contralateral hand).

    E. Look for lumbar hyperlordosis with walking or hunched-over gait due to hip flexion contracture.

II.   Range of motion:

    A. Limited hip motion:

        1. Hip rotation should be assessed at 90 degrees of flexion and compared with contralateral hip.

2. Pelvis should be stabilized to prevent lumbosacral motion with examination.

3. Difficulty with external rotation, hip extension, adduction, abduction, or hip flexion often with obligate external rotation.

4. Limited internal rotation: posterior capsular contracture, FAI.

5. Obligate external rotation (sits with legs crossed).

B. Hip flexion contracture (Thomas' test): both hips are flexed up and the affected side is allowed to extend until the end point or pelvic tilt is noted.

III. Provocative maneuvers:

A. Trochanteric tenderness may signal bursitis or abductor tendonitis and may occur simultaneously with hip OA.

B. Passive straight leg raise sign performed to rule out referred back symptoms.

C. Resisted straight leg raise (Stinchfield's test) with reproduction of pain.

D. Pain with "figure 4" position (Patrick's test).

IV. Leg length differences: noted at either the iliac crests, the tibial tubercles, or the malleoli:

A. This can be measured using calibrated blocks with subjective or radiographic assessment for length equality.

B. Direct palpation of the iliac crests in a neutral stance.

C. Measurement of the medial malleoli with respect to one another or by measuring from a fixed distance (such as anterosuperior iliac spine [ASIS]) to the malleoli:

1. Apparent leg length—measure from the umbilicus to the medial malleoli.

2. True leg length—measure from the ASIS to the medial malleoli.

Radiographic Evaluation[5]

I. Optimal X-rays views (**Fig. 19.2**):

A. Anteroposterior (AP) pelvis (weight bearing).

B. AP hip with leg in 15 degrees of internal rotation—optimizes visualization of the femoral neck.

C. Frog-leg lateral.

D. Additional views: may be used to assess signs of aspherical femoral head, acetabular retroversion, or signs of impingement:

1. Lumbar spine standing views—in conjunction with the AP pelvis view may indicate resting pelvic flexion or extension as well as lumbar flexibility.

2. Emerging radiographic technology may ultimately be predictive of functional pelvic position and risk factors for dislocation (EOS Imaging, Inc.).

3. Cross-table lateral.

4. Dunn's view—good to look for FAI with good visualization to detect femoral head–neck asphericity; patient's hip is flexed 45 or 90 degrees and abducted 20 degrees with a neutral pelvis.

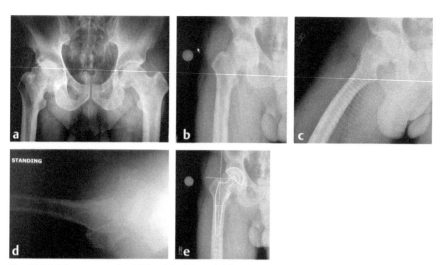

Fig. 19.2 (a) Anteroposterior (AP) pelvis. **(b)** AP, **(c)** frog-lateral, and **(d)** shoot-through lateral of the hip—part of the standard radiographs to assess hip osteoarthritis, along with a templating radiograph **(e)** prior to total hip arthroplasty.

5. False-profile view—obtained with the patient standing, pelvis rotated approximately 65 degrees in relation to the film holder, and the foot parallel to the cassette; helps with head coverage and acetabular depth.

II. Features to assess:

A. Joint line:

1. Marginal osteophytes.

2. Joint space loss.

3. Sclerosis of subchondral bone.

4. Cystic changes.

B. Pelvic morphology on standing view:

1. Inlet/outlet: indicates standing pelvic tilt.

2. Ischial spine prominence may indicate acetabular retroversion.

3. Lumbar spine hardware.

4. Acetabular coverage:

a. Lack of acetabular coverage over the femoral head can indicate subtle or overt hip dysplasia.

b. This can be assessed using center-edge angle measurements as well as assessing a plumb line from the lateral acetabular edge with respect to the femoral head.

C. Femoral morphology:

1. Prominent lesser trochanter reveals leg rotation/anteversion.

2. Canal width (Dorr's classification)[6]—described in categories (A, B, and C) to assess mismatch between the diaphyseal width and the metaphyseal width:

      a. Type A: "champagne flute" femur with a wide proximal metaphysis and narrow shaft.

      b. Type B is standard radiograph—essentially between an A and a B.

      c. Type C represents "stove pipe" femur with large proximal and distal cavities in the metaphysis and diaphysis.

      d. These may have surgical implications on implant choice—may mean you have to ream to prepare the femur with a tighter canal or consider cemented fixation.

D. Varus or valgus angulation of the neck:

    1. Normal range: 120 to 135 degrees.

    2. Coxa vara less than 120 degrees.

    3. Coxa valga greater than 135 degrees: can affect implant choice should surgery be required.

E. Flexed or neutral position may affect measurements: can affect magnification or apparent size of structures such as femoral canal width. It can be difficult to identify without clinical correlation.

F. Advanced imaging:

    1. CT: Three-dimensional imaging that can be used to assess femoral and acetabular morphology, adjacent bone loss, and adjacent neurovascular structures. Less valuable in assessing soft tissues such as cartilage or labral pathology.

    2. MRI: It may show features such as edema within the femoral head or acetabulum, cystic changes, labral tears, or cartilage thickness. It can also be used to assess bone morphology. It may also reveal edema within the proximal femur, subchondral collapse, or cartilage irregularities, which can aid in the diagnosis of avascular necrosis.

Treatment Options

I. Conservative:

A. Activity modification[7]:

    1. Avoiding activities that provoke pain, using shoe aids, decreasing stair climbing, adding toilet or chair lifts to minimize squatting.

    2. When carrying loads, they should be carried with equal distribution over both sides, or if unilateral loads are carried, then carried toward the affected hip.

B. Weight loss:

    1. Decreases joint reactive forces across diseased hip joint surface.

    2. Most reliable/safe way to improve symptoms.

C. Assistive devices to decrease joint reaction forces:

    1. Cane: used in the hand opposite the painful side:

      a. This decreases joint reactive forces by using the rotational force created by the cane to decrease needed forces on the affected "hip abductor moment" complex.

2. Crutches/walkers also function to decrease load across the affected hip by transferring load bearing to upper extremities.

D. Oral medications:

1. Nonsteroidal anti-inflammatory medications: function by suppressing prostaglandin generation by cyclooxygenase (COX) enzymes decreasing pain and inflammation:

a. Oral steroids: more potent form of anti-inflammatory effect that decreases cytokine production in the affected joint.

2. Acetaminophen—avoid concomitant liver toxic medications and be wary of those with alcohol abuse.

3. Tramadol/opioids: central nervous system blockade of pain perception.

E. Physical therapy[8]: questionable efficacy as disease progresses; can teach the patient body mechanics and educate the patient regarding safe exercises to stay active without worsening pain.

F. Injection therapy:

1. Corticosteroids: local anti-inflammatory effect within the diseased joint. Often placed with imaging adjunct such as ultrasound or radiography; can show short-term relief in moderate to severe disease.[9]

2. Hyaluronic acid: off-label use; nonspecific mechanism of action; thought to work via restoring joint homeostasis via introduction of more "normal" synovial fluid.

3. Alternative injections: stem cells, platelet-rich plasma (PRP) injections; role not clearly defined in treatment of arthroplasty with no supportive data at this point; thought to aid "regeneration" of articular surfaces by introduction of pluripotent cells capable of differentiation into cartilage, thus restoring normal anatomy:

a. Encouraging early data have been noted with PRP and stem cells, but long-term success and large studies have not been completed yet.

II. Surgical treatment:

A. Hip hemiarthroplasty for arthritis:

1. Indications: primarily historical use for OA with little utility in present treatment of arthritic conditions; currently used for displaced femoral neck fractures in patients with low functional demands.

2. Contraindications: active infection, highly functional patients.

B. Hip resurfacing:

1. Less frequently used given concerns for metal debris reactions; involves placement of acetabular shell with smooth metal bearing surface; femoral neck is maintained while cemented surface is applied to the prepared femoral side.

2. Indications include younger patients (typically male) who are physically active/demanding on their joint.

3. Contraindications: avascular necrosis, active infection, females of child-bearing age, those at risk of a hip fracture:

  a. Outcomes: Hunter et al reported on 121 hip resurfacing cases with a 91% 10-year survivorship.[10] Revisions were more common in the cases with smaller sized implants. (Note: this was a nondesigner study.)

C. Resection arthroplasty ("Girdlestone")[11]:

 1. Indications: severe hip disease in nonambulator, active infection, flail limb (**Fig. 19.3**).

 2. Contraindications: functionally ambulatory patients.

D. Hip fusion:

 1. Limited role in present treatment of OA.[12]

 2. Classic treatment for young manual male laborers.

 3. Unilateral disease: cannot fuse both.

 4. Can lead to earlier breakdown in adjacent joints.

 5. Position of function: approximately 20 degrees of flexion, slight external rotation, neutral abduction.

E. Total hip arthroplasty:

 1. Indications include advanced arthritic disease with failure of conservative treatment.

 2. Contraindications include presence of active infection, patients who are not medically fit for surgery.

 3. Gold standard of care with replacement of both femoral head with fixation into the remaining femur and resurfacing of acetabulum.

 4. Bearing surface options include hard on hard (metal on metal/ceramic on ceramic) or "hard on soft" (metal on polyethylene/ceramic on polyethylene).

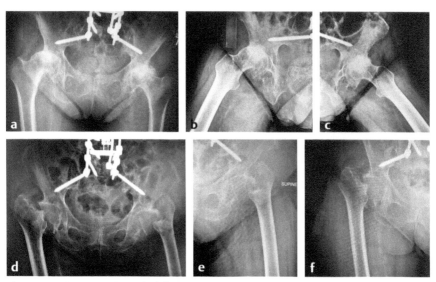

Fig. 19.3 (a–c) Preoperative and **(d–f)** postoperative radiographs of a nonambulatory patient with chronic, unrelenting hip pain that underwent a Girdlestone resection arthroplasty.

5. Implant fixation options include biologic fixation surfaces versus acrylic cement fixation:

   a. In-growth/on-growth surfaces use textured forms of metal that permit the body to primarily adhere to the implants with new bone growth. This design can be used on either the acetabular or the femoral side. Initial fixation provided via a "press fit" or additional fixation (such as screws placed into the acetabular component) until ingrowth fixation is achieved.

   b. Cement fixation, which was previously more commonplace, obtained immediate fixation to the host bone surface upon "curing" of the cement. This bonded the prosthesis of the femur or acetabulum to the prepared receiving bone. Longevity of this type of fixation is somewhat less due to its lack of ability to remodel; however, femoral cement fixation still stands as a reliable form of fixation especially with poor bone quality or for certain types of anatomy (i.e., Dorr's type C femur shape). Cement fixation for acetabular components is rarely used with currently available implant designs.

References

1. Fernández-Moreno M, Rego I, Carreira-Garcia V, Blanco FJ. Genetics in osteoarthritis. Curr Genomics 2008;9(8):542–547
2. Hunziker EB. Articular cartilage repair: basic science and clinical progress. A review of the current status and prospects. Osteoarthritis Cartilage 2002;10(6):432–463
3. Tetlow LC, Adlam DJ, Woolley DE. Matrix metalloproteinase and proinflammatory cytokine production by chondrocytes of human osteoarthritic cartilage: associations with degenerative changes. Arthritis Rheum 2001;44(3):585–594
4. Martin HD, Palmer IJ. History and physical examination of the hip: the basics. Curr Rev Musculoskelet Med 2013;6(3):219–225
5. Lim SJ, Park YS. Plain radiography of the hip: a review of radiographic techniques and image features. Hip Pelvis 2015;27(3):125–134
6. Dorr LD, Faugere MC, Mackel AM, Gruen TA, Bognar B, Malluche HH. Structural and cellular assessment of bone quality of proximal femur. Bone 1993;14(3):231–242
7. Neumann DA. Biomechanical analysis of selected principles of hip joint protection. Arthritis Care Res 1989;2(4):146–155
8. Roddy E, Zhang W, Doherty M, et al. Evidence-based recommendations for the role of exercise in the management of osteoarthritis of the hip or knee: the MOVE consensus. Rheumatology (Oxford) 2005;44(1):67–73
9. Kruse DW. Intraarticular cortisone injection for osteoarthritis of the hip. Is it effective? Is it safe? Curr Rev Musculoskelet Med 2008;1(3–4):227–233
10. Hunter TJA, Moores TS, Morley D, Manoharan G, Collier SG, Shaylor PJ. 10-year results of the Birmingham Hip Resurfacing: a non-designer case series. Hip Int 2018;28(1):50–52
11. Rubin LE, Murgo KT, Ritterman SA, McClure PK. Hip resection arthroplasty. JBJS Rev 2014;2(5):01874474-201402050-00003
12. Schafroth MU, Blokzijl RJ, Haverkamp D, Maas M, Marti RK. The long-term fate of the hip arthrodesis: does it remain a valid procedure for selected cases in the 21st century? Int Orthop 2010;34(6):805–810

20 Primary Total Hip Arthroplasty

Michael A. Flierl, Matthew Knedel, Brett R. Levine

History

I. Typical patient complaints:

    A. Pain located in the groin, anterior thigh, lateral thigh, and sometimes buttocks.

    B. Limitations in activities of daily living, such as ambulating longer distances, walking up and down the stairs, putting on socks and shoes, getting up from a sitting position, and getting in and out of a car.

    C. Limp sometimes necessitating assistive devices for ambulation.

    D. In later stages of degenerative joint disease of the hip, patients will awaken at night from pain.

    E. Presentation and duration of symptoms may vary somewhat based on the disease process leading to surgery.

Surgical Indications

I. Significant limitations in activities of daily living secondary to hip pain and dysfunction.

II. Failure of nonsurgical treatments: activity modification, weight loss, nonsteroidal anti-inflammatory drugs (NSAIDs), physical therapy, and use of assistive devices.

III. Typical disorders presenting for primary total hip arthroplasty (THA) include the following (expand as needed):

    A. Osteoarthritis.

    B. Inflammatory arthritides (rheumatoid arthritis, psoriatic arthritis, lupus, etc.).

    C. Osteonecrosis.

    D. Posttraumatic degenerative joint disease.

    E. Displaced subcapital femoral neck fracture in active and independent individuals.

    F. Acute THA for acetabular fractures with preexisting arthritis (evolving).

IV. Radiographic changes consistent with end-stage hip degenerative joint disease.

V. Medical optimization and complete preoperative risk assessment has been performed:

    A. All modifiable risk factors (BMI [body mass index], smoking cessation, diabetes, chronic opioid dependence, etc.) need to be optimized.

    B. Expectations, anticipated restrictions, and outcomes discussed preoperatively.

Radiographic Evaluation

I. Radiographic examination:

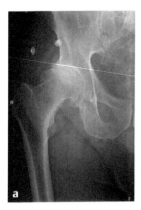
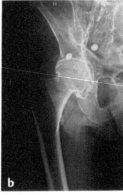

Fig. 20.1 Typical radiographic changes of degenerative joint disease. **(a)** Osteoarthritis: joint space narrowing, subchondral sclerosis, subchondral cysts, and osteophyte formation. **(b)** Rheumatoid arthritis: symmetric joint space narrowing, periarticular osteopenia, bony erosions, periarticular cysts, and protrusion acetabuli.

   A. Plain radiography:
      1. Low anteroposterior (AP) pelvis: assess leg lengths, offset, and compare with the other side.
      2. AP of affected hip: typically obtained with a marker for digital templating or to calibrate for acetate templating/planning.
      3. Lateral of affected hip: frog-leg lateral and shoot thru: can assess acetabular version, columns, and femoral deformities.
   B. Advance imaging:
      1. CT scan: rarely necessary unless there is the need to assess an acute fracture or acetabular anteversion.
      2. MRI: rarely necessary to plan for THA.
II. Degenerative joint disease:
   A. Osteoarthritis: joint space narrowing, subchondral sclerosis, subchondral cysts, osteophyte formation (**Fig. 20.1a**).
III. Inflammatory arthropathy:
   A. Rheumatoid and general inflammatory arthritis: symmetric joint space narrowing, periarticular osteopenia, bony erosions, periarticular cysts, and coxa profunda/protrusio acetabuli (**Fig. 20.1b**).
   B. Ankylosis spondylitis: symmetric joint space narrowing, protrusio acetabuli, and bony ankylosis.

Surgical Approaches

I. Direct anterior (Smith-Peterson) approach[1,2]:
   A. Interval: sartorius/tensor fascia latae, rectus femoris/gluteus medius.
   B. Dangers: lateral femoral cutaneous nerve, ascending branch of the lateral femoral circumflex artery.
   C. Advantages: extensile to anterior column of the pelvis and true internervous plane.

D. Disadvantages: difficult femoral exposure, technically demanding, specialized equipment needed, heterotopic ossification, periprosthetic femoral fractures, learning curve.

E. Can be performed supine on regular table (radiolucent) or on traction/fracture table.

F. Outcomes: no long-term differences in clinical outcome between direct anterior and posterior approaches[3,4] or direct anterior and the direct lateral approaches.[5,6] No statistical difference has been described in dislocation rates in direct anterior versus posterior approach (0.84 vs. 0.79%, respectively).[7]

II. Anterolateral (Watson–Jones) approach:

A. Interval: tensor fascia latae/gluteus medius.

B. Dangers: femoral nerve, branch of superior gluteal nerve, superior gluteal artery.

C. Advantages: lower dislocation rates, good acetabular and femoral exposure.

D. Disadvantages: abductor damage—postoperative limp, difficult femoral exposure, technically demanding.

E. Positioning can be lateral decubitus or supine.

F. Outcomes: no differences in clinical outcome between anterolateral, direct lateral, and posterior approaches.[8] Dislocation rates have been described as similar rates between anterolateral (3%) and posterior (4%) approaches. Rates of aseptic loosening are reported to be higher in the anterolateral approach (24%) compared to the posterior approach (20%).[9]

III. Lateral (Hardinge) approach:

A. Interval: none. Modified Hardige approach divides the anterior one-third from the posterior two-thirds of the gluteus medius: the split through the gluteus medius can be in line with its fibers straight superiorly, or may involve the anterior one-third of the gluteus medius to minimize muscle damage.

B. Dangers: femoral nerve, branch of superior gluteal nerve and artery.

C. Advantages: lowest dislocation rate out of all approaches, good exposure to acetabulum and femur.

D. Disadvantages: postoperative abductor weakness (Trendelenburg gait, up to 18%), high rate of heterotopic ossification (up to 47%).

E. Positioning can be lateral decubitus or supine.

F. Outcomes: no differences in clinical outcome between direct anterior, anterolateral, direct lateral, and posterior approaches.[6–8] No significant difference between dislocation rates between posterior (1.3%) and direct lateral surgical (4.2%) approaches has been describeD. The risk of nerve palsy appears to be significantly higher among the direct lateral approaches (20 vs. 2% for the posterior approach).[10]

IV. Posterolateral:

A. Interval: none: gluteus maximus split.

B. Dangers: sciatic nerve.

C. Advantages: abductor preservation, good exposure, easy to extend exposure, low overall complication rates, "workhorse approach."

D. Disadvantages: leg length discrepancy (to minimize dislocation risk), risk of foot drop and dislocation.

E. Outcomes: no differences in clinical outcome between the anterolateral, direct lateral, and posterior approaches. With the advent of a posterior capsular repair, dislocation rates of the posterior approach have been described as 0.79% (vs. 0.84% for direct anterior, vs. 4.2% for direct lateral vs. 3% for anterolateral approaches).[7-10]

Preoperative Templating

I. Goal: restore native hip biomechanics—offset, leg length, center of femoral head rotation.

II. Radiographic templating (**Fig. 20.2**)[11]:

A. Choose appropriate implants—Assess Dorr's classification[12]:

1. Dorr's classification forms the ratio of the inner canal diameter at midportion of the lesser trochanter divided by the diameter 10 cm distal to it.

a. Dorr A: ratio less than 0.5—consider uncemented stem , with a narrow distal geometry.

b. Dorr B: ratio 0.5 to 0.75—consider uncemented stem.

c. Dorr C: ratio greater than 0.75—consider cemented stem.

B. Determine component positioning:

1. Acetabulum usually set for 45 degrees of abduction and at the level of the inferior teardrop. Medialize to or near the teardrop.

2. Femoral neck cut length is measured, assure implant will wedge where coating exits, and assess the need for adjunct reamers.

C. Restore leg length, femoral offset—use other side if normal.

D. Assess for limb length and need for shortening osteotomy.

E. Evaluate any proximal femoral deformities that may need to be addressed.

Implant Fixation

I. Cemented THA[13]:

A. Utilizes polymethyl methacrylate (PMMA):

1. PMMA components[14]:

a. Liquid MMA monomer.

b. Powered MMA–styrene copolymer.

c. Stabilizer/inhibitor: hydroquinone (prevents premature polymerization).

d. Initiator: dibenzoyl peroxide.

e. Accelerator: N, N-dimethyl-p-toluidine (encourages polymer and monomer to polymerize at room temperature).

f. Opacifying agents: zirconium dioxide (ZrO_2) or barium sulfate ($BaSO_4$).

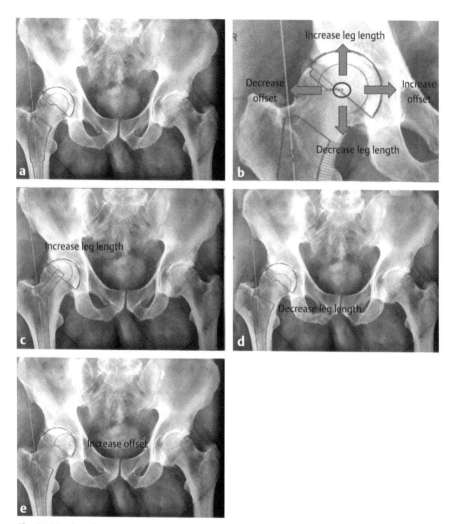

Fig. 20.2 Basics of preoperative templating a total hip arthroplasty. (**a**) Goal of templating: restore leg length and offset. Note how the center of rotation of the acetabular component and the femoral component matches. (**b**) If the center of rotation of the femoral component does not match the center of rotation of the acetabular component, then changes on leg length and offset result. (**c**) Example of increasing leg length: note how the center of femoral rotation is superior to the center of acetabular rotation. (**d**) Example of decreasing leg length: note how the center of femoral rotation is inferior to the center of acetabular rotation. (**e**) Example of increasing offset: note how the center of femoral rotation is medial to the center of acetabular rotation.

   g. Mixing of liquid MMA monomer and a powered MMA-styrene copoly-
    mer results in exothermic polymerization around the prepolymerized
    powder particles, generating a "PMMA grout."
  2. Stronger in compression than tension.
  3. Produces interlocking between surfaces ("grout").
 B. First described by Gluck in 1891 and popularized by Charnley in the 1950s.

C. Indications:
1. Dorr's type C femur (**Fig. 20.3**).
2. Elderly patients with osteoporotic bone.
3. Irradiated bone.
4. Controversial for acetabular component fixation due to higher rate of loosening at 9 to 12 years (31% cemented vs. 0% cementless).[15]

D. Technique:
1. Generations:
    a. First: hand mixed and finger packed.
    b. Second: cement restrictor, cement gun, and canal preparation.
    c. Third: vacuum mixing and cement pressurization.
    d. Fourth: heating the stem—greater interface shear strength of stem–cement interface, improvement of fatigue lifetimes, and decrease in interface porosity.[16]

2. Cement mantle:
    a. Avoid varus positioning of the stem.
    b. Increased rate of fracture with mantle less than 2 mm.
    c. Radiographic grading of the femoral cement technique[17]:
        i. Grade A: complete filling of medullary canal ("white out").
        ii. Grade B: minimal radiolucency at the bone–cement interface.
        iii. Grade C:
            (1) C1: radiolucency greater than 50% at the bone–cement interface.
            (2) C2: mantle less than 1 mm thick or stem touches bone.
        iv. Grade D: major defects in the mantle, or multiple large voids in the mantle, no cement distal to the stem tip.
        v. Significance: femoral cement mantle less than 1 mm, stem abutment against the femur and defects in the cement mantle → early loosening.[18,19]

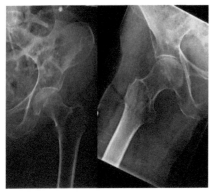

Fig. 20.3 Dorr's type C femur configuration. Note the wide canal with thin cortical walls ("stove pipe" femur).

3. Femoral stem:
   a. Surface morphology:
      i. Polished: Ra less than 1 μm, minimal abrasion, allows for stem subsidence and compressive loading of the cement mantle.
      ii. Matte: Ra less than 2 μm, no excessive abrasion unless micromotion, mechanical interlocking with cement.
      iii. Rough: Ra greater than 2 μm, excessive abrasion.
      iv. Outcomes: increased aseptic loosening with matte finish (10% at 10 years vs. 4% at 20 years with polished stem).[20]
   b. Implant design:
      i. Smooth surfaces without sharp edges to avoid stress concentration on implant–cement interface.
      ii. Wider laterally than medially to diffuse the compressive loads medially and tapered from proximal to distal to allow for subsidence within the cement mantle ("triple taper concept").
      iii. Mostly cobalt–chromium alloy stems → stiffer, generate less particulate debris than titanium implants (compared with mostly titanium implants in uncemented femoral stems).

II. Cementless THA stems and cups:
   A. Biologic fixation in which bone formation secures the implant:
      1. Bone ingrowth: bone grows into the porous coating.
      2. Bone ongrowth: bone grows onto the roughened surface (grit blasting vs. plasma spraying):
         a. Grit blasting: abrasive particles (aluminum oxide or corundum) create a textured surface.
         b. Plasma spraying: molten material is sprayed onto an implant to create a more textured surface.
         c. Hydroxyapatite (calcium phosphate compound): osteoconductive surface sprayed onto implant enhances bone growth.
   B. First FDA (Food and Drug Administration) approved implant in 1983 (anatomic medullary locking [AML] stem).
   C. In 2012, over 90% of THA in the United States were cementless.
   D. Technique:
      1. Press-fit: implant slightly larger than prepared surface (0.5–1 mm):
         a. Increased risk of fracture.
      2. Line-to-line: implant size equal to prepared surface.
   E. Biologic fixation and optimization (latest data show, for new implants is 60 to 70% porosity, interconnecting pores and pore sizes approximately 200 to 400 μm):
      1. Pore size: 50 to 150 μm.
      2. Porosity: 40 to 50%.
      3. Gaps: less than 50 μm.
      4. Micromotion: less than 150 μm.

5. Coefficient of friction: would like to be close to 1; it is ideal for the early fixation to have a coefficient of friction that will aid in limiting early micromotion.

F. Implant options:

1. Acetabular components:

a. Historically all-polyethylene cemented acetabular components were used.

b. It transitioned to noncemented acetabular components in the 1980s and has shown greater than 90% survivorship.

c. Contemporary components utilize a titanium porous coating:

i. Screw fixation is optional depending on stability.

ii. Hydroxyapatite coating may enhance bone ongrowth but use has been limited by cost.

2. Femoral components:

a. Names of sections of a femoral stem include:

i. Head, neck, trunnion, body.

b. Standard/primary femoral components:

i. Neck sparing stems: preserve bone and may limit stress shielding.

ii. Single taper stems (blade type): metaphyseal fixation.

iii. Double taper stems: metaphyseal fixation.

iv. Extensively porous-coated stems: metaphyseal/diaphyseal fixation:

(1) May increase stress shielding.

(2) Often laterality specific with anteversion built in to the prosthesis.

v. Anatomic stems: metaphyseal/diaphyseal fixation.

vi. Excellent clinical results with each subtype of noncemented femoral stems.

c. Modular/revision components:

i. In addition to modular heads, these implants incorporate at least one additional modular interface: may include stem, body, neck, and head.

ii. Allow for adjustment of femoral version, offset, length.

iii. Disadvantage: increased potential for motion, corrosion, and failure at additional interfaces, and price.

Bearing Surfaces

Bearing surfaces include the following[21]:

I. Metal on polyethylene:

A. Most common bearing surface with the longest track record.

B. Types of polyethylene:

1. Standard.

2. Ultra-high-molecular-weight polyethylene (high cross-linked): cross-linking provides improved wear properties but results in decreased toughness:

a. Free radicals are removed through remelting or annealing:

i. Remelting: thermal processing above the melting temperature (~150°C).

ii. Annealing: thermal processing just below melting temperature (~110°C).

b. Standard of care in most THAs.

3. Antioxidant impregnated: may decrease free radicals and improve wear characteristics but evidence is limited:

a. Vitamin-E-impregnated polyethylene has been used clinically since 2007:

i. Implanted at a rate of 1.6% of all THAs, according to the AJRR 2016 report.

ii. At 5 years, vitamin E–diffused highly cross-linked polyethylene liners had similar wear as previous generation medium cross-linked polyethylene.[22]

II. Ceramic on polyethylene:

A. Composition of ceramic heads:

1. Alumina (aluminum oxide).

2. Zirconia: improved burst strength and toughness.

3. Biolox delta: 17% zirconia and 82% alumina.

B. Improved wear characteristics:

1. Ceramic has excellent geometric form and wettable surface, enhances hardness, thereby maintaining lubrication, and increases resistance to third-body wear.

C. Increased cost of ceramic.

D. Outcomes:

1. When compared with metal-on-polyethylene bearings, ceramic-on-polyethylene bearings have reduced risk of infection (hazard ratio [HR]: 0.86) and reduced risk of dislocation (HR: 0.81) and mortality (HR: 0.92), but no significant difference in risk of revision 8 to 9 years after surgery.[23]

III. Metal-on-metal (MoM):

A. Cobalt chromium alloy, titanium alloy, and very early stainless steel.

B. Improved wear characteristics compared with metal-on-polyethylene bearings with lower volume of wear particles.

C. Increased metal ion level may lead to a delay type IV hypersensitivity reaction:

1. Cell-mediated, not antibody-mediated response.

2. CD4+ Th1 helper T cells recognize antigen/MHC (major histocompatibility complex) class II on the surface of antigen-presenting cells.

3. CD4⁺ T cells induce further release of other Th1 cell cytokines, triggering an immune response.

4. Activated CD8⁺ T cells destroy target cells on contact.

D. Pseudotumor formation.

E. No proven cancer link.

F. Potential for delayed hypersensitivity reactions and organ toxicity.

G. Metal particles may cross the placental barrier but no evidence of teratogenicity.

H. Largely abandoned due to "MoM" complications.

I. Metal particles can induce local tissue reactions:

1. Inflammatory responses, necrosis, and pseudotumor.

2. Aseptic lymphocyte-dominant vasculitis-associated lesion (ALVAL)/ adverse local tissue reaction (ALTR):

a. ALVAL: a 10-point histologic scoring system predicting the degree of ALVAL via examination of synovial lining, inflammatory cells, and tissue organization has been developed.[24]

b. ALTR: includes all adverse responses resulting from wear-related and biologic causes. Can occur in asymptomatic, well-functioning MoM hip arthroplasties.

c. Metal artifact reduction sequence MRI is used to detect ALTR.

IV. Ceramic on ceramic:

A. Lowest wear rate of all currently available bearing surfaces.

B. Risk of "squeaking":

1. Associated with malpositioned components (edge loading):

a. May be caused by abnormalities in fluid film lubrication.

2. Australian National Joint Registry demonstrated a 4.2% incidence of squeaking.

C. Risk of fracture: decreased with modern, fourth-generation, ceramic heads[25]:

1. Alumina ceramic heads: 0.021%.

2. Biolox delta heads: 0.003%.

3. Fracture risk of acetabular lines stable at 0.03%.

4. Fracture risk decreases as head diameter increases.

Hip Hemiarthroplasty

I. Replacement with femoral component only, with retention of native acetabulum.

II. Indications (controversial)[26]:

A. Femoral neck fractures in the elderly with low functional demands and activity level:

1. Lower dislocation rate than THA.

2. Contraindicated in the presence of acetabular disease:

a. Acetabular cartilage damage/wear may result in pain, requiring conversion to a THA.

Hip Resurfacing

I. Resurfacing of the femoral head without significant bone resection:

   A. MoM bearing surface.

   B. Increased femoral head size (improved stability).

II. Best outcomes in young males with good bone stock.

III. Contraindications:

   A. Absolute: advanced age, osteoporosis, bone stock deficiency (prior fracture/infection, osteonecrosis, rapidly progressive osteoarthritis), cystic changes, hip dysplasia, small acetabulum.

   B. Relative: female gender, coxa vara or leg length discrepancies.

IV. Complications:

   A. Periprosthetic fracture:

      1. Significantly higher than THA (up to 4%).

   B. Elevated metal ion levels and pseudotumor.

   C. Largely abandoned due to "MoM" complications.

Complications

I. Periprosthetic joint infection (PJI)[27]:

   A. Incidence: 1% primary THA; 3 to 5% revision THA.

   B. Risk factors: immunosuppression, prior wound infection, poor wound healing, rheumatoid arthritis, psoriasis, diabetes, smoking, obesity.

   C. Clinical presentation:

      1. Pain: every painful THA should be considered infected until proven otherwise.

      2. Acute onset swelling, erythema, tenderness, warmth.

      3. Draining wound or draining sinus.

   D. Workup:

      1. Serum screening tools:

         a. Erythrocyte sedimentation rate (normalizes 3 months after surgery).

         b. C-reactive protein (normalizes 3 weeks after surgery).

      2. If one or both are elevated: joint aspiration—greater than 3,000 WBC/μL and greater than 80% (PMN) differential concerning for infection.

      3. Radiographs can present with generalized bone resorption, periosteal reaction. In acute infection, often not helpful.

   E. Classification:

      1. Acute postoperative PJI: within 3 weeks of surgery. Often *Staphylococcus aureus*, β-hemolytic strep, gram-negative bacteria.

      2. Chronic PJI: 3 months to years after surgery. Often coagulase-negative Staphylococcus, gram-negative bacteria.

      3. Acute hematogenous PJI: acute onset pain in a previously well-functioning THA.

F. Treatment:

1. Irrigation and debridement with head/liner exchange: consider for acute postoperative PJI and acute hematogenous PJI. Depending on offending organism, approximately 50% success rate.

2. Two-stage exchange (initial resection arthroplasty with antibiotic spacer placement, 6 weeks of organism-directed iv antibiotics, revision THA when infection cleared): gold standard in the United States for chronic PJI; approximately 80% success rate.

3. Chronic antibiotic suppression: patients who are unfit for or refuse surgery. Success rate of 10 to 25%.

4. Hip disarticulation/Girdlestone's procedure: recalcitrant infections.

II. Dislocation:

A. Incidence: 1% after primary THA.

B. Risk factors:

1. Prior hip surgery, female gender, older than 80 years, drug/alcohol abuse, posterior approach.

2. Component positioning: acetabular component—40-degree abduction, 15-degree anteversion.

3. Component design: decreased head-to-neck ratio.

4. Soft-tissue tension: decreased offset.

5. Soft-tissue function: neuromuscular dysfunction (Parkinson's, multiple sclerosis, stroke, etc.), prior muscle trauma/injury.

C. Clinical presentation:

1. Often directly related to "at-risk" activities.

2. Anterior dislocation: external rotation and hip extension.

3. Posterior dislocation: internal rotation and hip flexion.

4. Infection parameters.

D. Imaging:

1. Diagnostic: AP pelvis, AP/frog-leg lateral/cross-table lateral hip.

E. Treatment:

1. Closed reduction: two-thirds of early hip dislocations are successfully treated with closed reduction.

2. Revision THA: indicated for recurrent dislocations due to component malpositioning (vertical and retroverted acetabular component), polyethylene wear.

3. Resection arthroplasty with antibiotic spacer: for PJI.

III. Neurovascular injuries:

A. Nerve injuries:

1. Incidence: up to 3%.

2. Causes: aberrant retractor placement, compression, excessive tension.

3. Peroneal branch of the sciatic nerve most commonly affected.

    4. Risk factors: revision THA, female, lengthening of extremity greater than 4 cm, congenital hip dysplasia.

    5. Outcome: one-third full recovery, one-third partial recovery, one-third permanent palsy.

B. Vascular injuries:

    1. Causes: during screw insertion, penetrating instruments/retractors.

    2. Incidence: less than 1%.

    3. Hip quadrant system for safe insertion of screws[28]:

        a. Posterosuperior quadrant: "safe zone."

        b. Posteroinferior quadrant: risks injury to sciatic nerve, inferior gluteal vessels/nerve, inferior pudendal vessels/nerve.

        c. Anteroinferior quadrant: risks injury to obturator vessels/nerve.

        d. Anterosuperior quadrant: "zone of death"—risks injury to external iliac vessels.

IV. Heterotopic ossification:

A. Traditionally common complication: up to 80%.

B. Risk factors: aggressive soft-tissue handling, traditional Hardinge approach, long surgical time.

C. Prophylaxis: NSAIDs (classically—indomethacin 25 mg three times a day for 6 weeks), single-dose postoperative radiation within 72 hour postoperative (700 Gy).

V. Venous thromboembolic events (VTE)[29]:

A. Up to 60% after THA WITHOUT any postoperative VTE prophylaxis.

B. Risk factors: Virchow's triad (venostasis, endothelial damage, hypercoagulable state), previous VTE, cancer, old age, oral contraceptives, hypercoagulable states, obesity.

C. Clinical presentation: leg swelling, redness, calf tenderness, shortness of breath, tachycardia, chest pain, hypotension, cyanosis.

D. Diagnosis: venography, ultrasonography, CT angiogram for pulmonary embolism.

E. Prophylaxis:

    1. Intraoperative: reduced surgical time, regional anesthesia/spinal.

    2. Postoperative: early mobilization, pneumatic leg compression devices, and chemical prophylaxis. Chemical prophylaxis may include aspirin, warfarin, LMWH (low-molecular-weight heparin), or novel factor X-inhibitors.

VI. Polyethylene wear/osteolysis:

A. Pathogenesis: particulate debris → macrophage activation → osteolysis → prosthesis micromotion → component loosening.

B. Risk factors: long shelf life of polyethylene liners, air sterilization, young age.

C. Diagnosis:

    1. Plain radiographs (often underestimate degree of osteolysis).

    2. MRI and CT with metal artifact reduction protocols have been developed to effectively visualize osteolytic lesions and measure wear.[30]

    D. Treatment: revision THA if symptomatic, imminent wear liner through, recurrent dislocations/instability.

VII. Corrosion reactions in metal-on-polyethylene THA[31,32]:

    A. Mechanically assisted corrosion at the trunnion → metallic debris → hypersensitivity reaction → joint effusion, ALTRs, pseudotumors, tissue destruction.

    B. Lymphocyte-driven reaction (vs. macrophage-driven reaction of polyethylene-associated osteolysis).

    C. Presentation: hip pain.

    D. Diagnosis:

        1. Radiographs: often lytic lesion medial calcar.

        2. Metal ion levels: cobalt and chromium:

            a. Cobalt levels greater than 1 parts per billion (ppb) concerning.

            b. Cobalt elevation greater than chromium elevation.

            c. MRI: assess for fluid collections, pseudotumors, abductor loss.

    E. Treatment: change Co-Cr head to ceramic head with titanium option taper.

Conclusion

THA continues to be one of the most successful procedures in orthopaedics. Thorough preoperative clinical/radiographic evaluation and preoperative planning optimize chances of a successful outcome. Several surgical approaches can be chosen to perform a THA with fairly similar outcomes. THA can be performed in either cemented or uncemented fashion; preoperative assessment of bone morphology can aid in decision-making. Numerous bearing surfaces are available for THA with intrinsic risks and benefits, with metal-on-polyethylene and ceramic-on-polyethylene bearings being the most commonly used surfaces. Complications following THA are rare but are potentially devastating and have to be carefully discussed with the patient preoperatively.

References

1. Lewallen D. Primary total hip arthroplasty: anterolateral and direct lateral approaches. In: Lieberman J, Berry D, eds. Advanced Reconstruction Hip. Rosemont, IL: American Academy for Orthopaedic Surgeons; 2005:11–16

2. Pelicci P, Su E. Primary total hip arthroplasty: posterolateral approach. In: Lieberman J, Berry D, eds. Advanced Reconstruction Hip. Rosemont, IL: American Academy for Orthopaedic Surgeons; 2005:3–10

3. Malek IA, Royce G, Bhatti SU, et al. A comparison between the direct anterior and posterior approaches for total hip arthroplasty: the role of an "enhanced recovery" pathway. Bone Joint J 2016;98-B(6):754–760

4. Poehling-Monaghan KL, Kamath AF, Taunton MJ, Pagnano MW. Direct anterior versus miniposterior THA with the same advanced perioperative protocols: surprising early clinical results. Clin Orthop Relat Res 2015;473(2):623–631

5. Parvizi J, Restrepo C, Maltenfort MG. Total hip arthroplasty performed through direct anterior approach provides superior early outcome: results of a randomized, prospective study. Orthop Clin North Am 2016;47(3):497–504

6. De Anta-Díaz B, Serralta-Gomis J, Lizaur-Utrilla A, Benavidez E, López-Prats FA. No differences between direct anterior and lateral approach for primary total hip arthroplasty related to muscle damage or functional outcome. Int Orthop 2016;40(10):2025–2030

7. Maratt JD, Gagnier JJ, Butler PD, Hallstrom BR, Urquhart AG, Roberts KC. No difference in dislocation seen in anterior vs posterior approach total hip arthroplasty. J Arthroplasty 2016;31(Suppl 9):127–130

8. Greidanus NV, Chihab S, Garbuz DS, et al. Outcomes of minimally invasive anterolateral THA are not superior to those of minimally invasive direct lateral and posterolateral THA. Clin Orthop Relat Res 2013;471(2):463–471

9. Lindgren V, Garellick G, Kärrholm J, Wretenberg P. The type of surgical approach influences the risk of revision in total hip arthroplasty: a study from the Swedish Hip Arthroplasty Register of 90,662 total hipreplacements with 3 different cemented prostheses. Acta Orthop 2012;83(6):559–565

10. Jolles BM, Bogoch ER. Posterior versus lateral surgical approach for total hip arthroplasty in adults with osteoarthritis. Cochrane Database Syst Rev 2006;(3):CD003828

11. Della Valle AG, Padgett DE, Salvati EA. Preoperative planning for primary total hip arthroplasty. J Am Acad Orthop Surg 2005;13(7):455–462

12. Dorr LD, Absatz M, Gruen TA, Saberi MT, Doerzbacher JF. Anatomic porous replacement hip arthroplasty: first 100 consecutive cases. Semin Arthroplasty 1990;1(1):77–86

13. Corten K, Bourne RB, Charron KD, Au K, Rorabeck CH. Comparison of total hip arthroplasty performed with and without cement: a randomized trial. A concise follow-up, at twenty years, of previous reports. J Bone Joint Surg Am 2011;93(14):1335–1338

14. Vaishya R, Chauhan M, Vaish A. Bone cement. J Clin Orthop Trauma 2013;4(4):157–163

15. Clohisy JC, Harris WH. Matched-pair analysis of cemented and cementless acetabular reconstruction in primary total hip arthroplasty. J Arthroplasty 2001;16(6):697–705

16. Iesaka K, Jaffe WL, Kummer FJ. Effects of preheating of hip prostheses on the stem-cement interface. J Bone Joint Surg Am 2003;85(3):421–427

17. Barrack RL, Mulroy RD Jr, Harris WH. Improved cementing techniques and femoral component loosening in young patients with hip arthroplasty. A 12-year radiographic review. J Bone Joint Surg Br 1992;74(3):385–389

18. Mulroy WF, Estok DM, Harris WH. Total hip arthroplasty with use of so-called second-generation cementing techniques. A fifteen-year-average follow-up study. J Bone Joint Surg Am 1995;77(12):1845–1852

19. Jasty M, Maloney WJ, Bragdon CR, Haire T, Harris WH. Histomorphological studies of the long-term skeletal responses to well fixed cemented femoral components. J Bone Joint Surg Am 1990;72(8):1220–1229

20. Howie DW, Middleton RG, Costi K. Loosening of matt and polished cemented femoral stems. J Bone Joint Surg Br 1998;80(4):573–576

21. Jacobs JJ. Bearing Surfaces. Rosemont, IL: American Academy for Orthopaedic Surgeons; 2005

22. Nebergall AK, Greene ME, Laursen MB, Nielsen PT, Malchau H, Troelsen A. Vitamin E diffused highly cross-linked polyethylene in total hip arthroplasty at five years: a randomised controlled trial using radiostereometric analysis. Bone Joint J 2017;99-B(5):577–584

23. Kurtz SM, Lau E, Baykal D, Springer BD. Outcomes of ceramic bearings after primary total hip arthroplasty in the Medicare population. J Arthroplasty 2017;32(3):743–749

24. Campbell P, Ebramzadeh E, Nelson S, Takamura K, De Smet K, Amstutz HC. Histological features of pseudotumor-like tissues from metal-on-metal hips. Clin Orthop Relat Res 2010;468(9):2321–2327

25. Massin P, Lopes R, Masson B, Mainard D; French Hip & Knee Society (SFHG). Does Biolox delta ceramic reduce the rate of component fractures in total hip replacement? Orthop Traumatol Surg Res 2014;100(6, Suppl):S317–S321

26. Baker RP, Squires B, Gargan MF, Bannister GC. Total hip arthroplasty and hemiarthroplasty in mobile, independent patients with a displaced intracapsular fracture of the femoral neck. A randomized, controlled trial. J Bone Joint Surg Am 2006;88(12):2583–2589

27. Della Valle C, Parvizi J, Bauer TW, et al; American Academy of Orthopaedic Surgeons. American Academy of Orthopaedic Surgeons clinical practice guideline on: the diagnosis of periprosthetic joint infections of the hip and knee. J Bone Joint Surg Am 2011;93(14):1355–1357

28. Wasielewski RC, Crossett LS, Rubash HE. Neural and vascular injury in total hip arthroplasty. Orthop Clin North Am 1992;23(2):219–235
29. Jacobs JJ, Mont MA, Bozic KJ, et al. American Academy of Orthopaedic Surgeons clinical practice guideline on: preventing venous thromboembolic disease in patients undergoing elective hip and knee arthroplasty. J Bone Joint Surg Am 2012;94(8):746–747
30. Ries MD, Link TM. Monitoring and risk of progression of osteolysis after total hip arthroplasty. Instr Course Lect 2013;62:207–214
31. Cooper HJ, Della Valle CJ, Berger RA, et al. Corrosion at the head-neck taper as a cause for adverse local tissue reactions after total hip arthroplasty. J Bone Joint Surg Am 2012;94(18):1655–1661
32. Jennings JM, Dennis DA, Yang CC. Corrosion of the head-neck junction after total hip arthroplasty. J Am Acad Orthop Surg 2016;24(6):349–356

21 Revision Total Hip Arthroplasty

Brett R. Levine

Etiology

I. Instability (22.5% of revision cases in 2005–2006[1] and 17.3% of revision cases in 2009–2013[2]):

    A. Dislocation is often reported to occur in 1 to 3% of cases of primary cases but is dependent on surgeon experience, approach, patient factors, and implants.

        1. Early—within the first 6 weeks to 6 months postoperative:

            a. Assess component position—combined anteversion of the stem and the cup:

                i. Recently, an emphasis has been placed on the total anteversion of the hip arthroplasty construct and not necessarily on one component in isolation.[3]

                ii. Lewinnek's safe zone: 40 ± 10 degrees for cup inclination and 15 ± 10 degrees of acetabular anteversion[4]:

                    (1) This so-called safe zone has been questioned in recent studies:

                        (a) Fifty-eight percent of dislocated total hip arthroplasties (THAs) were within the aforementioned "safe zone."[5]

                    (2) Proponents of combined anteversion have published on approximately 37 degrees as a safe number when combining that of the stem and the cup, with a range of 25 to 50 degrees.[3]

            b. Trauma—often an injury that extenuates the range of motion of the hip (extension and external rotation [ER] = anterior dislocation and flexion and internal rotation [IR] = posterior dislocation).

            c. Abductor insufficiency:

                i. Primary—failed repair, more common with direct lateral approach, denervation from superior gluteal nerve (SGN) injury.

                ii. Secondary—greater trochanter (GT) fracture.

            d. Exceed range-of-motion parameters—impingement of neck on cup (which is why the goal in primary abductor insufficiency is to maximize head-to-neck ratio when possible):

                i. Anterior dislocation—extension and ER.

                ii. Posterior dislocation—flexion, adduction and IR.

        2. Late—after 6 months; if it does not occur early, it typically occurs years later:

            a. Assess component position—pay attention to combined anteversion of the implants:

                i. Serial radiographs are important as dislocation may be the first symptoms of aseptic loosening of the implants.

      ii. Cups may migrate into more vertical and retroverted position.

      iii. Stem may have subsided, leading to impingement or abductor insufficiency.

      iv. Elevated rims or prominent liners may decrease the range of motion to impingement and lead to THA instability.

  b. Trauma—may be related to altered mental status, proprioception, or the development of neuromuscular disorders with age.

  c. Abductor insufficiency:

      i. Primary—muscle weakness, failed repair (with direct lateral approach or GT osteotomy), denervation from prior SGN injury.

      ii. Secondary—late GT fracture (can occur around stress-shielded proximal bone), progressive neuromuscular disease, due to the destruction caused by an adverse local tissue reaction (trunnion or articular surface–generated metal debris).

  d. Polyethylene (PE) wear—component fracture with highly cross-linked polyethylene (seen with vertical component positioning and thin liner [≤3 mm]);[6] sufficient wear to allow hip instability.

B. Subluxation:

  1. Sensation of instability without frank dislocation:

    a. Often a prelude to dislocation—feels a clunk or shifting inside.

    b. Watch patient closely and assess parameters above for early or late dislocation.

II. Infection[7] (14.8% of revision cases in 2005–2006[1] and 12.8% of revision surgeries in 2009–2013[2]):

A. Acute (within 3–4 weeks postoperative; controversial as far as time is concerned; many will suggest up to 6 weeks is still an acute infection):

  1. CDC (Centers for Disease Control and Prevention) suggest less than 90 days is considered an acute infection.

  2. Biofilms tend to form by 4 weeks and beyond on the surface of the implants, greatly impacting the success of component retention.

B. Chronic (>4 weeks postoperative; again controversial; many will consider infection chronic after 6 weeks):

  1. CDC suggest greater than 90 days as the cutoff for a chronic infection.

  2. Infection likely has invaded deeper and can penetrate the bone–prosthetic interface and even lead to osteomyelitis.

C. Acute hematogenous:

  1. Can occur after dental procedures.

  2. Any illness that may cause sepsis.

  3. Bacterial load then supersedes the body defenses and seeds the replaced joint.

III. Component loosening (19.7% of revision cases in 2005–2006[1] and 16.8% of revision surgeries in 2009–2013[2]): This is often associated with start-up pain in the groin (cup loosening) or the thigh (stem loosening).

A. Aseptic: failure of bone ingrowth/ongrowth—if osseointegration does not occur early, typically a fibrous layer will form, preventing future fixation and leaving, at best, a fibrous-stable implant:

1. Early micromotion—fixation failure, component subsidence.

2. Gap—not enough host bone–implant contact.

3. Fracture—acetabular or femoral fracture with loosening.

4. Osteolysis—wear-related bone loss leads to secondary loosening.

5. Poor bone quality—irradiated bone, osteonecrosis, pagetoid bone.

6. Poor material—not optimal ingrowth (pore: size [historically 50–150 μm, but more recently we see 200–400 μm], interconnectivity, strength)/ongrowth surface, low surface coefficient of friction, poor biocompatibility, higher modulus of elasticity.

B. Septic—chronic/acute infection leads to loss of fixation or prevents early fixation.

IV. PE wear ± osteolysis[8] (5.0% [bearing wear] and 6.6% [osteolysis] of revision cases in 2005–2006[1] and 4.7% [bearing wear] and 5.7% [osteolysis] of revision surgeries in 2009–2013[2]): This is often insidious in onset and can range from minor discomfort to pain and loss of abductor function.

A. Bearing wear often goes hand in hand with osteolysis; local particulate-induced synovitis can cause pain or wear can be bad enough to lead to metallosis (head wears into the metallic cup), dislocation, or subluxation:

1. Wear is defined as the loss of material associated with two surfaces sliding over each other during motion that involves loading:

a. Typically occurs through abrasion, adhesion, fatigue, and third-body debris.

b. Volumetric wear is typically the most significant indicator of particle quantity that is being generated.

c. Highly cross-linked PE has less wear, generates smaller but a greater quantity of particles, and results in less wear-associated osteolysis.[8]

B. Osteolysis is typically related to wear debris being removed by the body; it can lead to weakened bone and subsequent periprosthetic fracture or component loosening:

1. Lower degrees of annual wear lead to less osteolysis:

a. Typically wear less than 80 mm^3 per year does not lead to osteolysis, while greater than 140 mm^3 per year leads to significant osteolysis.[9]

2. Degree of bone loss is associated with the particle type, number, density, and size:

a. Particles of PE between 0.3 and 1.0 μm are the most potent simulators of local phagocytic cells; when smaller than 0.3 μm, they are eliminated via pinocytosis and not phagocytosis-related mechanisms.

b. Biological mechanisms associated with wear particles and removal follow a predictable pathway involving the following:

i. Macrophages, cell receptors, an inflammatory process, and release of cytokines—all resulting in the destructive process found with osteolysis.

V.   Modern bearing issues (i.e., metal-on-metal [MoM] bearings; ceramic-on-ceramic [CoC] bearings): Many times, this is a delayed diagnosis as radiographs and clinical examination could be benign initially.

  A. Metallosis can be due to component design, positioning, and stability:

   1. MoM—articular bearing surface debris is worse with a vertical cup, which can lead to edge loading; this can be further potentiated by head–neck corrosion/multiple trunnions; **Table 21.1**[10]):

    a. Many modern implants have been removed from the market due to adverse reactions to MoM debris.[11]

   2. Soft-tissue effects can occur with all bearing couples and is often related to metallic debris from bearing or associated with mechanically assisted crevice corrosion (MACC) or similar process (**Table 21.2**[10]):

    a. Adverse local tissue reaction (ALTR)/Aseptic lymphocyte–dominated immunologic response (ALVAL)—represents a spectrum of soft-tissue reactions, ranging from small masses to large fluid collections that can be locally destructive.

    b. Pseudotumor—among the worst manifestations of an adverse local tissue reaction as this mass is locally destructive and difficult to manage despite not being a malignancy.

   3. Systemic responses—elevated metal levels (namely, cobaltism) have been reported to have potential effects on end organs such as kidneys, central nervous system, heart, thyroid, and eyes.[12]

  B. Ceramic bearings: Fracture and squeaking are two etiologies for ceramic bearings that often can be diagnosed clinically or on follow-up radiographs.

   1. Component fracture—often related to trauma, component impingement, or incomplete seating of the femoral head or ceramic liner:

    a. More common with alumina bearings and metal-backed ceramic liners.

    b. Femoral head fracture—historically reported to be between 0.021 and 0.002%[13]:

     i. Incidence ranges from 0.009% with most modern Biolox Delta heads to 0.119% with the Biolox Forte heads[14]:

      (1) Risk factors include smaller head size (28-mm Biolox Forte heads with 0.382% fractures) and higher body mass index (BMI).[14]

    c. Acetabular liner fracture:

     i. Incidence ranges from 0.126% with Biolox Delta liners to 0.112% with Biolox Forte liners.[14]

     ii. Overall rates range from 0.028 to 2%, depending on the liner type and case series[15]:

      (1) Risk factors include smaller head size and higher BMI; liner thickness did not impact the fracture rate.[14]

      (2) Technical errors have been noted to cause these problems as well.[15]

   2. Squeaking—micro-separation and alterations led to a squeaking noise in specific designs; incidence: approximately 1.4[16] to 21%.[17,18]

Table 21.1 Metal-on-metal total hip arthroplasty classification for failures

Type	Description	Treatment Recommendations
1	Metal sensitivity: stable, well- aligned acetabular component, elevated metal ions, and pain	Revise bearing only to metal-polyethylene or ceramic-polyethylene if modular cup; if monoblock cup, revise cup with metal-polyethylene or ceramic-polyethylene bearing
2	Malpositioned cup: stable, malaligned acetabular component, elevated metal ions, and pain	Revise cup with metal-polyethylene or ceramic-polyethylene bearing
3	Loose cup	Revise cup with metal-polyethylene or ceramic-polyethylene bearing
4	Early failure cups: acetabular components with known high early failure rates	Revise cup with metal-polyethylene or ceramic-polyethylene bearing
5	Iliopsoas impingement: ion levels within normal limits, cup retroverted	Iliopsoas release or revise cup to optimal position with metal-polyethylene or ceramic- polyethylene bearing

Source: Adapted with permission from Fabi D, Levine B, Paprosky W, et al. Metal-on-metal total hip arthroplasty: Causes and high incidence of early failure. Orthopaedics 2012;35(7):1009–1016.

Table 21.2   Classification system for soft-tissue complications after metal-on-metal total hip arthroplasty

Type Intraoperative Description	Treatment Options
I. Intracapsular effusion, capsule intact	Revise bearing and/or cup if needed. Stability is less of an issue.
II. Extracapsular effusion, capsule affected, abductors intact	Revise bearing and/or cup if needed. Stability is more of an issue.
III. Capsule affected, abductors affected	Revise bearing and/or cup if needed. Stability severely compromised. Consider a constrained liner and other salvage options.

Source: Adapted with permission from Fabi D, Levine B, Paprosky W, et al. Metal-on-metal total hip arthroplasty: Causes and high incidence of early failure. Orthopaedics 2012;35(7):1009–1016.

3. In general, COC bearing–related revisions occur early (within 4 years of index procedure) and are related to squeaking or fracture. This represented 12.2% (23 cases of fracture and 6 cases of squeaking included) of the revision cases in the COC of cohort in a study by the French Society for Orthopaedic Surgery and Traumatology (SoFCOT) study group.[19]

4. Liner dissociation has been reported to be a problem as well, as these implants need to be correctly placed and fitted within a morse-type taper:

   a. Rates have been reported to be as high as 16%.[15]

VI. Soft-tissue impingement (i.e., iliopsoas impingement): hard to quantify percentage from large databases based on coding; reports up to 4.3% found in the literature[20]:

A. Iliopsoas impingement—large diameter femoral heads, retroverted cups, prominent acetabular rim.[21]

    B. Iliopsoas impingement is a potential cause for persistent groin pain after THA—typically found with pain on resisted hip flexion:

        1. Typical options to manage iliopsoas tendon impingement include injections, tenotomy, and acetabular revision.

        2. Recently, Chalmers et al reported more predictable groin pain resolution with ≥8 mm of anterior acetabular component overhang and revision THA surgery.[22]

VII. Catastrophic failure (9.9% of revision cases in 2005–2006[1] and 3.3% of revision surgeries in 2009–2013[2]—numbers may be underestimated as coding could overlap with other mechanical complication or problem):

    A. Stem fracture—typically a fatigue fracture related to the portion of a stem remaining well fixed, while there is motion to the rest of the implant:

        1. Often found with long, cylindrical, cobalt–chromium (CoCr) stems:

           a. Cemented or cementless stem that can be potted distally without significant support proximally.

           b. Not uncommon in the cases with stem diameter ≤13 mm (remember the strength of the stem is the radius to the fourth power in these scenarios).

    B. Liner fracture—more common with COC bearings and highly cross-linked PE with thin areas around locking mechanisms (see earlier sections).

    C. Modular component failure—difficult to put an exact number on these cases but typically involve an implant with a head–neck taper and a neck–body taper:

        1. Titanium modular necks associated with fractures in 0.5 to 6% cases.[23–25]

        2. CoCr modular necks associated with corrosion and ALTRs.

        3. Obesity, larger head diameters, and longer offset and length necks may be prone to fracture and/or corrosion processes.

        4. Could also be due to implant design or manufacture itself (0.2 vs. 1.5% fracture rate between two companies with the same design of implant).[26]

Diagnosis

Multiple modalities are available for making the correct diagnosis prior to revision THA and start with basic imaging and move to more advanced examinations and laboratory tests.

I. Plain radiography—standard radiographs are typically the first line in making the diagnosis after a complete history and physical examination; serial radiographs are critical to making the diagnosis and should include preoperative, immediate postoperative and any available follow-up radiographs[27]:

    A. Anteroposterior (AP) pelvis: A good AP pelvis is required to assess the pelvic ring and SI (sacroiliac) joints as well as the hip replacement components and contralateral hip.

        1. Important to assess the following regions/landmarks and lines:

           a. Shenton's line—look to see if this is intact, close, or at least comparable to the contralateral hip (if native); it can help judge offset and limb lengths.

           b. Measure component abduction angle using the interteardrop or obturator line.

c. Assess component migration from the line at the superior obturator foramen.

d. The ilioischial line helps determine medial migration and integrity of the medial wall.

e. A rough estimate of limb lengths can be assessed by the relative heights of the lesser trochanters on both sides of the hip compared with inter-teardrop, obturator, or transischial line.

f. The ischium and ileum should be assessed for bone quality, osteolysis, and overall integrity.

g. Assess for progressive osteolysis behind the acetabular component and radiolucent lines in the DeLee and Charnley zones[28]:

   i. Udomkiat et al reported on the following criteria for cementless acetabular loosening[29]:

   (1) Radiolucent line initially appearing ≥2 years after surgery.

   (2) Progressive radiolucent lines after year 2.

   (3) Circumferential radiolucent line.

   (4) Component migration.

   (5) Radiolucent line in any zone greater than 2 mm.

h. Acetabular defects can be graded based on the Paprosky classification[30] (**Table 21.3**).

Table 21.3 Paprosky's classification for acetabular defects[30]

	Radiographic findings	Anticipated bone defects
Type 1 Minimal bone loss	No migration Minimal osteolysis	Completely supportive bone
Type 2 Columns intact and supportive	2A: superomedial migration, no ischial osteolysis, and teardrop intact	Migration <2 cm superiorly Superior dome defect, but rim intact
	2B: superolateral migration, no ischial osteolysis, and teardrop intact	Migration <2 cm superiorly Superior dome defect with rim defect
	2C: straight medial migration, teardrop is lost, minimal ischial osteolysis	Migration <2 cm superiorly Medial wall defect or absent
Type 3 Columns nonsupportive	3A: "Up and out"—superior migration, teardrop partially intact, severe medial and ischial osteolysis	Migration >2 cm superiorly Kohler's line is intact 30–60% host bone–implant contact anticipated Severe loss of supportive acetabular rim
	3B: "Up and in"—superior migration, teardrop lost, severe medial and ischial osteolysis, possible pelvic discontinuity	Migration >2 cm superiorly Kohler's line is lost Up to 60% host bone–implant contact anticipated Severe loss of supportive acetabular rim

B. AP hip—if performed correctly, it should give a good look at the GT and the remainder of the femoral neck:

1. Along with the earlier findings on the AP pelvis, it is important to assess the following:

   a. The GT for evidence of osteolysis, stress shielding, and fracture.

   b. The femoral stem should be assessed for spot welds (usually at the area where the component coating ends), which signifies a well-fixed implant as does proximal stress shielding.

   c. Radiolucent lines particularly around the coated portion of the stem are concerning if circumferential or progressive:

      i. In portions of the stem without coating, it is not uncommon to see radiolucent lines surrounding this area.

      ii. Lines and areas of osteolysis are best described by the Gruen zones—seven on the AP and seven on the lateral radiograph (start lateral to medial and anterior to posterior).[31]

   d. Calcar resorption can signify stress shielding and wear-related osteolysis; presence of a pseudotumor versus calcar hypertrophy under a collared implant often means the bone is being inappropriately loaded by a loose stem.[32]

   e. Cemented stems are suspicious for loosening if you see subsidence, cement mantle fracture, implant–cement debonding (often at the shoulder of the implant), or progressive radiolucent lines between cement and stem, stem fracture.[33]

   f. Heterotopic ossification should be assessed and graded along the Brooker classification[34]:

      i. Stage I—bone islands seen within adjacent soft tissues.

      ii. Stage II—bone extending from the femur and/or the pelvis with at least 1 cm of space between them.

      iii. Stage III—bone extending from the femur and/or the pelvis with less than 1 cm of space between them.

      iv. Stage IV—bony ankylosis of the hip.

   g. Femoral remodeling is important to ascertain, as varus or valgus remodeling may make it hard to extract and/or implant a new femoral component.

   h. Pedestal formation is a dense area of bone often at the tip of a stem that is loose and pistons up and down against the reactive bone:

      i. It can be very difficult to get through and may require a femoral osteotomy to expose the pedestal.

   i. Femoral defects can be classified by the Paprosky classification[35] (**Table 21.4**).

C. Frog-leg lateral—good to assess the proximal femur for deformity and remodeling.

D. Shoot through lateral—can assess acetabular version (at least a relative estimate); femoral head prominence (in large diameter THAs); can evaluate ischial bone quality and possible discontinuity.

Table 21.4 Paprosky's classification of femoral defects[35]

Type	Characteristics	Treatment options
I	Minimal bone loss, intact metaphysis and diaphysis	Proximal or distal fixed stems can be utilized (primary or revision style implants are applicable)
II	Metaphyseal bone loss with an intact diaphysis and minimal bone remodeling	Distally fixed stems are preferred (modular or nonmodular implants are applicable)
IIIA	Metaphyseal and diaphyseal bone loss, significant proximal remodeling, >4 cm of intact diaphysis	Distally fixed stems are preferred (modular or nonmodular implants are applicable): Avoid using cylindrical cobalt–chromium (CoCr) stems with a diameter less than 14 mm or greater than 18 mm Avoid modular stems without proximal bony support
IIIB	Metaphyseal and diaphyseal bone loss, significant proximal remodeling, <4 cm of intact diaphysis	Distally fixed stems are preferred (modular or nonmodular implants are applicable): Avoid using cylindrical CoCr stems with a diameter less than 14 mm or greater than 18 mm Avoid modular stems without proximal bony support
IV	Metaphyseal and diaphyseal bone loss with a nonsupportive diaphysis (essentially complete "stove-pipe" femur)	Most often requires a megaprosthesis, allograft–prosthetic composite, or impaction grafting Distal fixation devices may be applicable

    E. Advanced imaging:

        1. Inlet/outlet views—can be used to look at the pelvic ring, not commonly ordered.

        2. Judet's views—good to look at the anterior and posterior columns; can help with better visualizing defects and/or pelvic discontinuity.

II. CT scan—typically used to look for component version or the extent of osteolysis surrounding the hip:

    A. Pelvis: It is good to assess the acetabular component version and overhang; it can also be used to look at the areas of osteolysis:

        1. One study showed that if less than 40% of the cup is surrounded by osteolysis then the component is likely not loose.[36]

    B. Femur: can assess femoral component version if it includes the distal femur as well; can monitor femoral osteolysis and pedestal presence and quality, evaluate femoral remodeling, and can clarify the presence of subtle periprosthetic fractures.

III. MRI:

    A. Metal artifact reduction sequence (MARS) MRI:

        1. Reduces the local distortion around THA components.

        2. Can assess local soft tissues for injuries (abductors, iliopsoas, etc.).

3. Excellent to detect ALTRs associated with metal debris.

4. When the appropriate sequences are obtained, with a well-trained radiologist, etiologies such as aseptic loosening, wear-induced synovitis, and MoM complications.[37]

IV. Nuclear medicine:

A. Technetium-99 labeled diphosphonate scan (^{99}Tc-MDP):

1. Used to assess implant loosening, HO maturity, or periprosthetic stress fractures.[38]

2. Overall nonspecific and can be positive in an uncomplicated THA for up to 2 years after the index procedure[39,40]:

   a. Lieberman et al found that this test is no more effective than serial radiographs in making a diagnosis.[41]

   b. It can also be positive with modulus mismatch, tumor, metabolic bone disease, complex regional pain syndrome, and infection.[39]

B. Indium 111 (^{111}In) labeled leukocyte scan has a good negative predictive value for ruling out infection as the source of THA pain:

1. It has now been combined with sulfur colloid scan (below) to reduce the number of false-positive results.

C. Gallium-67 (^{67}Ga) citrate scan can be used in conjunction with technetium scans to rule out infection; although this has typically been replaced by indium scans in the United States.

D. Technetium-99m sulfur colloid ^{111}In-labeled scintigraphy (TcSC-Ind bone marrow [BM]/white blood cell [WBC])—the combination of tests helps account for marrow packing that can occur in a normal scan that yields increased uptake.

E. Fluorodeoxyglucose positron emission topography (FDG-PET)—a newer imaging modality that detects energy consumption of tissues:

1. Pill et al compared TcSC-Ind BM/WBC with FDG-PET to rule out infection[42]:

   a. FDG-PET resulted in 95.2% sensitivity, 93% specificity, 80% positive predictive value, and 98.5% negative predictive value in diagnosing infection.

   b. TcSC-Ind BM/WBC resulted in 50% sensitivity, 95.1% specificity, 41.7% positive predictive value, and 88.6% negative predictive value.

V. Laboratory tests:

A. Blood work is typically used for screening test to determine likelihood for infection and need for aspiration:

1. Complete blood count is not very accurate in diagnosing prosthetic joint infection (PJI).[43]

2. Erythrocyte sedimentation rate (ESR) represents an increase in proteins (normal and abnormal) that enhances red cell aggregation and accelerates the settling of red blood cells, leading to an elevated sedimentation rate[44]:

   a. Sensitive but nonspecific marker for inflammation; measured in millimeter per hour; normal levels vary per laboratory; current recommendation is that greater than 30 mm/h is elevated.[45]

3. C-reactive protein (CRP) is an acute phase protein produced by the liver with maximum production within 36 hours of an inflammatory event[44]:

   a. Sensitive but non-specific marker (better than ESR), measured in mg/L, beware that unit of measure often varies between laboratories, current recommendation is that greater than 1 mg/dL is elevated[45]:

4. Interleukin-6 (IL-6) is an inflammatory cytokine produced by monocytes and macrophages leading to an increase in production of acute-phase proteins[44]:

   a. Conflicting data have been reported on the utility of this biomarker in detecting infection, with prospective studies affording ranges of 49 to 81% sensitivity and 58 to 95% specificity[44]; this is compared with a meta-analysis in which the sensitivity and specificity were 97 and 91%, respectively.[46]

5. D-dimer—a test that detects fibrinolytic activity in the body, which has recently been suggested to be a possible marker for PJI:

   a. Shahi et al reported on 245 patients, with 89% sensitivity and 93% specificity for PJI in this cohort, which was better than ESR and CRP.[47]

   b. Current recommendation is that greater than 860 ng/mL is elevated.[45]

6. Metal levels—assessing levels of particular metals such as titanium, cobalt, chromium, and nickel is difficult as laboratory detection is not always standardized and varies based on trunnion corrosion and MoM debris:

   a. Trunnionosis is often associated with 5:1, or greater, ratios of Co to Cr, often in the range of 8 to 11 parts per billion (ppb) for Co and 1 to 5 ppb for Cr; of note, a well-functioning metal on PE THA should result in less than 1 ppb of serum metal levels.[48–50]

   - Typically caused by mechanically assisted crevice corrosion—this involves fretting at the head–neck junction with debris formation and breakdown of the passivated layer of the trunnion, which undergoes a viscous cycle of reoxidation and corrosion.

   - Currently, greater than 1 ppb for Co has a sensitivity of 95% and specificity of 94% for ALTR, while a Co/Cr ratio greater than 2 has a sensitivity of 83% and specificity of 72%[51]:

     – MoM serum levels—surface debris of the articulation may be compounded by trunnion debris making levels less predictable but often at a higher level when associated with ALTR:

     – Seven ppb seems to be a reasonable number for determining excessive wear in MoM cases.

     – Co/Cr ratio of 1.4, Co ≥ 7 ppb, and continuous Co of 2.4 ppb were associated with ALTR in MoM patients.[52]

B. Aspiration[53]:

1. Cell count—aspirated fluid should be sent for a cell count and differential:

   a. In the setting of metal debris/corrosion, a manual cell count should be ordered as the necrotic tissue can falsely elevate the white blood cell count.

   b. Cutoffs have varied, but typically greater than 3,000 WBC/μL is indicative of a chronic prosthetic infection.[45]

    c. For acute infections, the numbers are quite a bit higher:

       i. Twelve thousand eight hundred WBC/μL (with CRP of 93 mg/L and differential of 89%).

2. Differential—when ordering a cell count, a differential should be included; varying levels have been used, but the recent cutoff in the diagnosis of infection is greater than 80% neutrophils on the differential.

3. Cultures—required to diagnose the offending organism:

    a. Remain negative in 20% of infected cases (poor sensitivity).

    b. Hold antibiotics for at least 2 weeks prior to an aspiration.

    c. Consider prolonged incubation in the cases with fastidious organisms.

4. Biomarkers[54]: It is thought that the body creates a predictable immune response to pathogens that can be recognized in the form of a unique gene expression signature:

    a. This has spawned the interest in utilizing biomarkers as a more sensitive, specific, and accurate means to diagnose PJI.

    b. Biomarkers of interest include the following:

       i. Human α-defensin 1–3, Interleukins (1α, 1β, 6, 8, 10, 17), granulocyte colon-stimulating factor, vascular endothelial growth factor, CRP, neutrophil elastase 2, lactoferrin, neutrophil gelatinase–associated lipocalin, resistin, thrombospondin 1, bactericidal/permeability increasing protein:

          (1) Five of these biomarkers had a sensitivity and specificity of 100% in a study by Deirmengian et al (α-defensin, neutrophil elastase 2, bactericidal/permeability increasing protein, neutrophil gelatinase-associated protein, and lactoferrin).[54]

          (2) Lee et al looked at 13 diagnostic tests and found that α-defensin was the best synovial marker based on the highest log diagnostic odds ratio.[55]

VI. Musculoskeletal Infection Society criteria for infection[45,56]

  A. Major criteria—one of the following is required:

    1. Sinus tract that communicates with joint/prosthesis (or visualization of the implant itself).

    2. A common pathogen isolated from two sets of tissue or fluid specimens from the joint in question.

  B. Minor criteria: new scoring system—(≥6 is infected, 2–5 possible infection and 0–1 not infected):

    1. Elevated D-dimer (>860 ng/mL) or CRP (>1 mg/dL) = 2 points.

    2. Elevated ESR (>30 mm/h) = 1 point.

    3. Elevated synovial fluid white blood cell count (>3,000 cells/μL) or leukocyte esterase (++) = 3 points.

    4. Positive α-defensin from synovial fluid (signal to cutoff ratio >1) = 3 points.

    5. Elevated synovial PMN (>80%) = 2 points.

6. Elevated synovial CRP (6.9 mg/L) = 1 point.

C. Inconclusive pre-op score or dry tap—move to intraoperative assessment (≥6 is infected, 4–5 possible infection, and ≤3 not infected):

1. Add preoperative score to the following:

2. Greater than 5 neutrophils per high-powered field in 5 high-power fields on histologic analysis at ×400 magnification = 3 points.

3. Positive purulence = 3 points.

4. Single positive culture = 2 points.

Management

I. Instability: covers a spectrum of disorders including subtle impingement, subluxation, and frank dislocation:

A. Impingement occurs when the neck of the prosthesis makes contact with the edge of the cup, prominence of the PE liner, or the adjacent anatomy (bone, tendon, soft tissues).

B. Recurrent episodes of impingement can lead to PE wear and fatigue fracture; metal debris and adverse local tissue reaction; pain from tendonitis, bone impaction and soft-tissue compression; or frank dislocation.

C. Subluxation is often a precursor to dislocation and should be treated as such and watched closely; often patients will feel a clunk or the hip moving; this should serve as a premonition of future dislocation.

II. Dislocation: Overall rate varies and is often quoted as 1% or less; however, Medicare data suggest this number is closer to approximately 4%[57]:

A. Early dislocation: within 6 weeks to 3 months after surgery.

B. Wera et al reported six categories for instability[58]:

1. Type I—malposition of the acetabulum (outside of 15 degrees of anteversion and 40 degrees of abduction ±10 degrees:

a. Treat with acetabular revision—address the problem at hand.

2. Type II: malposition of the femoral component—femoral anteversion of 20 ±10 degrees:

a. Treat with revision of the femoral component.

b. Type I and II instabilities treated with revision are associated with only 6% failure rate.

3. Type III: abductor deficiency—absence or compromise of the abductor-trochanter complex (gluteus tear, trochanter nonunion/absence, severe heterotopic ossification):

a. Treat with a constrained liner if components are in the correct position; modern day thinking is to possibly utilize dual mobility as well.

b. Twenty-two percent failure rate and the most difficult to manage.

4. Type IV: impingement—may be related to suboptimal head-to-neck ratio, failure to restore offset, elevated liners, retained osteophytes, and malpositioned implants:

    a. Treat by assessing the source of impingement and removing it.

    b. Maximize head-to-neck ratio.[59]

    c. Reposition implants as needed; remove bony osteophytes.

    d. Avoid elevated or prominent PE liners.

    e. Following these principles led to zero dislocations out of seven cases.

5. Type V: late wear of PE liner—prior well-functioning THA with eccentric PE wear:

    a. Modular headliner exchange recommended with maximum ball size.

    b. Eighty percent success rate—best if femoral head is upsized at the time of revision.

6. Type VI: unclear etiology of instability—diagnosis of exclusion:

    a. Often treated with a constrained liner or now dual mobility options as the source of instability is unclear at the time of surgery.

C. Treatment:

1. Begins with preoperative planning and prevention of dislocation.[60]

2. First time dislocation (typically in the first 6–12 weeks after surgery)→ treat with abduction brace and/or knee immobilizer, hip precautions, education, and muscle training:

    a. Dewal et al found no difference in recurrent dislocation rates with bracing acute dislocations versus no brace (61 vs. 64%); similarly chronic dislocators showed no difference with a brace either (55 vs. 56%).[61]

    b. Historically, Yuan and Shih found that only 15% of their primary THA dislocations required reoperation (out of 2,728 THAs),[62] while Joshi et al found a similar result with 81% of closed reductions being successful—most common causes of recurrent dislocation were component malposition and abductor failure.[63]

    c. A successful closed reduction typically results in functional results similar to those that have not dislocated, despite a trend toward the nondislocators being more satisfied with their surgery.[64]

3. Recurrent dislocation → two or more dislocations after THA → surgery is advised and recommended:

    a. Assess causation using classification above → often multifactorial in etiology:

        i. Cup malposition—assess cup position with a shoot-through lateral radiograph as an idea of version and a CT scan for a definitive measure of cup version:

            (1) Keep in mind that spinopelvic mobility must be accounted for, as there is a growing body of literature describing alterations in pelvic orientation with sitting, standing, and lying down in the setting of spinal degenerative joint disease/stiffness/fusion:

                (a) Forsythe et al found a dislocation rate of 5.2% in patients with a prior spinal fusion versus 1.7% for a control group;

multilevel fusion and those involving the sacrum were at greatest risk.[64]

(2) Revise cup to optimal position ± larger femoral head (maximize head size and/or consider dual mobility):

    (a) Assess impingement points intraoperatively and try to minimize.

    (b) Maximize head-to-neck ratio.

    (c) Elevated and offset liners can be utilized when necessary.

(3) Do not place a constrained liner into a malpositioned acetabular component.

(4) Enhanced capsular closure is recommended when possible via the posterior approach, as is abductor repair with direct lateral procedures.[65]

ii. Poor soft-tissue tension (i.e., decreased offset and/or short leg):

(1) PE exchange: increased offset liner ± larger femoral head with increased neck length.

(2) Trochanter advancement (with well-placed components).

(3) In the absence of adequate abductors, transfer of the gluteus maximus tendon can be performed.

iii. Multifactorial and acceptable component position → larger femoral head with possible elevated liner if possible:

(1) Large diameter femoral heads, dual mobility, or an unconstrained tripolar construct are also possible solutions.

(2) Constrained liners have a role in these cases.[66,67]

(3) If capsular repair or reinforcement is required, there are reports of using Achilles tendon allograft or a synthetic ligament prosthesis.[68,69]

D. Late dislocation:

1. Treatment (follow classification algorithm mentioned earlier):

a. Assess causation:

i. PE wear → catastrophic failure or eccentric wear can lead to impingement and dislocation:

(1) Liner exchange—can add an elevated lip or constrained liner as needed; may need to cement a liner in place if locking mechanism is compromised.[70]

(2) Utilize a larger head size.

(3) Revise the cup if necessary to enhance implant position, liner options, and increase femoral head options—more a last resort if above options do not work.

ii. Abductor dysfunction → often seen with ALTR/pseudotumor formation in MoM and trunnionosis cases, abductor repair failures, migration of trochanteric osteotomies, and with injury to the SGN:

(1) Similar to acute dislocation scenario, the goal is to restore abductor tension/function if possible.

(2) Maximize head-to-neck ratio with larger femoral head or dual mobility.

(3) Can resort to a constrained liner option.

(4) Revise cup to gain the ability to improve position and have more liner and head options.

(5) Gluteus maximus transfer or trochanteric advancement procedures when applicable.

iii. Multifactorial → need to make sure implant position is appropriate; may need to evaluate spine if changes have occurred after the initial THA:

(1) Dual mobility, PE exchange, and larger diameter femoral head or constrained liner remain viable options.[71]

Infection

I.   Acute: early infection within 4 to 6 weeks of the index procedure:

A.   Treatment options include the following:

1.   Irrigation and debridement with modular component exchange (debridement, antibiotics, irrigation, and retention [DAIR]):

a.   Success rates vary.

b.   de Vries et al reported on 109 THAs, 84 of which underwent DAIR; there was 74.3% component retention with acute infections compared with late infection, (84 vs. 46.6%).[72]

c.   Estes et al described a two-stage retention protocol where the wound is debrided and temporary cement beads are placed, followed by modular component exchange 7 days later—this led to infection control in 18/20 patients.[73]

2.   One-stage exchange revision—all components out and replaced at the same surgery:

a.   Hansen et al reported on 27 patients with a mean follow-up of 50 months[74]:

i.   They found 19/27 (70%) retained their hardware—4 did require a repeat debridement.

ii.   Overall success rate was 56%.

3.   Two-stage exchange—remove implants and place a spacer (dynamic or static), intravenous (IV) antibiotics given, drug holiday (minimum 2 weeks), followed by second-stage reimplantation if cultures are negative (occasionally requires a second spacer).

4.   Permanent Girdlestone without spacer—not great for function and does not afford the ability to deliver local antibiotics, but is only one procedure.

B.   There has been some recent thoughts that each case should be handled based on the host and the infecting organism:

1.   Methicillin-resistant Staphylococcus aureus (MRSA) → two-stage exchange.

2.   MSSA (methicillin-susceptible S. aureus) → highly consider stage exchange.

3. Other organisms → irrigation and debridement, head and poly exchange, and IV antibiotics.

II.   Chronic → late infection, typically occurs greater than 6 weeks after the index procedure:

A. Treatment options include the following:

1. Irrigation and debridement with modular component exchange (DAIR):

a. Bene et al have recently suggested that chronic suppression/long-term antibiotics will lead to a decreased risk of reoperation.[75]

b. For well-fixed cementless THA, DAIR can be successful if no draining sinus, healthy host, and a sensitive organism.[76]

c. Herman et al found a 59% infection eradication rate with DAIR, but the patients were very satisfied with the results when it worked (equivalent outcomes to those without an infection).[77]

2. One-stage exchange revision—all components out and replaced at the same surgery:

a. Typically done with cemented femoral stem and cementless cup in Europe; antibiotics directed toward infecting organism are placed in the cement:

i.   Offers the advantage of one surgery, less antibiotics, reduced hospitalization, reduced transfusions, and reduced overall costs.[78]

ii. With good selection criteria, one-stage procedures are successful—100% successful for one-stage versus 97.8% for two-stage in 84 infected THAs.[79]

iii. Worldwide data suggest one-stage revision may be as effective as 2-stage revision for infected THAs.[80]

b. Whiteside and Roy recently described a technique to remove cemented implants and revise in one stage to cementless implants coupled with catheter placement and intra-articular infusion of antibiotics for 6 weeks:

i.   They found a 95% infection eradication rate in 21 infected THAs with a mean follow-up of 63 months.[81]

3. Two-stage exchange:

a. This is the gold standard at the moment in the United States.

b. This may be more costly and involves two surgeries; however, there are reports of superior outcomes:

i.   Infection eradication of 94.5% compared with 56.8% with one-stage procedure.[82]

c. Whiteside et al now suggest a 3-month course of oral antibiotics after a two-stage exchange procedure, citing a 5 vs. 19% reinfection among those receiving extended antibiotic and those that do not.[81]

d. At times, the second stage may not be performed—if doing well with mobile spacer or patient not medically a candidate for reimplantation.

i.   Berend et al found a 4% 90-day mortality rate after the first stage and 76% survival and infection control rate after a two-stage procedure.[83]

e. Partial two-stage exchange—cup removed and stem retained with a cement ball placed on the trunnion:

i. Ekpo et al found an 89% infection eradication rate at 2-year follow-up with this technique.[84]

4. Permanent Girdlestone—not very functional, but good pain relief and rates of infection control; the next step is hemipelvectomy, which is severely disabling.

III. Acute hematogenous → occurs in recent proximity to a surgical procedure, remote infection, dental procedure, etc. (typically occurs many years after the index procedure but as an acute event with systemic transfer of the bacteria to the prosthetic joint); big difference with this infection is that the source has to be considered and treated appropriately.

A. Treatment options include the following:

1. Irrigation and debridement with modular component exchange:

a. The most common option for acute infection.

b. Konigsberg et al reported on 20 THAs with acute hematogenous infection treated with modular component exchange, with 76% survivorship at 2 years and greater success with nonstaphylococcal infections.[85]

c. Fink et al found only 57.1% success rate for acute hematogenous infection compared with 82.1% for early infections treated with the same protocol for modular component exchange.[86]

2. One-stage exchange revision—all components out and replaced at the same surgery.

3. Two-stage exchange—likely the best option with resistant and virulent organisms related to a hematogenous infection (studies show poor results with Staphylococcus aureus infections and resistant organisms); need to find the source of the infection and control it there.[87]

Aseptic Loosening

I. Acetabular loosening:

A. Epidemiology: advancements in technology, including osseointegration surfaces and PE, are lowering rates of aseptic loosening both as a primary problem and as a secondary condition related to particulate-induced osteolysis:

1. Monoblock CoCr cups have had varying rates of success based on implant design, with several models being recalled for not only wear concerns, but also high rates of aseptic loosening.[88]

2. Modern implants with and without adjunct fixation have extremely low rates of aseptic loosening.[89]

B. It can occur from failure of osseointegration, late PE wear sequelae, or metal-related pathology (i.e., ALTR).

C. Revise cup to cementless cup (highly consider highly porous components) with augments or triflange based on amount of bone loss; in severe defects cage, cup-cage and impaction grafting techniques can be called upon.

D. Acetabular defects[90]:
  1. Paprosky's classification[30] (**Table 21.3**):
    a. Based on a common pattern of bone loss in the acetabulum.
    b. Helps direct treatment based on classification type.
    c. Must distinguish if there is a pelvic discontinuity and if this is acute or chronic as that helps direct treatment[91]:
      i. Chronic discontinuity—no pelvic healing potential:
        (1) Pelvic distraction method—place 4- to 8-mm larger cup than the last reamer and rely on pelvic ligaments for stability.[92]
        (2) Stabilize the pelvis with a bridge plate and place a new cup.
        (3) Custom triflange—custom implant designed to address the defects on a preoperative CT scan[93,94]:
          (a) Multicenter study of 95 reconstructions reported good outcomes at 3.5-year follow-up, with 22% complications and only 1 case of aseptic loosening.
          (b) At a minimum of 10 years, Moore et al reviewed 37 patients with a custom triflange and found 91% were still functioning well at latest follow-up; they had two infections and no dislocations.[93]
        (4) Impaction grafting—defect is contained with mesh and allograft is packed into the defect with a cup that is cemented into this bony bed:
          (a) Abdullah et al reported on 47 THAs with impaction grafting and noted 100% survivorship at the mean follow-up of 10 years; however, they did note 8 cases of lysis and migration in 4 patients that have not been revised.[95]
        (5) Cup-cage technique—cage is placed over the top of a porous cup that spans the discontinuity or defect:
          (a) Hipfl et al reported on 35 hips at a mean of 47-month follow-up; they found 89% survivorship at 5 years with no cases of aseptic loosening.[96]
      ii. Acute discontinuity—may be trauma related or due to an unrecognized intraoperative fracture:
        (1) ORIF (open reduction and internal fixation) of the pelvis and revision of the cup:
          (a) Rogers et al reviewed nine patients with an acute pelvic discontinuity with eight requiring posterior column compression plating and revision of the cup at a mean of 34-month follow-up; no revisions were noted in this cohort.[91]
        (2) Less likely to do distraction technique or wait for a custom triflange to be made.

Femoral Component Loosening

I. Epidemiology: Aseptic loosening rates have decreased with modern cemented and cementless implants. Appropriate surgical technique is required to assure that the implant is placed so that the fixation is solid and the porous surface is securely against the host bone. When these principles are not respected, there is a higher risk for persistent thigh pain and component loosening.[97,98] Additionally, many cases of early loosening are related to missed intraoperative fractures.

II. Often recommended to revise to longer stem options:

    A. Can use long cemented stem with or without impaction grafting.

    B. Cementless stem options:

        1. Use shortest stem to bypass defect (any holes/stress risers should be bypassed by two cortical diameters) and get into good host bone.

        2. Splined, tapered stems have largely taken over this role, both in the monoblock and modular designs.

        3. Cylindrical, CoCr stems are not used as often and must be put in correctly to avoid late fatigue fractures (stems 13 mm in diameter or less), thigh pain (stems greater than 18 mm in diameter), and corrosion.

III. Femoral defects:

    A. Paprosky's classification[35]:

        1. Assesses bone defects based on location in the bone and preservation of the isthmus.

        2. Guides treatment options and directs overall management (**Table 21.4**).

        3. The greater the defect and more compromised the host is medically, the worse outcomes tend to be in these difficult cases.

Bearing Wear

PE wear and particulate-induced osteolysis are common historical problems for THA. Modern highly cross-linked and treated PEs have improved wear rates and have resulted in a substantial reduction in peri-implant osteolysis. The bearing surface has long been considered the weak link for a THA construct. With younger patients now receiving THA surgeries, the future will likely hold a large number of revision surgeries for bearing wear or implant loosening related to particulate sequelae.

I. Epidemiology—in some series, wear and loosening secondary to wear sequelae may be responsible for up to 40 to 60% of revision cases.

II. Wear rates—various wear rates are reported in the literature depending on the type of PE used.

    A. Median wear rates were reported at 0.024 to 0.41 mm/y with an irradiated and remelted highly cross-linked PE, regardless of femoral head size (26, 28, 32, 36, or 40 mm) and with only 14% osteolysis being found.[99,100]

    B. Vitamin E–infused PE has been found to have similar wear rates that are quite low compared with historical PE wear rates; with 32- and 36-mm heads, the annual wear was found to be 0.02 and 0.01 mm, respectively[101]

III. Treatment options:

    A. PE and femoral head exchange when possible:

        1. Assess trunnion for taper damage.

   2. Avoid mixing manufacture head–stem combinations for fear of slight trunnion mismatches.

   3. PE exchange when adequate options are available and locking mechanism remains intact.

B. Revise cup if:

   1. Unable to achieve adequate stability based on cup position and/or inability to achieve larger head.

   2. Occasionally, the femoral component has to be revised as well if instability is related to the position of the femur (version, height, offset).

   3. PE liners no longer manufactured—can cement PE in if cup is large enough to accept a liner and have room for 1 to 2 mm of cement.

   4. Locking mechanism damaged (can consider cementing in liner in these cases as well):

      a. Can cement an entire cup in place or a liner to avoid revising a well-fixed and appropriately positioned acetabular component.[71]

C. Bone graft osteolytic lesions when accessible.[102]

Metal-on-Metal and Trunnion Issues

This is a modern-day concern with alternative bearings and taper connections that have become more prevalent in the past 10 years. MoM implants have seen a significant reduction in utilization due to these concerns, as have dual-modular femoral components. Taper corrosion is multifactorial and is not isolated to MoM THAs.[103] A tremendous amount of ongoing research is targeted at investigating the etiology and prevention of such problems.

I. Epidemiology:

   A. MoM THA—revision rates of modern MoM THA have been reported to be 18 to 19% at 10 years[52]:

      1. Damage from metal debris can be dramatic and compromise revision outcomes.[104]

      2. Early detection and a low threshold to workup is important.

   B. Taper corrosion related to MACC is estimated to be the etiology of up to 3 to 4% of all current revisions.[105,106]

II. Workup:

   A. Assess component position:

      1. Vertical components can lead to edge loading and focused areas of wear.

      2. Excessive version can lead to impingement and metal debris.

   B. Identify known implants with early failure rates:

      1. There are known implants that have had trunnion or wear concerns that should be identified and trigger earlier suspicion and workup when warranted.

   C. Obtain metal ion levels:

      1. Greater than 5 to 7 ppb for chromium and/or cobalt should raise concern for MoM THA or resurfacing.

2. Greater than 1 ppb for a metal-on-PE THA should raise red flags.

3. Look at cobalt-to-chromium ratio to assess for corrosion.

D. Investigate plain radiographs for peri-implant osteolysis that is out of proportion or disproportionate to the time of implantation of the components.

E. Obtain further advance imaging such as MRI and/or ultrasound to assess for soft-tissue damage and pseudotumor.

III. Treatment:

A. Revise to a hard on soft bearing surface (ceramic with a titanium sleeve on PE is preferable).

B. Beware of possible instability due to soft-tissue damage (i.e., abductor injury).

C. The head size may need to be maximized.

D. Controversial to revise to dual mobility due to trying to remove the cobalt and chromium from the system.

IV. Taper corrosion:

A. Revise stem based on severity of corrosion.

B. If stem is salvageable, then use a ceramic head with a titanium sleeve at the time of revision.

Ceramic Issues

When COC bearings are utilized, we can anticipate incredibly low wear rates, but there have been reports of squeaking and implant fracture that can be quite difficult to manage.

I. Squeaking: In a recent study with modern COC THA, a 9.6% incidence of squeaking was found, with a historical range of 2 to 21% being reported[107]:

A. May occur from edge loading but is likely multifactorial in nature.

B. Revise to a hard-on-soft bearing (CoCr or ceramic-on-PE).

C. May require cup revision if acetabular cup is nonmodular or does not accept a softer bearing surface option.

II. Fracture:

Luo et al reported on a modern COC bearing and found a 0.76% incidence of ceramic liner fracture, with a historical range of 0 to 5.7% being reported in the literature[107]:

A. Clear debris and revise to a hard-on-soft bearing, preferably a new ceramic head on PE.

B. May need to avoid a metal head, as if there are remaining ceramic pieces, these will rapidly cut into the metal head and create a tremendous amount of debris.

C. Removing the ceramic debris is an incredibly tedious process and one must be careful as the shards are sharp and will penetrate surgical gloves easily.

Summary

Revision THA surgery can range from a relatively simple diagnosis and procedure to much more complex undertakings. It is important to follow an algorithmic approach in making the diagnosis, so nothing is missed and the etiology of failure is made in a timely fashion. Once a diagnosis is made, a treatment plan must be established taking into account bone defects, soft-tissue integrity, hip stability, patient comorbidities, and presurgery level of function.

References

1. Bozic KJ, Kurtz SM, Lau E, Ong K, Vail TP, Berry DJ. The epidemiology of revision total hip arthroplasty in the United States. J Bone Joint Surg Am 2009;91(1):128–133
2. Gwam CU, Mistry JB, Mohamed NS, et al. current epidemiology of revision total hip arthroplasty in the United States: national inpatient sample 2009 to 2013. J Arthroplasty 2017;32(7):2088–2092
3. Dorr LD, Malik A, Dastane M, Wan Z. Combined anteversion technique for total hip arthroplasty. Clin Orthop Relat Res 2009;467(1):119–127
4. Lewinnek GE, Lewis JL, Tarr R, Compere CL, Zimmerman JR. Dislocations after total hip-replacement arthroplasties. J Bone Joint Surg Am 1978;60(2):217–220
5. Abdel MP, von Roth P, Jennings MT, Hanssen AD, Pagnano MW. What safe zone? the vast majority of dislocated THAs are within the lewinnek safe zone for acetabular component position. Clin Orthop Relat Res 2016;474(2):386–391
6. Moore KD, Beck PR, Petersen DW, Cuckler JM, Lemons JE, Eberhardt AW. Early failure of a cross-linked polyethylene acetabular liner. A case report. J Bone Joint Surg Am 2008;90(11):2499–2504
7. Berríos-Torres SI, Umscheid CA, Bratzler DW, et al; Healthcare Infection Control Practices Advisory Committee. Centers for disease control and prevention guideline for the prevention of surgical site infection, 2017. JAMA Surg 2017;152(8):784–791
8. Sukur E, Akman YE, Ozturkmen Y, Kucukdurmaz F. Particle disease: a current review of the biological mechanisms in periprosthetic osteolysis after hip arthroplasty. Open Orthop J 2016;10:241–251
9. Oparaugo PC, Clarke IC, Malchau H, Herberts P. Correlation of wear debris-induced osteolysis and revision with volumetric wear-rates of polyethylene: a survey of 8 reports in the literature. Acta Orthop Scand 2001;72(1):22–28
10. Fabi D, Levine B, Paprosky W, et al. Metal-on-metal total hip arthroplasty: causes and high incidence of early failure. Orthopedics 2012;35(7):e1009–e1016
11. Bolognesi MP, Ledford CK. Metal-on-metal total hip arthroplasty: patient evaluation and treatment. J Am Acad Orthop Surg 2015;23(12):724–731
12. Bradberry SM, Wilkinson JM, Ferner RE. Systemic toxicity related to metal hip prostheses. Clin Toxicol (Phila) 2014;52(8):837–847
13. Massin P, Lopes R, Masson B, Mainard D; French Hip & Knee Society (SFHG). Does Biolox Delta ceramic reduce the rate of component fractures in total hip replacement? Orthop Traumatol Surg Res 2014;100(6, Suppl):S317–S321
14. Howard DP, Wall PDH, Fernandez MA, Parsons H, Howard PW. Ceramic-on-ceramic bearing fractures in total hip arthroplasty: an analysis of data from the National Joint Registry. Bone Joint J 2017;99-B(8):1012–1019
15. Baek SH, Kim WK, Kim JY, Kim SY. Do alumina matrix composite bearings decrease hip noises and bearing fractures at a minimum of 5 years after THA? Clin Orthop Relat Res 2015;473(12):3796–3802
16. Baek SH, Kim SY. Cementless total hip arthroplasty with alumina bearings in patients younger than fifty with femoral head osteonecrosis. J Bone Joint Surg Am 2008;90(6):1314–1320
17. McDonnell SM, Boyce G, Baré J, Young D, Shimmin AJ. The incidence of noise generation arising from the large-diameter Delta Motion ceramic total hip bearing. Bone Joint J 2013;95-B(2):160–165
18. Keurentjes JC, Kuipers RM, Wever DJ, Schreurs BW. High incidence of squeaking in THAs with alumina ceramic-on-ceramic bearings. Clin Orthop Relat Res 2008;466(6): 1438–1443

19. Migaud H, Putman S, Kern G, et al; SoFCOT Study Group. Do the reasons for ceramic-on-ceramic revisions differ from other bearings in total hip arthroplasty? Clin Orthop Relat Res 2016;474(10):2190–2199

20. Lachiewicz PF, Kauk JR. Anterior iliopsoas impingement and tendinitis after total hip arthroplasty. J Am Acad Orthop Surg 2009;17(6):337–344

21. Henderson RA, Lachiewicz PF. Groin pain after replacement of the hip: aetiology, evaluation and treatment. J Bone Joint Surg Br 2012;94(2):145–151

22. Chalmers BP, Sculco PK, Sierra RJ, Trousdale RT, Berry DJ. Iliopsoas impingement after primary total hip arthroplasty: operative and nonoperative treatment outcomes. J Bone Joint Surg Am 2017;99(7):557–564

23. Gofton WT, Illical EM, Feibel RJ, Kim PR, Beaulé PE. a single-center experience with a titanium modular neck total hip arthroplasty. J Arthroplasty 2017;32(8):2450–2456

24. Grupp TM, Weik T, Bloemer W, Knaebel HP. Modular titanium alloy neck adapter failures in hip replacement--failure mode analysis and influence of implant material. BMC Musculoskelet Disord 2010;11:3

25. Pour AE, Borden R, Murayama T, Groll-Brown M, Blaha JD. High risk of failure with bimodular femoral components in THA. Clin Orthop Relat Res 2016;474(1):146–153

26. Shah RR, Goldstein JM, Cipparrone NE, Gordon AC, Jimenez ML, Goldstein WM. Alarmingly high rate of implant fractures in one modular femoral stem design: a comparison of two implants. J Arthroplasty 2017;32(10):3157–3162

27. Chang CY, Huang AJ, Palmer WE. Radiographic evaluation of hip implants. Semin Musculoskelet Radiol 2015;19(1):12–20

28. DeLee JG, Charnley J. Radiological demarcation of cemented sockets in total hip replacement. Clin Orthop Relat Res 1976;(121):20–32

29. Udomkiat P, Wan Z, Dorr LD. Comparison of preoperative radiographs and intraoperative findings of fixation of hemispheric porous-coated sockets. J Bone Joint Surg Am 2001;83(12):1865–1870

30. Paprosky WG, Perona PG, Lawrence JM. Acetabular defect classification and surgical reconstruction in revision arthroplasty. A 6-year follow-up evaluation. J Arthroplasty 1994;9(1):33–44

31. Gruen TA, McNeice GM, Amstutz HC. "Modes of failure" of cemented stem-type femoral components: a radiographic analysis of loosening. Clin Orthop Relat Res 1979;(141):17–27

32. Engh CA, Massin P, Suthers KE. Roentgenographic assessment of the biologic fixation of porous-surfaced femoral components. Clin Orthop Relat Res 1990;(257):107–128

33. Harris WH, McGann WA. Loosening of the femoral component after use of the medullary-plug cementing technique. Follow-up note with a minimum five-year follow-up. J Bone Joint Surg Am 1986;68(7):1064–1066

34. Brooker AF, Bowerman JW, Robinson RA, Riley LH Jr. Ectopic ossification following total hip replacement. Incidence and a method of classification. J Bone Joint Surg Am 1973;55(8):1629–1632

35. Weeden SH, Paprosky WG. Minimal 11-year follow-up of extensively porous-coated stems in femoral revision total hip arthroplasty. J Arthroplasty 2002;17(4, Suppl 1):134–137

36. Egawa H, Ho H, Hopper RH Jr, Engh CA Jr, Engh CA. Computed tomography assessment of pelvic osteolysis and cup-lesion interface involvement with a press-fit porous-coated acetabular cup. J Arthroplasty 2009;24(2):233–239

37. Berkowitz JL, Potter HG. Advanced MRI techniques for the hip joint: focus on the postoperative hip. AJR Am J Roentgenol 2017;209(3):534–543

38. Mittal R, Khetarpal R, Malhotra R, Kumar R. The role of Tc-99m bone imaging in the management of pain after complicated total hip replacement. Clin Nucl Med 1997;22(9):593–595

39. Dangwal TR, Aggarwal V, Malhotra V, Baveja U, Mittal SK. Clinical spectrum of chronic liver disease in north Indian children. Trop Gastroenterol 1997;18(4):174–176

40. Oswald SG, Van Nostrand D, Savory CG, Callaghan JJ. Three-phase bone scan and indium white blood cell scintigraphy following porous coated hip arthroplasty: a prospective study of the prosthetic tip. J Nucl Med 1989;30(8):1321–1331

41. Lieberman JR, Huo MH, Schneider R, Salvati EA, Rodi S. Evaluation of painful hip arthroplasties. Are technetium bone scans necessary? J Bone Joint Surg Br 1993;75(3):475–478

42. Pill SG, Parvizi J, Tang PH, et al. Comparison of fluorodeoxyglucose positron emission tomography and (111)indium-white blood cell imaging in the diagnosis of periprosthetic infection of the hip. J Arthroplasty 2006;21(6, Suppl 2):91–97

43. Di Cesare PE, Chang E, Preston CF, Liu CJ. Serum interleukin-6 as a marker of periprosthetic infection following total hip and knee arthroplasty. J Bone Joint Surg Am 2005;87(9):1921–1927

44. Saleh A, George J, Faour M, Klika AK, Higuera CA. Serum biomarkers in periprosthetic joint infections. Bone Joint Res 2018;7(1):85–93

45. Parvizi J, Tan TL, Goswami K, et al. The 2018 definition of periprosthetic hip and knee infection: an evidence-based and validated criteria. J Arthroplasty 2018;33(5):1309–1314.e2

46. Berbari E, Mabry T, Tsaras G, et al. Inflammatory blood laboratory levels as markers of prosthetic joint infection: a systematic review and meta-analysis. J Bone Joint Surg Am 2010;92(11):2102–2109

47. Shahi A, Kheir MM, Tarabichi M, Hosseinzadeh HRS, Tan TL, Parvizi J. Serum D-dimer test is promising for the diagnosis of periprosthetic joint infection and timing of reimplantation. J Bone Joint Surg Am 2017;99(17):1419–1427

48. Hothi HS, Eskelinen AP, Berber R, et al. Factors associated with trunnionosis in the metal-on-metal pinnacle hip. J Arthroplasty 2017;32(1):286–290

49. Plummer DR, Berger RA, Paprosky WG, Sporer SM, Jacobs JJ, Della Valle CJ. Diagnosis and management of adverse local tissue reactions secondary to corrosion at the head-neck junction in patients with metal on polyethylene bearings. J Arthroplasty 2016;31(1):264–268

50. Levine BR, Hsu AR, Skipor AK, et al. Ten-year outcome of serum metal ion levels after primary total hip arthroplasty: a concise follow-up of a previous report*. J Bone Joint Surg Am 2013;95(6):512–518

51. Kwon YM, MacAuliffe J, Arauz PG, Peng Y. Sensitivity and specificity of metal ion level in predicting adverse local tissue reactions due to head-neck taper corrosion in primary metal-on-polyethylene total hip arthroplasty. J Arthroplasty 2018;33(9):3025–3029

52. Laaksonen I, Galea VP, Donahue GS, Matuszak SJ, Muratoglu O, Malchau H. The cobalt/chromium ratio provides similar diagnostic value to a low cobalt threshold in predicting adverse local tissue reactions in patients with metal-on-metal hip arthroplasty. J Arthroplasty 2018;33(9):3020–3024

53. Ting NT, Della Valle CJ. Diagnosis of periprosthetic joint infection: an algorithm-based approach. J Arthroplasty 2017;32(7):2047–2050

54. Deirmengian C, Kardos K, Kilmartin P, Cameron A, Schiller K, Parvizi J. Diagnosing periprosthetic joint infection: has the era of the biomarker arrived? Clin Orthop Relat Res 2014;472(11):3254–3262

55. Lee YS, Koo KH, Kim HJ, et al. Synovial fluid biomarkers for the diagnosis of periprosthetic joint infection: a systematic review and meta-analysis. J Bone Joint Surg Am 2017;99(24):2077–2084

56. Parvizi J, Zmistowski B, Berbari EF, et al. New definition for periprosthetic joint infection: from the Workgroup of the Musculoskeletal Infection Society. Clin Orthop Relat Res 2011;469(11):2992–2994

57. Phillips CB, Barrett JA, Losina E, et al. Incidence rates of dislocation, pulmonary embolism, and deep infection during the first six months after elective total hip replacement. J Bone Joint Surg Am 2003;85(1):20–26

58. Wera GD, Ting NT, Moric M, Paprosky WG, Sporer SM, Della Valle CJ. Classification and management of the unstable total hip arthroplasty. J Arthroplasty 2012;27(5):710–715

59. Waddell BS, Koch C, Trivellas M, Burket JC, Wright T, Padgett D. Have large femoral heads reduced prosthetic impingement in total hip arthroplasty? Hip Int 2019;29(1):83–88

60. Rowan FE, Benjamin B, Pietrak JR, Haddad FS. Prevention of dislocation after total hip arthroplasty. J Arthroplasty 2018;33(5):1316–1324
61. Dewal H, Maurer SL, Tsai P, Su E, Hiebert R, Di Cesare PE. Efficacy of abduction bracing in the management of total hip arthroplasty dislocation. J Arthroplasty 2004;19(6): 733–738
62. Yuan L, Shih C. Dislocation after total hip arthroplasty. Arch Orthop Trauma Surg 1999;119(5–6):263–266
63. Joshi A, Lee CM, Markovic L, Vlatis G, Murphy JC. Prognosis of dislocation after total hip arthroplasty. J Arthroplasty 1998;13(1):17–21
64. Forsythe ME, Whitehouse SL, Dick J, Crawford RW. Functional outcomes after nonrecurrent dislocation of primary total hip arthroplasty. J Arthroplasty 2007;22(2):227–230
65. Weeden SH, Paprosky WG, Bowling JW. The early dislocation rate in primary total hip arthroplasty following the posterior approach with posterior soft-tissue repair. J Arthroplasty 2003;18(6):709–713
66. Williams JT Jr, Ragland PS, Clarke S. Constrained components for the unstable hip following total hip arthroplasty: a literature review. Int Orthop 2007;31(3):273–277
67. Mäkinen TJ, Fichman SG, Rahman WA, et al. The focally constrained liner is a reasonable option for revision of unstable total hip arthroplasty. Int Orthop 2016;40(11): 2239–2245
68. Lavigne MJ, Sanchez AA, Coutts RD. Recurrent dislocation after total hip arthroplasty: treatment with an Achilles tendon allograft. J Arthroplasty 2001;16(8, Suppl 1):13–18
69. Barbosa JK, Khan AM, Andrew JG. Treatment of recurrent dislocation of total hip arthroplasty using a ligament prosthesis. J Arthroplasty 2004;19(3):318–321
70. Walmsley DW, Waddell JP, Schemitsch EH. Isolated head and liner exchange in revision hip arthroplasty. J Am Acad Orthop Surg 2017;25(4):288–296
71. Chalmers BP, Ledford CK, Taunton MJ, Sierra RJ, Lewallen DG, Trousdale RT. Cementation of a dual mobility construct in recurrently dislocating and high risk patients undergoing revision total arthroplasty. J Arthroplasty 2018;33(5):1501–1506
72. de Vries L, van der Weegen W, Neve WC, Das H, Ridwan BU, Steens J. The effectiveness of debridement, antibiotics and irrigation for periprosthetic joint infections after primary hip and knee arthroplasty. A 15 years retrospective study in two community hospitals in the Netherlands. J Bone Jt Infect 2016;1:20–24
73. Estes CS, Beauchamp CP, Clarke HD, Spangehl MJ. A two-stage retention débridement protocol for acute periprosthetic joint infections. Clin Orthop Relat Res 2010;468(8): 2029–2038
74. Hansen E, Tetreault M, Zmistowski B, et al. Outcome of one-stage cementless exchange for acute postoperative periprosthetic hip infection. Clin Orthop Relat Res 2013;471(10):3214–3222
75. Bene N, Li X, Nandi S. Increased antibiotic duration improves reoperation free survival after total hip arthroplasty irrigation and debridement. J Orthop 2018;15(2):707–710
76. Rahman WA, Kazi HA, Gollish JD. Results of single stage exchange arthroplasty with retention of well fixed cement-less femoral component in management of infected total hip arthroplasty. World J Orthop 2017;8(3):264–270
77. Herman BV, Nyland M, Somerville L, MacDonald SJ, Lanting BA, Howard JL. Functional outcomes of infected hip arthroplasty: a comparison of different surgical treatment options. Hip Int 2017;27(3):245–250
78. Zahar A, Gehrke TA. One-stage revision for infected total hip arthroplasty. Orthop Clin North Am 2016;47(1):11–18
79. Klouche S, Leonard P, Zeller V, et al. Infected total hip arthroplasty revision: one- or two-stage procedure? Orthop Traumatol Surg Res 2012;98(2):144–150
80. Kunutsor SK, Whitehouse MR, Blom AW, et al; Global Infection Orthopaedic Management Collaboration. One- and two-stage surgical revision of peri-prosthetic joint infection of the hip: a pooled individual participant data analysis of 44 cohort studies. Eur J Epidemiol 2018;33(10):933–946

81. Whiteside LA, Roy ME. One-stage revision with catheter infusion of intraarticular antibiotics successfully treats infected THA. Clin Orthop Relat Res 2017;475(2):419–429

82. Wolf M, Clar H, Friesenbichler J, et al. Prosthetic joint infection following total hip replacement: results of one-stage versus two-stage exchange. Int Orthop 2014;38(7):1363–1368

83. Berend KR, Lombardi AV Jr, Morris MJ, Bergeson AG, Adams JB, Sneller MA. Two-stage treatment of hip periprosthetic joint infection is associated with a high rate of infection control but high mortality. Clin Orthop Relat Res 2013;471(2):510–518

84. Ekpo TE, Berend KR, Morris MJ, Adams JB, Lombardi AV Jr. Partial two-stage exchange for infected total hip arthroplasty: a preliminary report. Clin Orthop Relat Res 2014;472(2):437–448

85. Konigsberg BS, Della Valle CJ, Ting NT, Qiu F, Sporer SM. Acute hematogenous infection following total hip and knee arthroplasty. J Arthroplasty 2014;29(3):469–472

86. Fink B, Schuster P, Schwenninger C, Frommelt L, Oremek D. A standardized regimen for the treatment of acute postoperative infections and acute hematogenous infections associated with hip and knee arthroplasties. J Arthroplasty 2017;32(4):1255–1261

87. Vilchez F, Martínez-Pastor JC, García-Ramiro S, et al. Efficacy of debridement in hematogenous and early post-surgical prosthetic joint infections. Int J Artif Organs 2011;34(9):863–869

88. Althuizen MN, V Hooff ML, v d Berg-v Erp SH, V Limbeek J, Nijhof MW. Early failures in large head metal-on-metal total hip arthroplasty. Hip Int 2012;22(6):641–647

89. Macheras GA, Lepetsos P, Leonidou AO, Anastasopoulos PP, Galanakos SP, Poultsides LA. Survivorship of a porous tantalum monoblock acetabular component in primary hip arthroplasty with a mean follow-up of 18 years. J Arthroplasty 2017;32(12):3680–3684

90. Volpin A, Konan S, Biz C, Tansey RJ, Haddad FS. Reconstruction of failed acetabular component in the presence of severe acetabular bone loss: a systematic review. Musculoskelet Surg 2019;103(1):1–13

91. Rogers BA, Whittingham-Jones PM, Mitchell PA, Safir OA, Bircher MD, Gross AE. The reconstruction of periprosthetic pelvic discontinuity. J Arthroplasty 2012;27(8):1499–1506.e1

92. Hasenauer MD, Paprosky WG, Sheth NP. Treatment options for chronic pelvic discontinuity. J Clin Orthop Trauma 2018;9(1):58–62

93. Moore KD, McClenny MD, Wills BW. Custom triflange acetabular components for large acetabular defects: minimum 10-year follow-up. Orthopedics 2018;41(3):e316–e320

94. Berend ME, Berend KR, Lombardi AV, Cates H, Faris P. The patient-specific Triflange acetabular implant for revision total hip arthroplasty in patients with severe acetabular defects: planning, implantation, and results. Bone Joint J 2018;100-B(1, Supple A):50–54

95. Abdullah KM, Hussain N, Parsons SJ, Porteous MJL, Atrey A. 11-year mean follow-up of acetabular impaction grafting with a mixture of bone graft and hydroxyapatite porous synthetic bone substitute. J Arthroplasty 2018;33(5):1481–1486

96. Hipfl C, Janz V, Löchel J, Perka C, Wassilew GI. Cup-cage reconstruction for severe acetabular bone loss and pelvic discontinuity: mid-term results of a consecutive series of 35 cases. Bone Joint J 2018;100-B(11):1442–1448

97. Park CW, Eun HJ, Oh SH, Kim HJ, Lim SJ, Park YS. Femoral stem survivorship in Dorr type A femurs after total hip arthroplasty using a cementless tapered wedge stem: a matched comparative study with type B femurs. J Arthroplasty 2019;34(3):527–533

98. White CA, Carsen S, Rasuli K, Feibel RJ, Kim PR, Beaulé PE. High incidence of migration with poor initial fixation of the Accolade stem. Clin Orthop Relat Res 2012;470(2):410–417

99. Lachiewicz PF, Soileau ES, Martell JM. Wear and osteolysis of highly crosslinked polyethylene at 10 to 14 years: the effect of femoral head size. Clin Orthop Relat Res 2016;474(2):365–371

100. Lachiewicz PF, O'Dell JA, Martell JM. Large metal heads and highly cross-linked polyethylene provide low wear and complications at 5-13 years. J Arthroplasty 2018;33(7):2187–2191

101. Lindalen E, Thoen PS, Nordsletten L, Hovik O, Rohrl SM. Low wear rate at 6-year follow-up of vitamin E-infused cross-linked polyethylene: a randomised trial using 32- and 36-mm heads. Hip Int 2019;29(4):355–362

102. Narkbunnam R, Amanatullah DF, Electricwala AJ, Huddleston JI III, Maloney WJ, Goodman SB. Outcome of 4 surgical treatments for wear and osteolysis of cementless acetabular components. J Arthroplasty 2017;32(9):2799–2805

103. Berstock JR, Whitehouse MR, Duncan CP. Trunnion corrosion: what surgeons need to know in 2018. Bone Joint J 2018;100-B(1, Supple A):44–49

104. Matharu GS, Judge A, Murray DW, Pandit HG. Outcomes after metal-on-metal hip revision surgery depend on the reason for failure: a propensity score-matched study. Clin Orthop Relat Res 2018;476(2):245–258

105. Sultan AA, Cantrell WA, Khlopas A, et al. Evidence-based management of trunnionosis in metal-on-polyethylene total hip arthroplasty: a systematic review. J Arthroplasty 2018;33(10):3343–3353

106. Marinier M, Edmiston TA, Kearns S, Hannon CP, Levine BR. A survey of the prevalence of and techniques to prevent trunnionosis. Orthopedics 2018;41(4):e557–e562

107. Luo Y, Sun XF, Chen J, Cui W, Wang T. Could larger diameter of 4th generation ceramic bearing increase the rate of squeaking after THA?: a retrospective study. Medicine (Baltimore) 2018;97(52):e13977

22 Hip Rehabilitation

David J. Kaufman

Assessment of Gait Abnormalities

I. A thorough physical examination and knowledge of anatomy are key to directing physical therapy (PT) for the painful hip.

    A. Discrete evaluation of the hip actions and their involved muscle groups is a necessary starting point:

        1. Flexors: psoas, iliacus, pectineus, and rectus femoris.

        2. Extensors: gluteus maximus and hamstrings.

        3. Abductors: gluteus medius and gluteus minimus.

        4. Adductors: adductor magnus, longus, and brevis.

        5. External rotators: gluteus maximus, superior/inferior gemellus, obturator internus/externus, and quadratus femoris.

        6. Internal rotators: tensor fascia lata, gluteus minimus, and gracilis.

II. Gait anomalies can arise from the following:

    A. Pain.

    B. Weakness.

    C. Structural abnormalities.

    D. Loss of motion.

    E. Combinations of the above.

III. Observation of gait and single leg stance provides important dynamic information regarding function of the hip and potential pathology.

    A. Key gait features include foot progression angle, pelvic motion, stance phase, stride length, truncal motion, and arm swing.

    B. Gait anomalies and their associated anatomic correlates are described in **Table 22.1**.

Rehabilitation Principles for the Painful Hip

I. Requires appropriate diagnosis and differentiating spinal etiology, referred pain, extra-articular muscle injury, intra-articular pathology, muscle imbalance, and stiffness.

    A. The hip is part of the kinetic chain extending from the lumbar spine to the feet.

        1. Dysfunction at any point along this chain can impact hip function.

        2. As the hip becomes more stiff, increased mobility demands are placed at the lumbar spine, knees, ankles, and/or feet, and can lead to secondary injuries.

Table 22.1 Gait assessment

Description	Clinical Correlate
Trendelenburg gait: contralateral pelvic drop in stance phase	Abductor weakness
Antalgic gait: shortened stance phase, lengthened swing time	Lower extremity pain
Coxalgic gait: truncal shift over painful side, contralateral pelvic elevation	Intra-articular hip pain
Externally rotated foot progression angle	Femoral retroversion, torsional anomaly, hip effusion
Internally rotated foot progression angle	Excess femoral anteversion, torsional anomaly
Quadriceps avoidance: increased knee extension	Quad weakness, knee pain, anterior cruciate ligament injury
Drop foot or steppage gait: increased hip and knee flexion with loss of ankle dorsiflexion	Sciatic nerve injury, ankle dorsiflexion weakness

II.   Goals of therapy include the following:

A. Improving range of motion (ROM):

1. Manual techniques to mobilize the joint with manipulation and distraction can stretch the capsule and surrounding muscles, and can help maintain mobility.[1]

B. Decreasing pain:

1. Modalities for muscle relaxation, pain relief, and anti-inflammation.

C. Improving muscle strength:

1. Strengthening the muscles around the hip, including core abdominal muscles and hip abductors, can be particularly useful to normalize gait.[2]

D. Minimizing detrimental effects of immobility or activity restriction:

1. Cane can be used in the contralateral hand.

i.   Allows for reciprocal arm swing.

ii. Widens base of support.

iii. Reduces joint reaction force on the affected side by up to 30%, with longer lever arm for abductor function.

E. Maintaining general fitness:

1. Weight reduction can significantly improve patient's symptoms and increase functional status, while decreasing the force on all joints.

2. Recreations such as swimming or cycling can provide fitness while minimizing forces across the hip.

F. Teaching home exercise program:

1. Education and empowerment can guide patients in activities, exercise programs, and footwear to reduce pain and optimize function.

Preoperative Considerations

I.   Comprehensive education to set patient expectations for surgery and rehabilitation course.

   A. Tailored to patient's baseline functional status, comorbidities, and postoperative goals.

   B. Preoperative education shows modest beneficial effect on anxiety before and after surgery.

      1. Effect on pain, functional outcome, and length of stay is inconclusive.[3]

   C. Address patient and family questions or concerns.

      1. Create realistic expectations.

II. Organize the home environment:

   A. Remove throw rugs.

   B. Address bathroom—toilet seats, shower bars, chairs.

   C. Stair management.

   D. Minimize obstacles that may cause injury or difficulty with recovery.

III. Arrange social support:

   A. Meals.

   B. Rides to PT or other doctor visits.

IV. A preoperative rehabilitation or "prehab" program of strengthening and gait training can improve postoperative pain control and function in the first few weeks after surgery.[4]

   A. Best evidence is to focus on patients with impaired mobility for preoperative strengthening, balance, and gait training.[5]

   B. Train patients on use of relevant durable medical equipment, including walking assistive devices.

V.   Set a hospital discharge plan, which may be subject to change after surgery.

   A. A prehab program before total hip arthroplasty (THA) has been shown to reduce rates of discharge to skilled nursing facilities and improve rates of discharge to home.[6]

Postoperative Rehabilitation after Hip Arthroscopy

I.   Protocols for PT and return to activity vary by the arthroscopy procedure performed.

   A. A hip abduction brace is frequently employed to limit postoperative hip motion.

   B. CPM (continuous passive motion) machine may be used to encourage ROM.

   C. Lying prone can help prevent the development of a flexion contracture.

   D. Protected weight bearing may be employed for a range of hip arthroscopy procedures.

II. Although there is no consensus rehabilitation protocol, specific precautions are based on the procedures performed.[7]

    A. Labral repair requires a period of restricted weight bearing, limited hip abduction, and no external rotation beyond neutral to protect the repair as it heals.

    B. Labral resection typically is followed by a 10- to 14-day period of partial weight bearing, and avoidance of excess flexion and abduction.

    C. Cheilectomy/osteoplasty requires a period of restricted weight bearing given risk of femoral neck fracture in the early postoperative period.

    D. Microfracture necessitates up to 6 weeks of restricted weight bearing.

    E. Capsular plication patients should have limited hip flexion, extension, and external rotation in the first 3 to 4 weeks after surgery to protect the anterior capsule.

III. Progressive ROM and strengthening is encouraged among all postoperative hip arthroscopy patients.[7]

    A. Gentle isometrics typically start around postoperative day 2, with gradual progression of active ROM (AROM) starting around the third week after surgery.

    B. It is important to avoid initiating activities that may lead to joint inflammation or tendinitis.

Postoperative Rehabilitation after Total Hip Arthroplasty

I. Inpatient setting:

    A. Typically first 0 to 3 days after surgery.

    B. Functional goals include the following:

        1. Early mobilization.

        2. Muscle activation.

        3. Gait training.

        4. Stair training.

        5. AROM and active-assisted ROM.

    C. Patients receiving earlier inpatient rehabilitation demonstrate shorter hospital stays and earlier independence.[8]

        1. "Fast track" clinical pathways encourage PT and mobilization on the day of surgery.[9]

        2. Early mobilization must balance benefits of rapid recovery with the need for a stable environment for implants to achieve osseointegration when cementless components are used.

    D. Early mobilization is strongly encouraged as a low-risk, low-cost strategy to reduce the risk of deep vein thrombosis (DVT).

        1. Early mobilization is a "consensus" recommended strategy for DVT prophylaxis from the American Academy of Orthopaedic Surgeons Board of Directors, reflecting expert opinion of the utility of this strategy.

E. Assistive devices improve biomechanical stabilization and somatosensory feedback:

1. Include crutches, walker, or cane depending on patient needs and surgeon-imposed restrictions.

F. Weight-bearing:

1. Full weight bearing is usually permitted after primary cementless or hybrid fixation:

   a. Historically, protected weight bearing was required for 6 weeks.

   b. Modern studies suggest this is not necessary but is still employed by some surgeons.

2. Restricted weight bearing may be employed after trochanteric osteotomy, complex revisions, or fracture.

G. Stair training before discharge is important for safe disposition, and to avoid torsional forces across the hip in the early postoperative period.[11]

1. Going up stairs: lead with nonoperative leg.

2. Going down stairs: lead with operative leg.

II. Hip precautions:

A. Standard posterior hip precautions involve limiting hip flexion, hip adduction, and internal rotation, particularly in the first 6 weeks after surgery as the soft-tissue repair heals.

1. Hip flexion beyond 90 degrees should be avoided during this time period.

2. Patients are encouraged to use an elevated toilet seat, "reacher," and "sock aid" to avoid excess hip flexion in the early postoperative period.

3. When reaching toward the floor, patients should keep the hip externally rotated by reaching between their legs, not out to the side.

4. The use of abduction bracing has not been shown to decrease dislocation rate after revision THA.[12]

B. Standard anterior hip precautions involve limiting hip extension and external rotation:

1. Commonly occurs with quick pivot-type movements or with turning in bed (foot rotates and relatively extends, while going from supine to prone).

C. There is some evidence that hip precautions are of limited utility after anterior THA.[13,14]

1. In a randomized study of 630 patients undergoing anterior THA, the authors found the following additional hip precautions did not reduce dislocation rate: use of abduction pillow, use of elevated toilet seat, avoidance of lying on the side, and avoidance of driving or riding in an automobile.[15]

III. Outpatient setting:

A. The majority of postoperative rehabilitation occurs after hospital discharge.

B. New payment methods for hip and knee replacement are driving a trend for shorter inpatient stays and minimizing use of therapy services.[16]

1. Acute postoperative rehabilitation can safely take place in multiple settings:
   a. Outpatient PT.
   b. Home PT.
   c. Skilled nursing facility.
   d. Inpatient rehabilitation facility.
2. No difference in functional status is conferred by inpatient versus home-based rehab.[17]
3. Patients with good baseline mobility and social supports are ideal candidates for early transition to outpatient PT.

C. Among certain patients undergoing THA, self-directed therapy may be as effective as formal PT in restoring function.[18]

Postacute Rehabilitation Therapy after Total Hip Arthroplasty

I. Quality of evidence:
   A. Controlled trials on post-THA therapy regimens are limited in scope design, and by variation in outcome assessment tools.
   B. Detailed protocols including frequency, duration, and equipment needs tend to be based on anecdotal or limited evidence rather than strict guidelines.[19]
   C. Multiple reviews show consensus for a progressive functional exercise program, supervised by the surgeon or other health professionals.[20,19]
      1. Includes training in the first 6 to 8 weeks after surgery with progressive resistance and body-weight support training.
      2. As function improves, exercise program should address specific impairments to include hip abductors, gait training, and core strengthening.
   D. Transition from bilateral support, such as walker or crutches, to cane, with goal of weaning off all assistive devices.
      1. Allows for a gradual progression to normal stride length and cadence.
   E. These devices bear partial body weight and decrease joint reactive forces:
      1. Alleviate pain, compensate for weakness, and minimize fall risk.

II. Components of a post-THA rehab program:
   A. Progressive resistance training:
      1. Low-intensity stimulation of skeletal muscle to lift lighter loads at frequent repetitions, with early focus on the quadriceps.
      2. Straight leg raises are often deferred in the first few weeks after surgery, as these are associated with elevated joint reactive forces and can cause a painful tendonitis that delays progress.
   B. Abductor strengthening:
      1. Crucial to normalizing gait and posture after surgery.

2. Tend to be tight in the first 4 to 6 weeks, can cause a "leaning" stance, and a false sense of a limb length discrepancy.

C. Core strengthening.

D. Active-assisted ROM:

1. Manual assistance is provided by the therapist as the hip is brought through a full ROM, decreases the muscle force applied by the patient.

E. Passive ROM:

1. Primarily indicated for patients with preoperative hip flexion contractures or other tightness around abductors, adductors.

2. Knee flexion contracture is not uncommon on the contralateral side due to compensation for preoperative limb length discrepancies.

3. May be delayed for 6 to 12 weeks in the setting of a trochanteric osteotomy or abductor repair.

F. Nonstandard adjuncts:

1. Neuromuscular electrical stimulation:

a. Some evidence that low-frequency electrical stimulation used in conjunction with conventional PT may improve strength and balance.[13]

Postrehabilitation

I. Begins when patients are discharged from formal, guided therapy:

A. May be from 6 weeks to 3 months after surgery, depending on baseline functional status, patient comorbidities, and technical factors:

1. Includes a gradual return to more physical activities and sports.

2. Long-term exercise program to maintain body weight and general health.

II. Return to driving is predicated on discontinuation of narcotics and ability to perform evasive maneuvers.

A. Depends on patient functions of strength, reaction time, ability to sit for prolonged periods, and confidence level.

B. In one review of 130 THA patients, 81% were able to resume driving at 6 weeks.[21]

III. Patients may progressively return to recreational activity, and low- to moderate-impact activities are encouraged.

A. There is no limitation to walking, cycling, swimming, and golf; however, moderation is always recommended.

IV. High-impact activity is generally discouraged, with theoretic concerns for increased revision risk from bearing surface wear or fracture, implant loosening, periprosthetic fracture, or dislocation.

A. In a 2009 survey of 139 American Association for Hip and Knee Surgeons members, 71% discouraged jogging, 83% discouraged difficult skiing, and 49% discouraged singles tennis.[22]

V. Resumption of sexual activity is rarely addressed with patients, as 86% of surgeons state they rarely or never discuss this topic, and 45 to 60% of patients desire more information.[23]

A. Patients return to sexual activity 2 to 3 months after THA, and counseling on safe positions is advised to reduce dislocation risks.[24]

References

1. MacDonald CW, Whitman JM, Cleland JA, Smith M, Hoeksma HL. Clinical outcomes following manual physical therapy and exercise for hip osteoarthritis: a case series. J Orthop Sports Phys Ther 2006;36(8):588–599
2. Weigl M, Angst F, Stucki G, Lehmann S, Aeschlimann A. Inpatient rehabilitation for hip or knee osteoarthritis: 2 year follow up study. Ann Rheum Dis 2004;63(4):360–368
3. McDonald S, Hetrick S, Green S. Pre-operative education for hip or knee replacement. Cochrane Database Syst Rev 2004;(1):CD003526
4. Wallis JA, Taylor NF. Pre-operative interventions (non-surgical and non-pharmacological) for patients with hip or knee osteoarthritis awaiting joint replacement surgery: a systematic review and meta-analysis. Osteoarthritis Cartilage 2011;19(12):1381–1395
5. Nankaku M, Tsuboyama T, Akiyama H, et al. Preoperative prediction of ambulatory status at 6 months after total hip arthroplasty. Phys Ther 2013;93(1):88–93
6. Cabilan CJ, Hines S, Munday J. The impact of prehabilitation on postoperative functional status, healthcare utilization, pain, and quality of life: a systematic review. Orthop Nurs 2016;35(4):224–237
7. Enseki KR, Martin RL, Draovitch P, Kelly BT, Philippon MJ, Schenker ML. The hip joint: arthroscopic procedures and postoperative rehabilitation. J Orthop Sports Phys Ther 2006;36(7):516–525
8. Munin MC, Rudy TE, Glynn NW, Crossett LS, Rubash HE. Early inpatient rehabilitation after elective hip and knee arthroplasty. JAMA 1998;279(11):847–852
9. Berger RA, Sanders SA, Thill ES, Sporer SM, Della Valle C. Newer anesthesia and rehabilitation protocols enable outpatient hip replacement in selected patients. Clin Orthop Relat Res 2009;467(6):1424–1430
10. American Academy of Orthopaedic Surgery (AAOS). Preventing Venous Thromboembolic Disease in Patients Undergoing Elective Hip and Knee Arthroplasty: Evidence-based guideline and evidence report. Rosemont, IL: AAOS; 2011
11. Dutton M. Orthopaedic Examination, Evaluation, and Intervention. 2nd ed. New York, NY: McGraw-Hill; 2008:1695
12. Murray TG, Wetters NG, Moric M, Sporer SM, Paprosky WG, Della Valle CJ. The use of abduction bracing for the prevention of early postoperative dislocation after revision total hip arthroplasty. J Arthroplasty 2012;27(8, Suppl):126–129
13. Cheng TE, Wallis JA, Taylor NF, et al. A prospective randomized clinical trial in total hip arthroplasty comparing early results between the direct anterior approach and the posterior approach. J Arthroplasty 2017;32(3):883–890
14. Tamaki T, Oinuma K, Miura Y, Higashi H, Kaneyama R, Shiratsuchi H. Epidemiology of dislocation following direct anterior total hip arthroplasty: a minimum 5-year follow-up study. J Arthroplasty 2016;31(12):2886–2888
15. Peak EL, Parvizi J, Ciminiello M, et al. The role of patient restrictions in reducing the prevalence of early dislocation following total hip arthroplasty. A randomized, prospective study. J Bone Joint Surg Am 2005;87(2):247–253
16. Iorio R, Clair AJ, Inneh IA, Slover JD, Bosco JA, Zuckerman JD. Early results of Medicare's bundled payment initiative for a 90-day total joint arthroplasty episode of care. J Arthroplasty 2016;31(2):343–350
17. Galea MP, Levinger P, Lythgo N, et al. A targeted home- and center-based exercise program for people after total hip replacement: a randomized clinical trial. Arch Phys Med Rehabil 2008;89(8):1442–1447
18. Austin MS, Urbani BT, Fleischman AN, et al. formal physical therapy after total hip arthroplasty is not required: a randomized controlled trial. J Bone Joint Surg Am 2017;99(8):648–655

19. Okoro T, Lemmey AB, Maddison P, Andrew JG. An appraisal of rehabilitation regimes used for improving functional outcome after total hip replacement surgery. Sports Med Arthrosc Rehabil Ther Technol 2012;4(1):5

20. Di Monaco M, Vallero F, Tappero R, Cavanna A. Rehabilitation after total hip arthroplasty: a systematic review of controlled trials on physical exercise programs. Eur J Phys Rehabil Med 2009;45(3):303–317

21. Abbas G, Waheed A. Resumption of car driving after total hip replacement. J Orthop Surg (Hong Kong) 2011;19(1):54–56

22. Swanson EA, Schmalzried TP, Dorey FJ. Activity recommendations after total hip and knee arthroplasty: a survey of the American Association for Hip and Knee Surgeons. J Arthroplasty 2009;24(6, Suppl):120–126

23. Issa K, Pierce TP, Brothers A, Festa A, Scillia AJ, Mont MA. Sexual activity after total hip arthroplasty: a systematic review of the outcomes. J Arthroplasty 2017;32(1):336–340

24. Charbonnier C, Chagué S, Ponzoni M, Bernardoni M, Hoff meyer P, Christofi lopoulos P. Sexual activity after total hip arthroplasty: a motion capture study. J Arthroplasty 2014;29(3):640–647

23 Synovial Proliferative Disorders

Hassan Alosh

Synovial Chondromatosis

I. Demographics:

    A. Intra-articular cartilaginous bodies that break off into individual nodules that can calcify.

    B. A 2:1 male-to-female occurrence.[1,2]

    C. The hip is the second most commonly affected joint (knee is first).

    D. Monoarticular.

    E. Usually occurs between age 30 and 50 years.

II. Presentation:

    A. Clinical manifestation:

        1. History: Most often patients will complain of groin and buttocks pain, which is worsened with activity. They can also complain of mechanical symptoms, including stiffness, grinding, and catching with motion. Most commonly presents as pain, limited motion, and mechanical symptoms.

        2. Physical examination: Provocative hip maneuvers such FABER (flexion, abduction, and external rotation) or flexion, adduction, and internal rotation (FADIR) will often illicit pain. Patients may also present with restricted motion in the hip, especially internal rotation.

    B. Imaging studies:

        1. Radiographs: Loose bodies visible if calcified. In late stages, concurrent signs of osteoarthritis are evident, that is, joint space narrowing, subchondral sclerosis, and osteophyte formation[3,4] (**Fig. 23.1**).

        2. Computed tomography (CT): Osteochondral bodies may or may not be visible.

        3. MRI: Noncalcified loose bodies are low signal T1 and high signal T2. Calcified bodies are low signal on T1 and T2 (**Fig. 23.2**).

        4. Little role for histology; findings include cartilaginous nodules in various stages of calcification.

III. Management:

    A. Surgical management:

        1. Arthroscopic debridement has been described with the goal of less morbidity and faster recovery. Potential disadvantages include incomplete synovectomy and inadequate visualization of loose bodies. It also requires advanced proficiency in hip arthroscopy, which may not be readily available.

            i. A recent meta-analysis of 197 patients demonstrated a recurrence rate of 7.1% at last follow-up. Conversion to THA at follow-up was most strongly predicted by the presence of full-thickness cartilage defects at arthroscopy.[1,2,4]

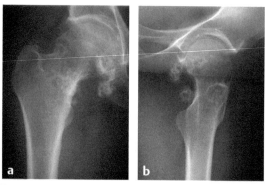

Fig. 23.1 (a, b) Calcified synovial chondromatosis evident on plain film. (Source: Discussion. In: Munk P, Ryan A, eds. Teaching Atlas of Musculoskeletal Imaging. New York, NY: Thieme; 2007.)

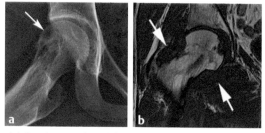

Fig. 23.2 (a, b) Synovial chondromatosis nodules evident on MRI in two different patients. (Source: Jaremko JL, Teh J, Weidekamm C, et al. Hip Inflammatory Conditions: A Practical Differential Diagnosis Algorithmic Approach in Adults and Children. Seminars in Musculoskeletal Radiology 2019;23(03):1-16)

2. Open debridement and synovectomy without femoral head dislocation has a greater recurrence rate than synovectomy with femoral head dislocation.

    a. A modified Hardinge approach with care to avoid the posterior capsule has been described to avoid compromising vascularity to the femoral head.

    b. The recurrence rate has been reported as high as 15% with open debridement without dislocation.[5,6]

3. Open synovectomy with femoral head dislocation demonstrated no recurrence in one series but resulted in a greater than 20% complication rate including avascular necrosis of the femoral head, nerve palsy, and intraoperative femur fracture. A trochanteric osteotomy may be utilized to facilitate dislocation.[5]

B. Complications/pitfalls:

1. Risk of progression of degenerative joint disease exists after synovectomy.

2. Greater severity of preoperative degenerative disease joint predicts progression of osteoarthritis.

3. Hip arthroplasty with synovectomy is indicated for those with severe degenerative joint disease and concomitant chondromatosis.[5]

Pigmented Villonodular Synovitis

I. Demographics:

1. Villous proliferation of synovium with hemosiderin deposition.

2. Associated with 5q33 chromosomal rearrangement.[7,8]

3. Presents as isolated area of hypertrophic synovium or diffuse disease.

4. Hip the second most commonly affected joint (after knee).[9]

5. Usually monoarticular but can present as polyarticular disease.

6. Affects both genders equally, usually in third or fourth decades of life.[10]

II. Presentation:

A. Clinical manifestation:

1. History: Isolated patches of PVNS in the hip will be described at discrete mechanical symptoms with catching or locking sensations during hip motion. Diffuse disease may also present with mechanical symptoms but can also be described as dull and diffuse groin and buttocks pain, which is worsened with activity.

2. Physical examination: Hip motion will often be restricted with positive provocative hip maneuvers. Stinchfield's (resisted hip flexion) and FADIR tests will often illicit pain in the groin. Patients may also present with a fixed hip flexion contracture in diffuse disease.

3. Aspiration may contain hemosiderin-laden fluid and giant cells, but may be normal.[10]

B. Imaging studies:

1. Plain films often normal, though hip PVNS often presents with concomitant arthritis.

2. CT scan: PVNS appears as mass that is higher density than skeletal muscle.[9]

3. MRI: Most often contains areas of low and high signals on T1 and T2 sequences[10] (**Fig. 23.3**):

a. Low signal demonstrates areas of hemosiderin deposition.

b. High signal on T1 indicates hemorrhage or fat deposition.

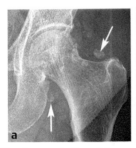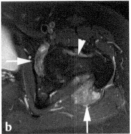

Fig. 23.3 (a, b) Hip pigmented villonodular synovitis demonstrating diffuse enhancement on contrast MRI in the sagittal plane. (Source: Jaremko JL, Teh J, Weidekamm C, et al. Hip Inflammatory Conditions: A Practical Differential Diagnosis Algorithmic Approach in Adults and Children. Seminars in Musculoskeletal Radiology 2019;23(03):1-16)

      c. High signal on T2 indicates joint effusion.

      d. Appearance on MRI may be confused for hemophilia, synovial hemangioma, or lipoma arborescens.

  C. Additional workup:

    1. Definitive diagnosis is by biopsy: percutaneous, arthroscopic, or open.

    2. Pathology: Mononuclear stromal cells infiltrating synovium with hemosiderin laden multinucleated giant cells.[9]

III. Management:

  A. Nonoperative management:

    1. Minimal role for symptomatic patients.

    2. Cortisone injections can provide transient relief but are not curative.

  B. Surgical management:

    1. Localized PVNS may be excised arthroscopically, though long-term data regarding recurrence are lacking.[11,12]

    2. Diffuse PVNS requires complete synovectomy with or without arthroplasty.

    3. Hip PVNS treated with complete synovectomy has a higher recurrence rate (35%), when combined with arthroplasty rate declines to 8%[8] (**Fig. 23.4**):

      a. Extent of degenerative joint disease is associated with higher risk of recurrence.

      b. Arthroplasty allows for dislocation of femoral head and more complete synovectomy:

        i. In several series reporting on hip arthroplasty, there were no recurrences reported of PVNS after hip arthroplasty. However, aseptic loosening has been reported as a complication with cemented THA.

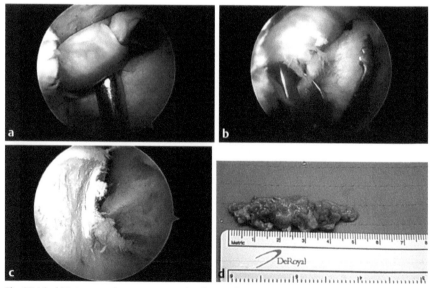

Fig. 23.4 (a–b) Intraoperative appearance of arthroscopic hip synovectomy for pigmented villonodular synovitis.

ii. A more recent series employing cementless prosthesis demon-strated successful outcomes with revisions only required for polyethylene wear.[13]

4. Adjuvant therapy with radiation or radioactive isotopes may be effective[14]:

a. May be used as an adjunct following surgical resection.

b. Can also be used for recurrent disease instead of surgery.

c. Series have demonstrated low recurrence rates when low-dose radiation has been applied after radiation[15]:

i. Low-dose radiation can be initiated 6 weeks after surgery.

ii. Radiation carries risk of skin breakdown, joint stiffness, and theoretical risk of malignancy.

d. Intra-articular radioactive isotopes can also be used to control diffuse disease and prevent recurrence[16]:

i. Yttrium-90 (Y-90) and dysprosium-165 (Dy-165) also have been used as adjuvant therapies.

ii. A series of patients who failed previous synovectomy and underwent repeat synovectomy with intra-articular radioactive isotopes demonstrated an 18% recurrence rate.

C. Complications/pitfalls:

1. Synovial sarcoma or synovial hemangioma may present with similar presentation and imaging.

2. Recurrence after resection is common and routine postoperative MRI monitoring may assist in detecting early recurrence.

Synovial Hemangioma

I. Demographics:

1. Vascular proliferation in the synovium.

2. Rare entity in the hip.

3. Most commonly seen in children and adolescents.

4. Can present with localized or diffuse lesions.

5. Polyarticular involvement suggests a genetic syndrome such as Maffucci's syndrome[17,18]:

a. Multiple enchondromas and hemangiomas.

b. High risk of malignant transformation (greater than 30%).

II. Presentation:

A. Clinical manifestation:

1. History: Isolated or small lesion may be relatively asymptomatic and not cause mechanical symptoms or pain. Diffuse disease will present with a history of stiffness, pain, and limited motion.

2. Physical examination: May reveal limited motion, hip flexion contracture, and groin/buttocks with provocative maneuvers.

B. Imaging studies:

1. Plain films often negative.

2. CT scan often unremarkable.

3. MRI can often mimic findings of PVNS[17,19]:

   a. Decreased signal on T1 and T2 demonstrates hemosiderin deposition.

   b. Increased signal on T1 demonstrates regions of hemorrhage.

   c. Can help distinguish extra-articular involvement.

C. Additional workup:

1. Histology and history can help distinguish from PVNS.[17,18] In ambiguous cases, intraoperative specimens and histology can distinguish PVNS and synovial hemangioma.

2. Hemangioma typically presents in younger patients.

3. Histology will demonstrate random distribution of blood vessels with capillary and cavernous architecture with diffuse hemosiderin deposits.

III. Management:

A. Nonoperative management:

1. Little role for nonoperative management.

2. Nonsteroidal anti-inflammatories provide some relief of symptoms.

3. Observation of patients with genetic conditions (such as Maffucci's syndrome) and polyarticular involvement may be indicated if surgical resection is not feasible.

B. Surgical management:

1. Arthroscopic resection has been described for isolated lesions successfully in case reports.[19]

2. Persistent bleeding can complicate arthroscopic resection and require open approach.[17]

3. Diffuse joint destruction requires total hip arthroplasty in addition to resection.

C. Complications/pitfalls:

1. Presentation and imaging very similar to PVNS.

2. History and histology can distinguish from other clinic entities.

3. Risk of sarcomatous transformation in patients with genetic syndromes is high and should be monitored appropriately.

References

1. Boyer T, Dorfmann H. Arthroscopy in primary synovial chondromatosis of the hip: description and outcome of treatment. J Bone Joint Surg Br 2008;90(3):314–318

2. de Sa D, Horner NS, MacDonald A, et al. Arthroscopic surgery for synovial chondromatosis of the hip: a systematic review of rates and predisposing factors for recurrence. Arthroscopy 2014;30(11):1499–1504.e2

3. Duif C, von Schulze Pellengahr C, Ali A, et al. Primary synovial chondromatosis of the hip - is arthroscopy sufficient? A review of the literature and a case report. Technol Health Care 2014;22(5):667–675

4. Ferro FP, Philippon MJ. Arthroscopy provides symptom relief and good functional outcomes in patients with hip synovial chondromatosis. J Hip Preserv Surg 2015;2(3):265–271

5. Lim S-J, Chung HW, Choi YL, Moon YW, Seo JG, Park YS. Operative treatment of primary synovial osteochondromatosis of the hip. J Bone Joint Surg Am 2006;88(11):2456–2464

6. Lim S-J, Park Y-S. Operative treatment of primary synovial osteochondromatosis of the hip. Surgical technique. J Bone Joint Surg Am 2007;89(Suppl 2, Pt.2):232–245

7. González Della Valle A, Piccaluga F, Potter HG, Salvati EA, Pusso R. Pigmented villonodular synovitis of the hip: 2- to 23-year followup study. Clin Orthop Relat Res 2001;(388):187–199

8. Vastel L, Lambert P, De Pinieux G, Charrois O, Kerboull M, Courpied JP. Surgical treatment of pigmented villonodular synovitis of the hip. J Bone Joint Surg Am 2005;87(5):1019–1024

9. Mankin H, Trahan C, Hornicek F. Pigmented villonodular synovitis of joints. J Surg Oncol 2011;103(5):386–389

10. Startzman A, Collins D, Carreira D. A systematic literature review of synovial chondromatosis and pigmented villonodular synovitis of the hip. Phys Sportsmed 2016;44(4):425–431

11. Lee S, Haro MS, Riff A, Bush-Joseph CA, Nho SJ. Arthroscopic technique for the treatment of pigmented villonodular synovitis of the hip. Arthrosc Tech 2015;4(1):e41–e46

12. Byrd JWT, Jones KS, Maiers GP II. Two to 10 years' follow-up of arthroscopic management of pigmented villonodular synovitis in the hip: a case series. Arthroscopy 2013;29(11):1783–1787

13. Yoo JJ, Kwon YS, Koo KH, Yoon KS, Min BW, Kim HJ. Cementless total hip arthroplasty performed in patients with pigmented villonodular synovitis. J Arthroplasty 2010;25(4):552–557

14. Shabat S, Kollender Y, Merimsky O, et al. The use of surgery and yttrium 90 in the management of extensive and diffuse pigmented villonodular synovitis of large joints. Rheumatology (Oxford) 2002;41(10):1113–1118

15. Berger B, Ganswindt U, Bamberg M, Hehr T. External beam radiotherapy as postoperative treatment of diffuse pigmented villonodular synovitis. Int J Radiat Oncol Biol Phys 2007;67(4):1130–1134

16. Chin KR, Barr SJ, Winalski C, Zurakowski D, Brick GW. Treatment of advanced primary and recurrent diffuse pigmented villonodular synovitis of the knee. J Bone Joint Surg Am 2002;84(12):2192–2202

17. Demertzis JL, Kyriakos M, Loomans R, McDonald DJ, Wessell DE. Synovial hemangioma of the hip joint in a pediatric patient. Skeletal Radiol 2014;43(1):107–113

18. Adelani MA, Wupperman RM, Holt GE. Benign synovial disorders. J Am Acad Orthop Surg 2008;16(5):268–275

19. Kim S-J, Cho S-H, Ko D-H. Arthroscopic excision of synovial hemangioma of the hip joint. J Orthop Sci 2008;13(4):387–389

24 Primary and Metastatic Tumors of the Hip

Yale A. Fillingham, Matthew Colman

Benign

I. Enneking staging system for benign bone tumors[1]:

 A. The staging system for benign bone tumors utilizes an Arabic numerical, which differentiates the staging system from the malignant bone tumor staging system based on Roman numerical.

 B. Stages 1 to 3 of the Enneking staging system:

 1. Stage 1 (latent):

 a. Defined as a benign bone tumor that maintains a consistent size or has a natural history of spontaneous resolution. Examples: enchondroma and nonossifying fibroma (NOF).

 2. Stage 2 (active):

 a. Defined as a benign bone tumor that has progressively grown in size but will be confined by anatomic barriers. Examples: unicameral bone cyst (UBC) and aneurysmal bone cyst (ABC).

 3. Stage 3 (locally invasive):

 a. Defined as a benign bone tumor that has progressively grown in size without being confined by anatomic barriers. Examples: giant cell tumor (GCT).

II. Synovial lesions:

 A. Pigmented villonodular synovitis (PVNS)[2]:

 1. Clinical presentation:

 a. Most common age group is middle-aged adults with a higher incidence among males than females.

 b. Typically only a single joint will be involved, most commonly the hip or knee.

 c. Patients will commonly have joint pain along with intermittent joint effusion and stiffness. A joint aspiration will typically be bloody in nature.

 2. Diagnostics:

 a. Radiographs:

 i. Plain film radiographs can show swollen soft tissue or juxtacortical erosions and sclerotic margins.

 b. MRI:

 i. Intra-articular lesion with low intensity (dark) on both T1- and T2-weighted images secondary to the large quantity of hemosiderin in the tumor.

   c. Histopathology:

   i. Disease will commonly be diffused throughout the joint, but it is possible to have only a localized area within the joint.

   ii. Histopathology will demonstrate highly cellular tissue with lipid-laden histiocytes, giant cells, and areas of chronic inflammation. The high cellularity will mimic sarcoma.

   iii. Due to the high vascularity, the tissue will classically have large amounts of hemosiderin.

3. Treatment and prognosis:

   a. Total synovectomy is the treatment of choice.

   b. Due to the difficulty of achieving a total synovectomy, the rates of recurrence can be greater than 50%.

   c. Often the natural history of PVNS will cause premature degenerative joint disease leading to definitive management with a total hip arthroplasty.

B. Synovial chondromatosis[3]:

1. Clinical presentation:

   a. Presents in a wide age range of typically 20 to 70 years. Most cases are isolated to large joints with a relatively even split between the hip and knee.

   b. Common complaints include an insidious onset of pain and swelling of the joint. Patients often report mechanical symptoms secondary to the presence of loose bodies.

2. Diagnostics:

   a. Radiographs:

   i. Plain film radiographs will have areas of calcifications around the joint of varying sizes representing the loose bodies (**Fig. 24.1**).

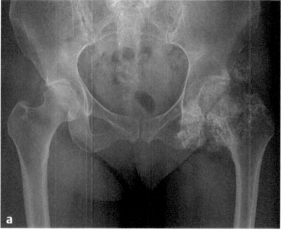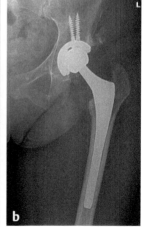

Fig. 24.1 Anteroposterior pelvis of a patient with synovial chondromatosis and severe degenerative joint disease of the left hip (**a**) that was treated with a total hip arthroplasty (**b**).

  b. Histopathology:

   i. The origin of synovial chondromatosis is the development of hyaline cartilage nodules from undifferentiated mesenchymal cells embedded in the synovium.

   ii. The loose bodies will have areas of hyaline cartilage with varying degrees of calcification secondary to endochondral ossification.

 3. Treatment and prognosis:

  a. Total synovectomy with removal of the loose bodies is the treatment of choice. Due to size limitations of arthroscopic removal of loose bodies, it can often necessitate an open synovectomy and removal of loose bodies.

  b. Due to the difficulty of achieving a total synovectomy, recurrence of the disease is common.

  c. Despite removal of the loose bodies, the high rates of recurrence can cause early degenerative joint disease requiring a total hip arthroplasty.

III. Fibrous lesions of the bone:

 A. UBC[4]:

  1. Clinical presentation:

   a. Common among individuals younger than 20 years with a propensity to occur in the proximal femur and humerus.

   b. UBC is usually discovered incidentally or as the result of a pathologic fracture.

  2. Diagnostics:

   a. Radiographs:

    i. Plain film radiographs will show a centrally located single metaphyseal cyst (possible for cyst to appear multilobulated).

    ii. Cyst will initially be located adjacent to the physis and gradually migrate away from the epiphysis. Although the cyst can appear expansile, it will rarely expand beyond the width of the physis.

    iii. Pathognomonic symbol on plain film radiographs is the "fallen leaf" sign that represents a fractured fragment of cortical bone that has fallen into the cyst (**Fig. 24.2**).

   b. MRI:

    i. The cyst will have a homogeneous high intensity on T2-weighted images. It can mimic the fluid–fluid levels of an ABC following a pathologic fracture of the cyst.

   c. Histopathology:

    i. The cystic fluid will appear similar to synovial fluid with the cyst having a thin fibrous membrane that can contain occasional giant cells.

  3. Treatment and prognosis:

   a. Lesions will typically regress spontaneously with physeal closure.

   b. Pathologic fractures are treated no different than a traumatic fracture.

   c. Impending pathologic fractures can be treated with prophylactic fixation.

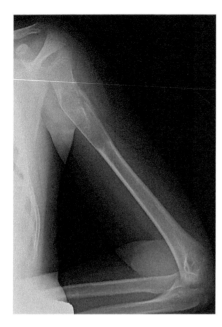

Fig. 24.2 Radiograph of the humerus demonstrates a fallen leaf sign representing the fractured cortex of the unicameral bone cyst.

B. ABC[5]:

1. Clinical presentation:

    a. Usually present in patients younger than 20 years, with the proximal femoral metaphysis, proximal tibia, and distal femur being the three most common locations.

    b. It is possible for the lesion to be discovered incidentally, but patients will often complain of vague pain in the hip.

2. Diagnostics:

    a. Radiographs:

        i. Plain film radiographs will show an eccentrically located single multilobulated expansile metaphyseal cyst (can have internal trabeculae).

    b. MRI:

        i. Classically described as having fluid–fluid levels representing the mixed blood and fluid composite of the cyst (**Fig. 24.3**).

    c. Histopathology:

        i. The cyst will have no endothelial, but the septa will have giant cells and immature osteoid matrix.

        ii. The multilobulated structures will have blood-filled areas representing the classically described "lakes of blood."

3. Treatment and prognosis:

    a. Because the lesion is considered locally aggressive, it is treated in the proximal femur with curettage, bone grafting, and prophylactic fixation.

    b. Recurrence rates are approximately 20% with higher rates of 50% in young children with open physes.

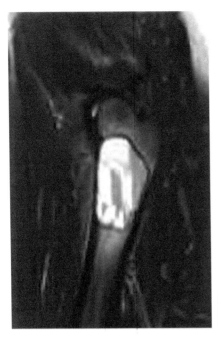

Fig. 24.3 Coronal T2 MRI image of a left proximal femur demonstrating the multiple fluid–fluid levels characteristic of aneurysmal bone cyst lesions.

C. Fibrous dysplasia[6]:

1. Clinical presentation:

   a. Presents in patients younger than 30 years, most commonly in the proximal femur.

   b. Most lesions are asymptomatic and found as incidental lesions on plain film radiographs.

   c. McCune–Albright syndrome is a combination of fibrous dysplasia, coast of Maine café au lait spots, and endocrinopathy (usually precocious puberty).

   d. Mazabraud's syndrome is a clinical entity of polyostotic fibrous dysplasia associated with intramuscular myxomas.

2. Diagnostics:

   a. Radiographs:

      i. Lesions can be present in the proximal femur metaphysis or diaphysis with a "ground-glass" appearance secondary to the small-disseminated bony islands.

      ii. The resultant weakening of the bone causes repeated microfractures leading to the classically described "shepherd's crook" deformity.

   b. Histopathology:

      i. Irregular woven bone described as having an "alphabet soup" or "Chinese letter" appearance.

      ii. Unlike most benign tumors with osteoid matrix, fibrous dysplasia will have minimal or no osteoblastic rimming of the bone.

    c. Genetics:

      i. The Gs alpha protein is a transmembrane cytokine signaling protein. Fibrous dysplasia is characterized by a mutation of chromosome 20q13 causing an activation of Gs alpha protein leading to an increased production of cyclic adenosine monophosphate (cAMP).

      ii. The mutation will cause an increased production of fibroblast growth factor 23 (FGF-23), leading to renal wasting of phosphate.

  3. Treatment and prognosis:

    a. Asymptomatic lesions are treated with observation because the lesion will stop growing after the patient reaches skeletal maturity.

    b. Deformity or pathologic fractures of the proximal femur are treated with curettage, bone grafting, correction of the deformity, and internal fixation.

    c. Patients are considered to have a 1% risk of malignant transformation.

IV. Benign cartilage lesions:

  A. Chondroblastoma[7,8]:

    1. Clinical presentation:

      a. Most patients presenting with a chondroblastoma will be younger than 25 years.

      b. Typically a patient will present with hip pain and limp, with the lesion being discovered during routine radiographs.

    2. Diagnostics:

      a. Radiographs:

        i. Chondroblastoma is one of the characteristic lesions found in the epiphysis. Plain film radiographs will show a well-circumscribed lytic lesion.

        ii. Frequently, the lesion will involve both epiphysis and metaphysis.

        iii. In the proximal femur, the lesion can be located in either the capital epiphysis or the greater trochanter apophysis.

      b. Histopathology:

        i. The lesions will have proliferating chondroblasts. The cells are classically described as having a "cobblestone" or "chicken wire" pattern.

        ii. Giant cells will be scattered within the field of mononuclear chondroblasts.

    3. Treatment and prognosis:

      a. Symptomatic patients are treated with curettage and bone grafting.

      b. Despite the benign classification of the lesion, it is known to have pulmonary metastases that are treated with surgical resection.

  B. Enchondroma[8]:

    1. Clinical presentation:

      a. A solitary enchondroma will typically be an incidental finding on plain film radiographs.

    b. The peak incidence of an enchondroma is during the third decade of life. Although the vast majority occurs in the hand, the most common location in a long bone is the proximal femur.

    c. Ollier's disease is a nonheritable disease characterized by multiple intramedullary enchondroma lesions.

    d. Maffucci's syndrome is a condition consisting of multiple enchondroma lesions with the presence of soft-tissue angiomas.

2. Diagnostics:

    a. Radiographs:

       i. Lesions will have variable patterns of calcifications often described as rings, stipples, or punctate, but these patterns will have a uniform distribution.

       ii. Scalloping that involves more than 50% of the cortical width is a characteristic of malignant transformation to a chondrosarcoma.

       iii. Enchondromas are classically observed as "hot" lesions on a bone scan.

    b. Histopathology:

       i. These lesions will be hypocellular with an abundance of hyaline matrix.

3. Treatment and prognosis:

    a. Observation is the mainstay of treatment with painful lesions necessitating curettage and bone grafting for concern of malignant transformation.

    b. A solitary enchondroma carries a 1% risk of malignant transformation.

    c. Approximately one-third of patients with Ollier's disease will have malignant transformation to chondrosarcoma.

    d. All patients with Maffucci's syndrome will have a malignant transformation to chondrosarcoma with risks of other visceral organ cancers.

Malignant

I. Staging of malignant tumors[1,9]:

1. The staging system for malignant bone tumors utilizes the Roman numerical system.

2. Determination of the assigned stage is based on tumor grade, location, and presence or absence of metastatic disease.

3. It includes stages I, II, and III, whereby stage I is low-grade tumors, stage II is high-grade tumors, and stage III is either low- or high-grade tumors with the presence of metastatic disease. Stages I and II are further broken down into an "A" and "B" stage, which is based on the tumor being intracompartmental (A) or extracompartmental (B; see **Table 24.1**).

II. Malignant cartilage lesions:

A. Conventional and dedifferentiated chondrosarcoma[8]:

1. Clinical presentation:

    a. Presents in a wide age range of typically 30 to 70 years with a slightly higher incidence in males than females. Nearly 75% of cases are isolated to the trunk, hip, and shoulder.

Table 24.1. Stages of Malignant Tumors

Stage	Tumor grade	Location	Metastasis
Stage IA	Low	Intracompartmental	Absent
Stage IB	Low	Extracompartmental	Absent
Stage IIA	High	Intracompartmental	Absent
Stage IIB	High	Extracompartmental	Absent
Stage III	Either	Either	Present

   b. Patients will usually present with a subjective complain of pain at the location of the lesion.

   c. Given the common location and size chondrosarcoma can reach before the onset of symptoms, patients can present with mass effect complains due to neurovascular or genitourinary issues.

2. Diagnostics:

   a. Radiographs:

      i. Lesion will be located in the metaphysis or diaphysis with lytic defects in the bone.

      ii. Axial and proximal lesions typically follow a more aggressive pattern of disease.

      iii. The larger tumor will appear as a soft-tissue mass with punctuated or stippled calcification.

      iv. Conventional and dedifferentiated chondrosarcoma cannot be distinguished on plain film radiographs.

   b. Histopathology:

      i. There will be an abundant amount of blue-gray chondroid matrix and variable amounts of cellularity and binucleated chondrocytes.

      ii. Dedifferentiated chondrosarcoma will differ from conventional chondrosarcoma by being dimorphic with a juxtaposed demarcated area of low-grade chondrosarcoma neighboring an area of high-grade mesenchymal spindle cells.

      iii. Due to the size of chondrosarcoma tumors, it is possible to misclassify the tumor as conventional instead of dedifferentiated due to histopathology sampling error.

3. Treatment and prognosis:

   a. Conventional and dedifferentiated chondrosarcomas are typically treated with wide resection.

   b. Chondrosarcoma tumors poorly respond to adjuvant therapies of radiation and chemotherapy.

   c. If chondrosarcoma metastasizes, it will often hematogenously spread to the lungs.

   d. Conventional chondrosarcoma has 5-year survival based on histologic grade: grade I—80 to 90%; grade II—50 to 80%; and grade III—0 to 40%.

e. Dedifferentiated chondrosarcomas have a 5-year survival rate of approximately 10%.

f. Rates of recurrence are higher when chondrosarcoma has increased telomerase activity on reverse transcriptase polymerase chain reaction testing.

B. Clear cell chondrosarcoma[8]:

1. Clinical presentation:

a. Presents among a wide range of ages with the peak incidence during the third decade. Males have a higher incidence at a rate of 2:1 compared with females.

b. Lesions are commonly found in the epiphysis of the proximal femur.

c. The most common presenting symptom is hip pain.

2. Diagnostics:

a. Radiographs:

i. Initially, the lesion will appear benign in the epiphysis well marginated and peripheral sclerosis similar to aseptic necrosis.

ii. Later appearance will be more malignant that is poorly marginated and lytic.

b. Histopathology:

i. The cellular makeup will appear similar to conventional chondrosarcomas, but cells will have abundant clear cytoplasm.

3. Treatment and prognosis:

a. Because clear cell chondrosarcoma is considered a low-grade tumor, it is commonly treated with wide resection alone.

b. Survival following clear cell chondrosarcoma is good with 10-year survival rates of 80 to 85%.

III. Bone tumors:

A. Osteosarcoma[10]:

1. Clinical presentation:

a. Osteosarcoma is vastly more common in the distal femur and proximal tibia, but it can still be diagnosed in the proximal femur and acetabulum.

b. Primary conventional osteosarcoma is usually noted in patients younger than 30 years. Secondary osteosarcomas from radiation exposure or Paget's disease occur in the adult population.

c. Initial presenting symptoms will typically be a painful mass around the joint. One differentiating characteristic of the pain is the presence of pain at night that is unresponsive to anti-inflammatory medications.

d. Patients with a mutation of the retinoblastoma tumor suppressor gene will have a predisposition to developing osteosarcoma.

2. Diagnostics:

a. Radiographs:

i. Lesions will usually be located in the metaphysis with a mixed lytic and sclerotic appearance. The radiographs can have matrix

mineralization in a sunburst pattern and periosteal reaction forming Codman's triangle.

b. MRI:

i. Advanced imaging should include the entire femur to investigate
for the presence of skip lesions.

ii. The extent of soft-tissue involvement will be better seen on the MRI.
Due to the soft-tissue involvement, most conventional osteosarcomas are a stage IIB.

c. Histopathology:

i. There will be characteristics of malignant cells with cellular atypia
and high rates of mitotic figures.

ii. The tumor cells are spindle shaped with formation of osteoid
matrix. The osteoid will not have any osteoblastic riming, which is
a differentiating feature of nonmalignant osteoid matrix.

3. Treatment and prognosis:

a. After completion of a complete oncological workup, patients are treated with neoadjuvant chemotherapy, followed by wide surgical resection with adjuvant chemotherapy after surgery.

b. Historically, wide surgical resection was limited to amputation, but
significant advances in reconstructive implant designs now allow for
limb salvage. Expendable bones are never reconstructed following
wide surgical resection.

c. Localized conventional osteosarcoma will have a 75% long-term dis-
ease-free survival with metastatic osteosarcoma having a much lower
survival rate of 25%.

d. The most common location for metastatic disease is the lungs with
other bones being the second most common location. Due to the risk
of pulmonary metastases, patients will get a CT scan of the chest.

Metastatic

I. General considerations[11,12]:

1. Typically metastatic disease occurs in patients older than 40 years.

2. Patients will not always present with a prior malignancy or history of an at-
risk activity for malignancy. The most common presenting symptom is pain.

3. Radiographic findings are described based on the number, size, location,
and type of lesion.

4. Histology of the lesion will depend on the primary source of the malignancy.

II. Diagnostic workup for metastatic disease of an unknown primary[12,13]:

1. Obtain a thorough history to assess for prior malignancies or activities that
place the patient at risk for a particular malignancy.

2. Perform a focused physical examination of the breast, prostate, thyroid,
and abdomen.

Table 24.2. Mirel's Criteria

Variable	1 point	2 points	3 points
Lesion site	Upper extremity	Lower extremity	Peritrochanteric
Pain	Mild	Moderate	Functional
Type of lesion	Blastic	Mixed	Lytic
Size	>1/3 diameter	1/3–2/3 diameter	>2/3 diameter

3. Laboratory tests should include alkaline phosphatase, basic metabolic panel (BMP), complete blood count (CBC), erythrocyte sedimentation rate (ESR), liver function, prostate-specific antigen (PSA), and serum protein electrophoresis.

4. Plain film radiographs should include a chest X-ray and any painful extremities or joints. A whole-body bone scan should be performed to investigate for the presence of multiple skeletal lesions.

5. Advanced imagining should include a CT scan of the chest, abdomen, and pelvis.

6. Biopsy should be performed to confirm lesion is not a primary bone malignancy.

III. Prophylactic fixation[14]:

1. Mirel's criteria[15]:

    a. Twelve-point system based on the lesion site, type of pain, type of lesion, and size (**Table 24.2**).

    b. The indication for prophylactic fixation is a Mirel criteria score of greater than 8.

2. Recommend whole-bone postoperative radiation therapy:

    a. Myeloma, lymphoma, and germ cell tumors are considered very radiation sensitive.

    b. Renal, melanoma, and non–small cell lung carcinomas are not considered radiation sensitive.

3. If the patient has a prognosis of less than 3 months to survive, then nonoperative management can be considered.

References

1. Kakhki VR, Anvari K, Sadeghi R, Mahmoudian AS, Torabian-Kakhki M. Pattern and distribution of bone metastases in common malignant tumors. Nucl Med Rev Cent East Eur 2013;16(2):66–69
2. Messerschmitt PJ, Garcia RM, Abdul-Karim FW, Greenfield EM, Getty PJ. Osteosarcoma. J Am Acad Orthop Surg 2009;17(8):515–527
3. Bickels J, Dadia S, Lidar Z. Surgical management of metastatic bone disease. J Bone Joint Surg Am 2009;91(6):1503–1516
4. Kaila R, Ropars M, Briggs TW, Cannon SR. Aneurysmal bone cyst of the paediatric shoulder girdle: a case series and literature review. J Pediatr Orthop B 2007;16(6):429–436
5. Lin PP, Thenappan A, Deavers MT, Lewis VO, Yasko AW. Treatment and prognosis of chondroblastoma. Clin Orthop Relat Res 2005;438(438):103–109
6. Parekh SG, Donthineni-Rao R, Ricchetti E, Lackman RD. Fibrous dysplasia. J Am Acad Orthop Surg 2004;12(5):305–313

7. Rougraff BT. Evaluation of the patient with carcinoma of unknown origin metastatic to bone. Clin Orthop Relat Res 2003;(415, Suppl):S105–S109
8. Chin KR, Barr SJ, Winalski C, Zurakowski D, Brick GW. Treatment of advanced primary and recurrent diffuse pigmented villonodular synovitis of the knee. J Bone Joint Surg Am 2002;84(12):2192–2202
9. Wilkins RM. Unicameral bone cysts. J Am Acad Orthop Surg 2000;8(4):217–224
10. Marco RA, Gitelis S, Brebach GT, Healey JH. Cartilage tumors: evaluation and treatment. J Am Acad Orthop Surg 2000;8(5):292–304
11. Rougraff BT, Kneisl JS, Simon MA. Skeletal metastases of unknown origin. A prospective study of a diagnostic strategy. J Bone Joint Surg Am 1993;75(9):1276–1281
12. Shpitzer T, Ganel A, Engelberg S. Surgery for synovial chondromatosis. 26 cases followed up for 6 years. Acta Orthop Scand 1990;61(6):567–569
13. Mirels H. Metastatic disease in long bones. A proposed scoring system for diagnosing impending pathologic fractures. Clin Orthop Relat Res 1989;(249):256–264
14. Enneking WF. A system of staging musculoskeletal neoplasms. Clin Orthop Relat Res 1986;(204):9–24
15. Enneking WF, Spanier SS, Goodman MA. A system for the surgical staging of musculoskeletal sarcoma. Clin Orthop Relat Res 1980; (153):106–120

25 Osteonecrosis of the Hip

Matthew W. Tetreault, Roshan P. Shah

Epidemiology

I. Osteonecrosis of the femoral head (ONFH) is synonymous with avascular necrosis (AVN).

II. Incidence:

    A. Twenty thousand to 30,000 new cases per year in the United States.[1]

    B. Approximately 10% of total hip arthroplasties in the United States are for ONFH.[2]

III. Demographics[3]:

    A. Male-to-female ratio depends upon/varies with etiology, for example, males predominate alcohol-associated ONFH and females predominate lupus-associated ONFH.

    B. Average age at presentation is younger than 50 years.

IV. Location:

    A. Usually occurs in the anterolateral femoral head.[3]

    B. Fifty percent to 70% have bilateral hip involvement.[1,3]

    C. Three percent of patients have multifocal osteonecrosis involving ≥3 joints.[4]

    D. The hip should be evaluated in patients with osteonecrosis of the knee, shoulder, or other joints throughout the body.

V. Risk factors[5]:

    A. Traumatic:

        1. Fractures about the hip can disrupt the local blood supply to the femoral head.

        2. Hip dislocation:

            a. Anterior dislocations are associated with an ONFH event rate of 0.09 to 0.3.

            b. Posterior dislocations are associated with an ONFH at a rate of 0.1 to 0.4.

            c. Delay of reduction of greater than 12 hours has an odds ratio of ONFH of 5.6.[6]

        3. In children, osteonecrosis can occur following a slipped capital femoral epiphysis (SCFE) injury:

            a. ONFH has been reported in 25% of cases after an unstable SCFE.[7]

    B. Atraumatic:

        1. Steroids (exogenous or endogenous) are responsible for 10 to 30% of ONFH cases.[8–10]

        2. Alcohol intake of up to 320-g ethanol per week (five bottles of wine) raises risk by a factor of 2.8[10–12]:

            a. Excessive alcohol intake and use of glucocorticoids are associated with greater than 80% of atraumatic cases.[13]

3. Sickle cell anemia (SS) and sickle cell hemoglobin C (SC) have high rates of ONFH, with SC occurring later in life. Sickle cell trait (S) has an intermediate risk of ONFH.[14]

4. Dysbaric disorders (decompression sickness, "the bends," Caisson's disease).[15]

5. Systemic lupus erythematosus (SLE).[16,17]

6. Marrow-replacing diseases (e.g., Gaucher's disease[18]).

7. Chronic renal failure or hemodialysis.[19]

8. Pancreatitis.[3]

9. Pregnancy.[20]

10. Hyperlipidemia.[3]

11. Hyperuricemia.[3]

12. Radiation.[21]

13. Transplant patients (solid organ[22] or hematopoietic cell transplantation[23,24]).

14. Coagulation factor abnormalities (e.g., genetic defects resulting in hypofibrinolysis or thrombophilia, like factor V Leiden, an autosomal dominant condition with incomplete penetrance that predisposes to excessive clotting[25-27]).

15. Cigarette smoking.[11]

16. Hematologic diseases (leukemia, lymphoma).[28,29]

17. Human immunodeficiency virus (HIV) infection with or without antiretroviral treatment.[10,30]

18. Idiopathic:

   a. In children, idiopathic ONFH occurs as Legg–Calvé–Perthes (LCP) disease with an incidence of around 15 per 100,000 children.[31]

   b. Multiple epiphyseal dysplasia (MED) is distinguished from LCP by its symmetric disease, bilateral involvement, early acetabular changes, and lack of metaphyseal cysts.

Anatomy

I.   Pertinent vasculature:

   A.   Extracapsular arterial ring:

      1.   At the base of the femoral neck.

      2.   Consists of:

         a.   Ascending branch of the medial femoral circumflex artery (MFCA) posteriorly.

         b.   Ascending branch of the lateral femoral circumflex artery (LFCA) anteriorly.

         c.   Superior and inferior gluteal arteries have minor contributions.

3. MFCA[32]:

   a. *Principal blood* supply to the weight-bearing portion of the femoral head in adults.[33]

   b. Arises from the profunda femoris artery.

   c. Travels posteriorly from its origin and gives off five consistent branches (superior, ascending, acetabular, descending, and deep). Preservation of the *deep branch* is most important in prevention of ONFH.

   d. This branch courses between the iliopsoas and pectineus, along the inferior border of the obturator externus (toward the intertrochanteric crest).

   e. When viewed posteriorly, the deep branch can be located in the space between the quadratus femoris and the inferior gemellus (**Fig. 25.1**).

   f. The main division of the deep branch continues its course superiorly by crossing posterior to the obturator externus tendon and then anterior to the conjoint tendon.

   g. The deep branch then perforates the hip capsule just cranial to the insertion of the superior gemellus tendon (and distal to the piriformis tendon).

B. Ascending cervical vessels:

   1. Arise from the extracapsular ring.

   2. Comprised of four retinacular vessels: anterior, posterior, medial, and lateral.

   3. These vessels are subsynovial in location beginning at the capsular attachment to the femoral neck (anteriorly at the intertrochanteric line and posteriorly at the intertrochanteric crest).

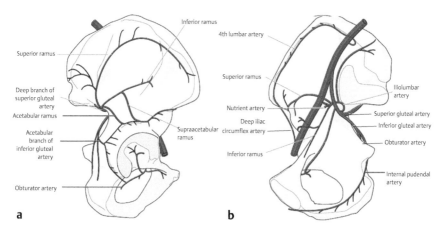

Fig. 25.1 (a-b) The extracapsular course of the medial femoral circumflex artery (MFCA). The area immediately adjacent to the medial border of the greater trochanter is at risk of vascular injury, representing the vascular danger zone. (Source: Anatomy of the acetabulum. In: Tile M, Helfet D, Kellam J, et al., eds. AO TRAUMA Fractures of the Pelvis and Acetabulum: Principles and Methods of Management. 4th Edition. Thieme; 2015.)

    4. Lateral vessels supply the greatest volume of the femoral head.

    5. LFCA gives rise to anterior vessels and MFCA often gives rise to the others.

C. Subsynovial intra-articular ring (of Chung[34]):

    1. Arises from the retinacular vessels as a ring on the surface of the neck at the articular cartilage border.

    2. Epiphyseal arteries enter the head from here, perforating into bone 2 to 4 mm distal to the bone–cartilage junction (**Fig. 25.2**):

        a. *Lateral epiphyseal artery*, which enters the head posterosuperiorly, is most important.

D. Artery of the ligamentum teres:

    1. Usually originates from the obturator artery, occasionally the MFCA.

    2. Forms the medial epiphyseal vessels.

    3. Supplies the femoral head more consistently in young children; a small and variable amount of the femoral head is nourished in adults.

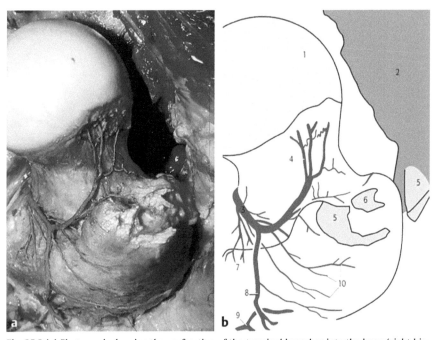

Fig. 25.2 (a) Photograph showing the perforation of the terminal branches into the bone (right hip, posterosuperior view). The terminal subsynovial branches are located on the posterosuperior aspect of the neck of the femur and penetrate the bone 2 to 4 mm lateral to the bone–cartilage junction. **(b)** Diagram showing (1) the femoral head, (2) gluteus medius, (3) the deep branch of the medial femoral circumflex artery (MFCA), (4) the terminal subsynovial branches of the MFCA, (5) insertion and tendon of gluteus medius, (6) insertion of tendon of piriformis, (7) the lesser trochanter with nutrient vessels, (8) the trochanteric branch, (9) the branch of the perforating artery, and (10) the trochanteric branches. (Source: Anatomy of the acetabulum. In: Tile M, Helfet D, Kellam J, et al., eds. AO TRAUMA Fractures of the Pelvis and Acetabulum: Principles and Methods of Management. 4th Edition. Thieme; 2015.)

E. Intraosseous vessels:

1. Intraosseous cervical vessels (within the medullary cavity) provide a relatively small portion of the femoral head blood supply.

II. Age-related changes:

A. The blood supply of the femoral head changes with age[35]:

1. *Birth to 4 years*: primary MFCA and LFCA, artery of the ligamentum teres.

2. *Four years to adult*: posterosuperior and posteroinferior retinacular vessels from MFCA. Minimal amount from LFCA or ligamentum teres:

a. *Corollary*: using a piriformis starting point for antegrade nailing of pediatric femur fractures can disrupt the posterosuperior retinacular vessels and cause ONFH.[36]

3. *Adult*: MFCA to lateral epiphyseal artery.

Pathophysiology

I. ONFH is the result of derangements that compromise blood supply to the femoral head resulting in cell death, fracture, and collapse of the articular surface.[1]

A. Atraumatic osteonecrosis:

1. Pathogenesis likely multifactorial, including genetic, metabolic, and local factors.[2,13,37]

2. Proposed pathways include:

a. Vascular occlusion:

i. Lipids:

(1) Increased glucocorticoids seen in systemic diseases such as SLE and alcohol abuse associated with changes in circulating lipids, triggering microemboli in arteries supplying the bone.[38]

(2) Increased risk of fat emboli has also been attributed to an increase in bone marrow fat cell size (adipocyte hypertrophy), which blocks venous flow.[1]

ii. Intravascular coagulation and thrombus formation:

(1) Antiphospholipid antibodies, inherited thrombophilia, and hypofibrinolysis affect the coagulation and fibrinolytic pathways.[1]

(2) Sickling of red blood cells and bone marrow hyperplasia as seen in sickle cell conditions can cause vascular occlusion.[1]

(3) Accumulation of cerebroside-filled cells within the bone marrow can occlude vessels in conditions like Gaucher's disease.[18]

(4) Decompression sickness associated with increased pressure incites nitrogen bubble formation, which can cause arteriolar occlusion and necrosis. This also leads to elevated plasma levels of plasminogen activator inhibitor, increasing coagulation.[39]

b. Direct cellular toxicity:

i. Damage to cells may be caused by irradiation, chemotherapy, or oxidative stress.

ii. This may lead to a reduction in osteogenic differentiation with diversion of mesenchymal stem cells to a fat-cell lineage.[40]

B. Trauma-related osteonecrosis:

1. Due to direct mechanical damage by rupture, compression, or kinking of the extraosseous vessels as a result of injury. The location of these vessels along the course of the femoral neck makes them susceptible to direct injury in the setting of trauma.[21,41]

2. Intracapsular hip fractures (femoral head and neck) are at greater risk of osteonecrosis than extracapsular hip fractures (intertrochanteric and subtrochanteric) secondary to potential to disrupt the blood supply described earlier[5] (**Fig. 25.3**) and risk of intracapsular hematoma:

a. Femoral head fracture: incidence of osteonecrosis varies from 6 to 23%[42–46]:

i. Reported after both surgical and nonsurgical treatments.

b. Femoral neck fracture:

i. Per recent meta-analysis, overall incidence of osteonecrosis is 14.3% (range, 10–25%).[47]

ii. Higher risk of osteonecrosis with greater initial fracture displacement[48–50] and malreduction.[48,51]

iii. Fractures in the subcapital region of the femoral neck at particular risk; trauma at this location disrupts the anastomosis between the lateral epiphyseal vessels (from the MFCA) and the artery of the ligamentum teres.[1]

iv. Relationship between time to fixation of intracapsular femoral neck fractures and risk of osteonecrosis is controversial. One retrospective study reported a lower rate of ONFH when operative

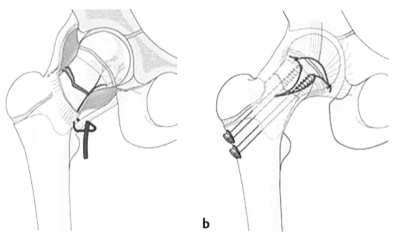

a   b

Fig. 25.3 (a-b) The prognosis of hip fractures varies by anatomic location. Intracapsular fractures are more likely to disrupt the blood supply to the femoral head, thereby increasing the risk of avascular necrosis, compared with extracapsular (i.e., intertrochanteric) fractures. (Source: Pediatric fractures. In: Rüedi T, Buckley R, Moran C, eds. AO Principles of Fracture Management. 2nd Edition. Thieme; 2007.)

fixation was performed within 12 hours of injury. Other studies have failed to demonstrate a significant difference between timing of fracture fixation and incidence of ONFH.[52]

v.   Decompression of the intracapsular hematoma has been proposed to reduce the risk of osteonecrosis by minimizing extraosseous compression of vessels supplying the femoral head. There is a paucity of clinical evidence evaluating this theory,[53] with conflicting results; at least one retrospective study found no relationship,[4] while another found a reduced risk of osteonecrosis with hip decompression in Garden type II and III fractures.[55]

3.   Extracapsular fractures of the trochanteric region have a significantly lower incidence of osteonecrosis as they are distal to the entry of the arterial branches that supply the femoral head.[56]

4.   Hip dislocations may also interrupt the extraosseous vascular supply of the femoral head[57–59]:

a.   Deep branch of the MFCA can be injured during a posterior dislocation as it courses posterior to obturator externus and anterior to quadratus femoris.[32,60]

b.   Rate of osteonecrosis associated with posterior dislocation between 5 and 60% depending on time to reduction and severity of associated fractures and other injuries.[57–69]

c.   In one case control study, 4.8 versus 52.9% rate of osteonecrosis in patients with a posterior hip dislocation reduced before versus after 6 hours, respectively.[57]

d.   Lack of data on long-term outcomes of anterior hip dislocations; limited literature suggests an osteonecrosis rate of roughly 10%.[61,62]

Evaluation

I.   Clinical:

A.   Symptoms:

1.   Pain: the most common presenting symptom of osteonecrosis[4,63]:

a.   Groin pain most common, followed by thigh and buttock pain.

b.   Weight-bearing or motion-induced pain in majority of cases.

c.   Rest pain present in about two-thirds of patients and night pain in one-third.

d.   Although rare, pain in multiple jointis suggestive of a multifocal process.

2.   A small proportion of patients are asymptomatic and the diagnosis of osteonecrosis is an incidental finding. Meanwhile, asymptomatic involvement contralateral to a symptomatic side is frequently noted.[3]

B.   Examination[3,13]:

1.   Physical findings largely nonspecif ic.

    2. May have pain with, and eventually (as the disease progresses with secondary acetabular involvement) limitations to, range of motion, particularly forced internal rotation and abduction:

        a. Often maintain a better range of motion than patients with chronic degenerative joint disease.

    3. Positive Stinchfield's test: pain with resisted hip flexion in the supine position.

    4. Flexion contracture of the hip joint and resultant limp may be present in the later courses of the disease.

II. Imaging:

  A. Radiographs:

    1. Recommend anteroposterior (AP) and frog-leg lateral views of the affected hip, and AP and lateral views of the contralateral hip.

    2. Lateral films are necessary to evaluate the superior portion of the femoral head in which subchondral abnormalities are often seen.

    3. Plain radiographs can remain normal for months after symptoms of osteonecrosis begin.

        a. Earliest findings are mild density changes.

        b. Followed by concomitant areas of sclerosis and cystic formation in the femoral head as the disease progresses.

        c. The pathognomonic crescent sign (subchondral radiolucency) is evidence of subchondral collapse.

        d. Later stages include loss of sphericity or collapse of the femoral head. Ultimate, joint space narrowing and acetabular-sided degenerative changes are seen (refer to "Classification" section for imaging examples).[64]

  B. Magnetic resonance imaging (MRI):

    1. Superior to X-ray or bone scan with studies reporting sensitivity and specificity greater than 99%.[37,65–70] More accurate than radiographs in evaluating the size of osteonecrotic lesions.[71,72]

    2. Advised when osteonecrosis is suspected but radiographs appear normal to rule out or stage osteonecrosis. Importantly, MR changes can be seen early in the course of disease when other studies are negative.[3]

    3. "Double-line sign" is pathognomonic[3]:

        a. T1: Focal lesions are well demarcated and inhomogeneous on T1. Earliest finding is dark/low-intensity band representing decreased signal from ischemic bone.

        b. T2: A second high-intensity line appears on T2 (within the line seen on T1 images), representing hypervascular granulation tissue. This is the double-line sign (**Fig. 25.4**).

    4. Presence of bone marrow edema (as evidenced by high signal intensity on T2-weighted MRI; **Fig. 25.5**) is not always seen; this finding is predictive of worsening pain and future disease progression.[73]

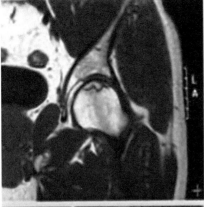

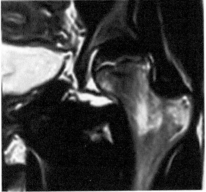

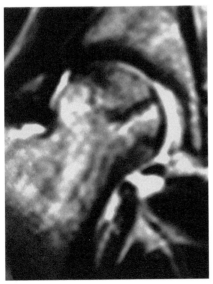

Fig. 25.4 Double-line sign on MR imaging of a femoral head, pathognomonic for osteonecrosis. On the T1-weighted coronal MR image (*top*), a serpiginous line of low signal is seen anterosuperiorly, demarcating ischemic from fatty marrow. On the T2-weighted coronal MR image (*bottom*), a hypodense line is paralleled by an inner and outer hyperintense line, representing hypervascular granulation tissue at the interface between necrotic and viable bone.

Fig. 25.5 A coronal T2-weighted MR image of a right hip with osteonecrosis of the femoral head and high signal intensity within the femoral neck indicative of bone marrow edema.

C. Bone scan:

1. Technetium-99 m bone scan: increased bone turnover at the junction of dead and reactive bone results in increased uptake surrounding a cold area; this has been called the "doughnut sign."[74]

2. While moderately sensitive, bone scan is nonspecific. It is both less sensitive and specific than MRI and its sensitivity is least in patients with early-stage lesions.[67] Thus, bone scan is not generally recommended for diagnosis of or screening for osteonecrosis.[3]

Diagnosis

I.   A clinical diagnosis is appropriately made in a symptomatic patient when MRI or radiographic findings are compatible with osteonecrosis and when other causes of pain and bony abnormalities either are unlikely or have been excluded by appropriate testing.[3]

II. MRI without contrast continues to be the "gold standard" for diagnosis in symptomatic and asymptomatic patients, especially in early-stage disease.[75,76] It has largely replaced measurement of bone marrow pressure, venography, and bone biopsy as a means of diagnosing early-stage disease.[3] For end-stage disease, MRI may be unnecessary.

Differential Diagnosis[3]

I.   The differential diagnosis of pain with characteristics suggestive of an osteoarticular origin and with imaging features compatible with osteonecrosis includes:

A. Transient osteopenia of the hip (also known as bone marrow edema syndrome):

1. May occur in isolation or along with injuries that result in neurologic damage, for example, chronic pain and transient osteopenia are features of complex regional pain syndrome.

2. When the hip is affected, MRI findings suggestive of transient osteopenia (decreased signal on T1-weighted images and increased intensity on T2-weighted images) may extend from the femoral head into the femoral neck. An effusion may also be present.

3. Absence of fever, leukocytosis, or elevated acute phase reactants (erythrocyte sedimentation rate and/or C-reactive protein) is typical of both osteonecrosis and transient osteopenia of the hip and helps exclude infectious etiology.

B. Subchondral fracture:

1. Typically occurs in patients with preexisting osteopenia and is often thought to represent an insufficiency fracture.

2. Such fractures may be difficult to appreciate on plain radiographs. Subtle flattening is sometimes present with early lesions, as collapse is progressive.

3. These rare fractures are characterized by linear regions of low signal on both T1- and T2-weighted MRI in the subchondral area paralleling the articular surface.[77,78]

Classification

I.   Several classification systems describe clinical and radiological severity/progression of disease (of note many of these are for research purposes and in reality it comes down to the etiology of ONFH and whether or not the femoral head is collapsed to determine treatment options).

   A. Ficat and Arlet's classification[41,79] (**Table 25.1**):

      1. Early classification that is still commonly used.

      2. Does not consider the extent of necrosis and therefore inadequate to assess progression.

Table 25.1 Ficat and Arlet's classification

Stage	Pain	Radiographs
0: Preclinical and preradiographic[a]	No	Normal
1: Preradiographic	Yes	Normal
2: Precollapse	Yes	Femoral head has normal sphericity but signs of bone remodeling (porosis, sclerosis, cysts)

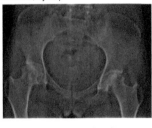

3: Early collapse	Yes	Subchondral collapse (crescent sign) or flattening of the femoral head

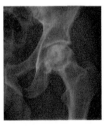

4: Osteoarthritis	Yes	Degenerative change in acetabulum with reduction in joint space

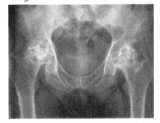

[a]Added later to initial classification system.

3. Stage 0 (preclinical and preradiographic "silent hip") added to the original four-stage classification to describe patients with contralateral ONFH.

B. Steinberg's staging system[80] (**Table 25.2**):

1. Incorporated MRI and percent involvement of the femoral head.

C. The Association Research Circulation Osseous (ARCO) staging system (**Table 25.3**):

1. Developed in an attempt to bring uniformity to clinical trials.

2. Combines features of the Ficat and Arlet and the Steinberg systems.

3. Modified to include an early and late stage 3.[81]

Prognosis

I. Kerboul's angle (**Fig. 25.6**)[82]:

A. Estimates extent of femoral head necrosis radiographically in early stages.

B. Measured as sum of the angles formed by the arc of the femoral head necrosis on AP and lateral hip radiographs.

C. Clinical outcomes better if value less than 200 degrees.

II. Modified Kerboul combined necrotic angle (**Fig. 25.6**)[83]:

A. Concept of angular summation applied to MRI; calculated by adding the arc of the femoral head necrosis on midsagittal and midcoronal MRI.

B. Predicts risk of femoral head collapse:

1. Low risk: less than 190 degrees.

2. Moderate risk: 190 to 240 degrees.

3. High risk: greater than 240 degrees.

Treatment options include nonsurgical options, joint-preserving surgery, and hip replacement surgery. The treatment is tailored to the individual as there is no gold standard, and patient factors like age, comorbidities, and function influence recommendations. The main aim of nonsurgical or joint-preserving treatment is to prevent collapse of the femoral head and delay progression of disease.

I. Nonsurgical:

A. Pharmacologic agents (bisphosphonates, vasodilators, statins, anticoagulants):

1. Bisphosphonates: Counteract collapse in ONFH by reducing osteoclast activity. Alendronate has been reported to prevent early collapse in Steinberg stage II and III nontraumatic ONFH at 24- to 28-month follow-up, and to reduce

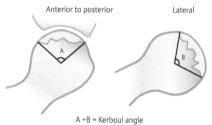

Anterior to posterior   Lateral

A +B = Kerboul angle

Fig. 25.6 The Kerboul angle is the sum of the angles formed by the extent of the femoral head lesion and the center of the femoral head on anteroposterior and lateral radiographs. The modified Kerboul angle uses this concept of angular summation and applies it to the midcoronal and midsagittal magnetic resonance images.

Table 25.2 Steinberg's staging system

Stage	Features
0	Normal radiograph, bone scan, and magnetic resonance imaging
I	Normal radiograph, abnormal bone scan, and/or magnetic resonance imaging
	A. Mild (involves <15% of femoral head)
	B. Moderate (involves 15–30% of femoral head)
	C. Severe (involves >30% of femoral head)
II	Cystic and sclerotic changes in the femoral head
	A. Mild (involves <15% of femoral head)
	B. Moderate (involves 15–30% of femoral head)
	C. Severe (involves >30% of femoral head)
III	Subchondral collapse (crescent sign) without flattening of the femoral head
	A. Mild (involves <15% of femoral head)
	B. Moderate (involves 15–30% of femoral head)
	C. Severe (involves >30% of femoral head)
IV	Flattening of the femoral head/femoral head collapse
	A. Mild (involves <15% of femoral head)
	B. Moderate (involves 15–30% of femoral head)
	C. Severe (involves >30% of femoral head)
V	Joint space narrowing and/or acetabular changes
	A. Mild
	B. Moderate
	C. Severe
VI	Advance degenerative joint disease

Table 25.3 Association Research Circulation Osseous (ARCO) staging system

Stage	Findings
0	All diagnostic studies normal and diagnosis by histology only
1	Plain radiographs and CT normal, scintigraph or MRI positive, and biopsy positive, with extent of femoral head involvement 15% (A), 15–30% (B), or >30% (C), and the location medial (A), central (B), or lateral (C)
2	Radiographs positive but no collapse (no crescent sign), with extent of involvement A, B, or C and location A, B, or C
Early 3	Crescent sign on the radiograph and/or flattening of articular surface of the femoral head. No collapse. Location (A, B, or C) and extent of involvement (A, B, or C)
Late 3	Collapse on the radiograph and/or flattening of articular surface of the femoral head. Location (A, B, or C) and extent of involvement (A, B, or C)
4	Joint space narrowing on plain radiography and acetabular involvement, as well as other signs of osteoarthritis

pain at 1-year follow-up relative to placebo.[84,85] It may also be beneficial as an adjunct to core decompression in early stages of ONFH.[85] However, evidence for slowing the progression of ONFH and preventing the need for total hip replacement remains controversial.[86]

2. Vasodilators: Prostacyclin may improve blood flow via a vasodilatory effect on terminal vessels. While improvements in clinical and radiographic outcomes have been reported for early stages of ONFH, long-term benefits are yet to be determined.[87]

3. Statins: Lipid lowering agents are potentially beneficial given the increase in number and size of circulating fat cells associated with ONFH.[1,38] Statins are shown to have protective effects in patients taking steroids, but capacity to reverse steroid-induced ONFH changes remains uncertain.[88,89]

4. Anticoagulants: May increase blood flow to ischemic areas of bone. Primarily beneficial in patients with underlying coagulopathy disorders.[90,91]

B. Other nonoperative modalities (extracorporeal shock wave therapy, electrical stimulation, hyperbaric O2)[92]:

1. Randomized clinical trials with long-term follow-up are lacking.

II. Joint-preserving procedures:

A. Core decompression:

1. Most common procedure currently performed to treat early stages of ONFH.[93]

2. Goal is decompression of femoral head pressure to restore vascular flow and relieve pain.

3. Small-diameter drilling with multiple passes proposed as alternative to large bore drilling given better ability to reach the anterior portion of the femoral head (most commonly involved region) and lesser morbidity, including risk of weakening the bone and predisposing to subtrochanteric fracture.[94]

4. Shown to slow progression of ONFH, but ability to cause reconstitution of a necrotic region has not yet been established.

5. Efficacy continues to be debated, but the larger, better-controlled series report a low rate of complications and superior outcomes compared with conservative therapy,[95] including symptomatic relief,[96] preservation of the femoral head, and delay of arthroplasty.[97]

B. Free vascularized fibular graft (FVFG):

1. Theorized to augment the benefit of a core decompression with the delivery of a supportive osteoinductive and osteoconductive graft.[1]

2. In certain centers, outcomes of FVFG, particularly in young patients, have been positive; however, its role in light of favorable modern arthroplasty outcomes is controversial.[98-100]

3. Extensive surgical time, donor-site morbidity,[101,102] and risk of proximal femoral fracture[103] have limited its widespread use.

C. Nonvascularized bone grafting:

1. Used to fill necrotic area in the femoral head.

    2.   Can be performed through core decompression tract or through a window in the femoral head or neck (trapdoor procedure).[104] The latter requires a surgical hip dislocation.

D. Tantalum implants:

    1.   Porous tantalum rods can theoretically provide structural support at the time of core decompression.

        a. Limited data exist regarding the success of this technique and it is no longer routinely performed.

    2.   Concerns including the added complexity in the event of hip replacement have limited the widespread adoption of this technique.

E. Cell-based therapy:

    1.   Recent enthusiasm for biological therapies that may enhance core decompression results with delivery of osteogenic (mesenchymal stem cells) and/or osteoinductive agents (bone morphogenic protein).[105]

    2.   Targets the hypothesis that ONFH is characterized by an insufficient supply of progenitor cells required for remodeling.[106]

    3.   Double-blind comparison of core decompression with and without bone marrow aspirate found reduced size of necrotic lesions at 24 months and protection against collapse at 5 years with bone marrow augmentation.[107,108]

    4.   Subsequent prospective randomized trials comparing core decompression with and without bone marrow aspirate have demonstrated equivalent or improved pain relief and functional scores at 2 years.[109–112] Superior protection against progression on imaging was noted in three of four studies,[109–111] with the fourth noting no benefit in bone regeneration or head survival.[112]

    5.   Data on biological therapies are preliminary with significant variations in cell harvesting, processing, and delivery methods.[105] Further investigation is needed.

F. Proximal femoral osteotomy:

    1.   Multiple proximal femoral osteotomies have successfully treated ONFH.[113,114]

    2.   Generally angular intertrochanteric or rotational transtrochanteric osteotomies designed to shift affected areas of femoral head away from the weight-bearing zone.[1]

    3.   Technically challenging.[96]

    4.   Subsequent conversion to a total hip arthroplasty (THA) is more complicated and has poorer longevity than primary THA.[113,115]

    5.   Should be done only by experienced surgeons in carefully selected patients in whom total hip replacement is not appropriate patient[96] (e.g., <45 years old with a Kerboul angle <200 degrees and no longer taking steroids[1]).

III. Joint replacement and hemijoint replacement:

A. Hip resurfacing:

    1.   Controversial for osteonecrosis. Some authors report acceptable results in strictly selected patients,[116] while others report poorer cumulative

survival compared with other diagnoses and view ONFH as a relative contraindication for resurfacing.[117]

B. Hemiarthroplasty:

1. Poorer results than total hip replacement in young patients with osteonecrosis, possibly from the lack of degenerative acetabular sclerosis.[118,119]

2. Concerns include development of protrusio and polyethylene wear particles leading to osteolysis and femoral component loosening.[120,121]

C. THA:

1. Generally reserved for late-stage symptomatic ONFH or older patients.[122]

2. ONFH accounts for over 10% of THAs performed in the United States.[2]

3. Procedure that most reliably reduces pain and improves mobility.[1]

4. Outcomes of THA for ONFH have improved compared with early studies reporting failure rates between 37 and 53%[123-125]; in the past 20 years, use of modern implants and improved surgical techniques have yielded encouraging results at midterm follow-up.[126,127]

   a. Ninety-eight percent stem survivorship and 85% cementless cup survivorship recently reported at mean follow-up of 17.3 years. Most common reason for revision was cup wear or loosening.[128]

   b. Dual-mobility acetabular components have demonstrated excellent stability and outcomes at 10 years.[129]

5. While outcomes after THA for ONFH are very good, they may still be inferior to outcomes of THA for osteoarthritis.[130]

   a. Renal failure and/or transplant and sickle cell disease have been associated with poorer outcomes.[131]

   b. In general, the underlying etiology for ONFH impacts the outcomes, complication rates and survivorship of THA.

6. Patients with ONFH are typically younger at the time of surgery than patients with osteoarthritis[96]:

   a. THA for ONFH in patients younger than 35 years had a 66% survival at 20 years. Implant survival significantly better in patients ≥25 years of age at the time of surgery compared with younger patients.[126]

References

1. Moya-Angeler J, Gianakos AL, Villa JC, Ni A, Lane JM. Current concepts on osteonecrosis of the femoral head. World J Orthop 2015;6(8):590–601

2. Mankin HJ. Nontraumatic necrosis of bone (osteonecrosis). N Engl J Med 1992;326(22):1473–1479

3. Jones LC, Mont MA. Osteonecrosis (avascular necrosis of bone). UpToDate Web site. Updated 2016. Accessed November 2016</bok>

4. LaPorte DM, Mont MA, Mohan V, Jones LC, Hungerford DS. Multifocal osteonecrosis. J Rheumatol 1998;25(10):1968–1974

5. Shah KN, Racine J, Jones LC, Aaron RK. Pathophysiology and risk factors for osteonecrosis. Curr Rev Musculoskelet Med 2015;8(3):201–209

6. Kellam P, Ostrum RF. Systematic review and meta-analysis of avascular necrosis and post-traumatic arthritis after traumatic hip dislocation. J Orthop Trauma 2016;30(1):10–16

7.   Zaltz I, Baca G, Clohisy JC. Unstable SCFE: review of treatment modalities and prevalence of osteonecrosis. Clin Orthop Relat Res 2013;471(7):2192–2198

8.   Dilisio MF. Osteonecrosis following short-term, low-dose oral corticosteroids: a population-based study of 24 million patients. Orthopedics 2014;37(7):e631–e636

9.   Shigemura T, Nakamura J, Kishida S, et al. Incidence of osteonecrosis associated with corticosteroid therapy among different underlying diseases: prospective MRI study. Rheumatology (Oxford) 2011;50(11):2023–2028

10.   Arbab D, König DP. Atraumatic femoral head necrosis in adults. Dtsch Arztebl Int 2016;113(3):31–38

11.   Matsuo K, Hirohata T, Sugioka Y, Ikeda M, Fukuda A. Influence of alcohol intake, cigarette smoking, and occupational status on idiopathic osteonecrosis of the femoral head. Clin Orthop Relat Res 1988;(234):115–123

12.   Fukushima W, Fujioka M, Kubo T, Tamakoshi A, Nagai M, Hirota Y. Nationwide epidemiologic survey of idiopathic osteonecrosis of the femoral head. Clin Orthop Relat Res 2010;468(10):2715–2724

13.   Mont MA, Hungerford DS. Non-traumatic avascular necrosis of the femoral head. J Bone Joint Surg Am 1995;77(3):459–474

14.   Milner PF, Kraus AP, Sebes JI, et al. Sickle cell disease as a cause of osteonecrosis of the femoral head. N Engl J Med 1991;325(21):1476–1481

15.   Sharareh B, Schwarzkopf R. Dysbaric osteonecrosis: a literature review of pathophysiology, clinical presentation, and management. Clin J Sport Med 2015;25(2):153–161

16.   Dimant J, Ginzler EM, Diamond HS, et al. Computer analysis of factors influencing the appearance of aseptic necrosis in patients with SLE. J Rheumatol 1978;5(2):136–141

17.   Abeles M, Urman JD, Rothfield NF. Aseptic necrosis of bone in systemic lupus erythematosus. Relationship to corticosteroid therapy. Arch Intern Med 1978;138(5):750–754

18.   Goldblatt J, Sacks S, Beighton P. The orthopedic aspects of Gaucher disease. Clin Orthop Relat Res 1978;(137):208–214

19.   Boechat MI, Winters WD, Hogg RJ, Fine RN, Watkins SL. Avascular necrosis of the femoral head in children with chronic renal disease. Radiology 2001;218(2):411–413

20.   Steib-Furno S, Luc M, Pham T, et al. Pregnancy-related hip diseases: incidence and diagnoses. Joint Bone Spine 2007;74(4):373–378

21.   Aaron RK, Gray R. Osteonecrosis: etiology, natural history, pathophysiology, and diagnosis. In: Callaghan JJ, Rosenberg AG, Rubash HE, eds. The Adult Hip. 2nd ed. Philadelphia, PA: Lippincott Williams & Wilkins; 2007:465–476

22.   Lopez-Ben R, Mikuls TR, Moore DS, et al. Incidence of hip osteonecrosis among renal transplantation recipients: a prospective study. Clin Radiol 2004;59(5):431–438

23.   Tauchmanovà L, De Rosa G, Serio B, et al. Avascular necrosis in long-term survivors after allogeneic or autologous stem cell transplantation: a single center experience and a review. Cancer 2003;97(10):2453–2461

24.   Schulte CM, Beelen DW. Avascular osteonecrosis after allogeneic hematopoietic stem-cell transplantation: diagnosis and gender matter. Transplantation 2004;78(7):1055–1063

25.   Zalavras CG, Vartholomatos G, Dokou E, Malizos KN. Genetic background of osteonecrosis: associated with thrombophilic mutations? Clin Orthop Relat Res 2004;(422):251–255

26.   Hadjigeorgiou G, Dardiotis E, Dardioti M, Karantanas A, Dimtroulias A, Malizos K. Genetic association studies in osteonecrosis of the femoral head: mini review of the literature. Skeletal Radiol 2008;37(1):1–7

27.   Glueck CJ, Freiberg RA, Boppana S, Wang P. Thrombophilia, hypofibrinolysis, the eNOS T-786C polymorphism, and multifocal osteonecrosis. J Bone Joint Surg Am 2008;90(10):2220–2229

28.   Karimova EJ, Rai SN, Howard SC, et al. Femoral head osteonecrosis in pediatric and young adult patients with leukemia or lymphoma. J Clin Oncol 2007;25(12):1525–1531

29.   Niinimäki R, Hansen LM, Niinimäki T, et al. Incidence of severe osteonecrosis requiring total joint arthroplasty in children and young adults treated for leukemia or lymphoma: a nationwide, register-based study in Finland and Denmark. J Adolesc Young Adult Oncol 2013;2(4):138–144

30. Miller KD, Masur H, Jones EC, et al. High prevalence of osteonecrosis of the femoral head in HIV-infected adults. Ann Intern Med 2002;137(1):17–25

31. Barker DJ, Hall AJ. The epidemiology of Perthes' disease. Clin Orthop Relat Res 1986;(209):89–94

32. Gautier E, Ganz K, Krügel N, Gill T, Ganz R. Anatomy of the medial femoral circumflex artery and its surgical implications. J Bone Joint Surg Br 2000;82(5):679–683

33. Dewar DC, Lazaro LE, Klinger CE, et al. The relative contribution of the medial and lateral femoral circumflex arteries to the vascularity of the head and neck of the femur: a quantitative MRI-based assessment. Bone Joint J 2016;98-B(12):1582–1588

34. Chung SM. The arterial supply of the developing proximal end of the human femur. J Bone Joint Surg Am 1976;58(7):961–970

35. Shuler FD, Schmitz MR. Anatomy: lower extremity and pelvis. In: Miller MD, Thompson SR, Hart JA, eds. Review of orthopaedics. 6th ed. Philadelphia, PA: Elsevier Saunders; 2012:185

36. Townsend DR, Hoffinger S. Intramedullary nailing of femoral shaft fractures in children via the trochanter tip. Clin Orthop Relat Res 2000;(376):113–118

37. Chang CC, Greenspan A, Gershwin ME. Osteonecrosis: current perspectives on pathogenesis and treatment. Semin Arthritis Rheum 1993;23(1):47–69

38. Jones JP Jr. Fat embolism and osteonecrosis. Orthop Clin North Am 1985;16(4):595–633

39. Miyanishi K, Kamo Y, Ihara H, Naka T, Hirakawa M, Sugioka Y. Risk factors for dysbaric osteonecrosis. Rheumatology (Oxford) 2006;45(7):855–858

40. Zalavras CG, Lieberman JR. Osteonecrosis of the femoral head: evaluation and treatment. J Am Acad Orthop Surg 2014;22(7):455–464

41. Assouline-Dayan Y, Chang C, Greenspan A, Shoenfeld Y, Gershwin ME. Pathogenesis and natural history of osteonecrosis. Semin Arthritis Rheum 2002;32(2):94–124

42. Roeder LF Jr, DeLee JC. Femoral head fractures associated with posterior hip dislocation. Clin Orthop Relat Res 1980;(147):121–130

43. Epstein HC, Wiss DA, Cozen L. Posterior fracture dislocation of the hip with fractures of the femoral head. Clin Orthop Relat Res 1985;(201):9–17

44. Stannard JP, Harris HW, Volgas DA, Alonso JE. Functional outcome of patients with femoral head fractures associated with hip dislocations. Clin Orthop Relat Res 2000;(377):44–56

45. Kloen P, Siebenrock KA, Raaymakers E, Marti RK, Ganz R. Femoral head fractures revisited. Eur J Trauma 2002;28(4):221–233

46. Marchetti ME, Steinberg GG, Coumas JM. Intermediate-term experience of Pipkin fracture-dislocations of the hip. J Orthop Trauma 1996;10(7):455–461

47. Slobogean GP, Sprague SA, Scott T, Bhandari M. Complications following young femoral neck fractures. Injury 2015;46(3):484–491

48. Barnes R, Brown JT, Garden RS, Nicoll EA. Subcapital fractures of the femur. A prospective review. J Bone Joint Surg Br 1976;58(1):2–24

49. Nikolopoulos KE, Papadakis SA, Kateros KT, et al. Long-term outcome of patients with avascular necrosis, after internal fixation of femoral neck fractures. Injury 2003;34(7):525–528

50. Wang T, Sun JY, Zha GC, Jiang T, You ZJ, Yuan DJ. Analysis of risk factors for femoral head necrosis after internal fixation in femoral neck fractures. Orthopedics 2014;37(12):e1117–e1123

51. Garden RS. Malreduction and avascular necrosis in subcapital fractures of the femur. J Bone Joint Surg Br 1971;53(2):183–197

52. Papakostidis C, Panagiotopoulos A, Piccioli A, Giannoudis PV. Timing of internal fixation of femoral neck fractures. A systematic review and meta-analysis of the final outcome. Injury 2015;46(3):459–466

53. Doak J, Schiller J, Eberson C. Circulation of the pediatric and adolescent hip. In: Aaron RK, ed. Skeletal circulation in Clinical Practice. Singapore: World Scientific; 2015:296–321

54. Shrader MW, Jacofsky DJ, Stans AA, Shaughnessy WJ, Haidukewych GJ. Femoral neck fractures in pediatric patients: 30 years experience at a level 1 trauma center. Clin Orthop Relat Res 2007;454(454):169–173

55. Ng GP, Cole WG. Effect of early hip decompression on the frequency of avascular necrosis in children with fractures of the neck of the femur. Injury 1996;27(6):419–421

56. Barquet A, Mayora G, Guimaraes JM, Suárez R, Giannoudis PV. Avascular necrosis of the femoral head following trochanteric fractures in adults: a systematic review. Injury 2014;45(12):1848–1858

57. Hougaard K, Thomsen PB. Traumatic posterior dislocation of the hip: prognostic factors influencing the incidence of avascular necrosis of the femoral head. Arch Orthop Trauma Surg 1986;106(1):32–35

58. Dwyer AJ, John B, Singh SA, Mam MK. Complications after posterior dislocation of the hip. Int Orthop 2006;30(4):224–227

59. McKee MD, Garay ME, Schemitsch EH, Kreder HJ, Stephen DJ. Irreducible fracture-dislocation of the hip: a severe injury with a poor prognosis. J Orthop Trauma 1998;12(4):223–229

60. Zlotorowicz M, Czubak J, Caban A, Kozinski P, Boguslawska-Walecka R. The blood supply to the femoral head after posterior fracture/dislocation of the hip, assessed by CT angiography. Bone Joint J 2013;95-B(11):1453–1457

61. Bastian JD, Turina M, Siebenrock KA, Keel MJ. Long-term outcome after traumatic anterior dislocation of the hip. Arch Orthop Trauma Surg 2011;131(9):1273–1278

62. Dreinhöfer KE, Schwarzkopf SR, Haas NP, Tscherne H. Isolated traumatic dislocation of the hip. Long-term results in 50 patients. J Bone Joint Surg Br 1994;76(1):6–12

63. Zizic TM, Marcoux C, Hungerford DS, Stevens MB. The early diagnosis of ischemic necrosis of bone. Arthritis Rheum 1986;29(10):1177–1186

64. Mazieres B. Osteonecrosis. In: Hochberg MC, Silman AJ, Smolen JS, Weinblatt ME, Weisman MH, eds. Rheumatology. 3rd ed. London: Mosby; 2003:1877

65. Mont MA, Ulrich SD, Seyler TM, et al. Bone scanning of limited value for diagnosis of symptomatic oligofocal and multifocal osteonecrosis. J Rheumatol 2008;35(8):1629–1634

66. Markisz JA, Knowles RJ, Altchek DW, Schneider R, Whalen JP, Cahill PT. Segmental patterns of avascular necrosis of the femoral heads: early detection with MR imaging. Radiology 1987;162(3):717–720

67. Bassett LW, Gold RH, Reicher M, Bennett LR, Tooke SM. Magnetic resonance imaging in the early diagnosis of ischemic necrosis of the femoral head. Preliminary results. Clin Orthop Relat Res 1987;(214):237–248

68. Coleman BG, Kressel HY, Dalinka MK, Scheibler ML, Burk DL, Cohen EK. Radiographically negative avascular necrosis: detection with MR imaging. Radiology 1988;168(2):525–528

69. Hauzeur JP, Pasteels JL, Schoutens A, et al. The diagnostic value of magnetic resonance imaging in non-traumatic osteonecrosis of the femoral head. J Bone Joint Surg Am 1989;71(5):641–649

70. Miller IL, Savory CG, Polly DW Jr, Graham GD, McCabe JM, Callaghan JJ. Femoral head osteonecrosis. Detection by magnetic resonance imaging versus single-photon emission computed tomography. Clin Orthop Relat Res 1989; (247):152–162

71. Gillespy T III, Genant HK, Helms CA. Magnetic resonance imaging of osteonecrosis. Radiol Clin North Am 1986;24(2):193–208

72. Glickstein MF, Burk DL Jr, Schiebler ML, et al. Avascular necrosis versus other diseases of the hip: sensitivity of MR imaging. Radiology 1988;169(1):213–215

73. Ito H, Matsuno T, Minami A. Relationship between bone marrow edema and development of symptoms in patients with osteonecrosis of the femoral head. AJR Am J Roentgenol 2006;186(6):1761–1770

74. Dumont M, Danais S, Taillefer R. "Doughnut" sign in avascular necrosis of the bone. Clin Nucl Med 1984;9(1):44

75. Amanatullah DF, Strauss EJ, Di Cesare PE. Current management options for osteonecrosis of the femoral head: part 1, diagnosis and nonoperative management. Am J Orthop 2011;40(9):E186–E192

76. Etienne G, Mont MA, Ragland PS. The diagnosis and treatment of nontraumatic osteonecrosis of the femoral head. Instr Course Lect 2004;53:67–85

77. Davies M, Cassar-Pullicino VN, Darby AJ. Subchondral insufficiency fractures of the femoral head. Eur Radiol 2004;14(2):201–207

78. Yamamoto T, Bullough PG. The role of subchondral insufficiency fracture in rapid destruction of the hip joint: a preliminary report. Arthritis Rheum 2000;43(11):2423–2427

79. Ficat RP, Arlet J. Ischemia and necrosis of bone. Baltimore, MD: Williams and Wilkins; 1980:171–182

80. Steinberg ME, Hayken GD, Steinberg DR. A quantitative system for staging avascular necrosis. J Bone Joint Surg Br 1995;77(1):34–41

81. Gardeniers JWM, Gosling-Gardeniers AC, Rijnen WHC. The ARCO staging system: generation and evolving since 1991. In: Koo KH, Mont MA, Jones LC, eds. Osteonecrosis. Berlin: Springer-Verlag; 2014:215

82. Kerboul M, Thomine J, Postel M, Merle d'Aubigné R. The conservative surgical treatment of idiopathic aseptic necrosis of the femoral head. J Bone Joint Surg Br 1974;56(2):291–296

83. Ha YC, Jung WH, Kim JR, Seong NH, Kim SY, Koo KH. Prediction of collapse in femoral head osteonecrosis: a modified Kerboul method with use of magnetic resonance images. J Bone Joint Surg Am 2006;88(Suppl 3):35–40

84. Lai KA, Shen WJ, Yang CY, Shao CJ, Hsu JT, Lin RM. The use of alendronate to prevent early collapse of the femoral head in patients with nontraumatic osteonecrosis. A randomized clinical study. J Bone Joint Surg Am 2005;87(10):2155–2159

85. Nishii T, Sugano N, Miki H, Hashimoto J, Yoshikawa H. Does alendronate prevent collapse in osteonecrosis of the femoral head? Clin Orthop Relat Res 2006;443(443):273–279

86. Kang P, Pei F, Shen B, Zhou Z, Yang J. Are the results of multiple drilling and alendronate for osteonecrosis of the femoral head better than those of multiple drilling? A pilot study. Joint Bone Spine 2012;79(1):67–72

87. Chen CH, Chang JK, Lai KA, Hou SM, Chang CH, Wang GJ. Alendronate in the prevention of collapse of the femoral head in nontraumatic osteonecrosis: a two-year multicenter, prospective, randomized, double-blind, placebo-controlled study. Arthritis Rheum 2012;64(5):1572–1578

88. Jäger M, Tillmann FP, Thornhill TS, et al. Rationale for prostaglandin I2 in bone marrow oedema: from theory to application. Arthritis Res Ther 2008;10(5):R120

89. Wang GJ, Cui Q, Balian G. The Nicolas Andry award. The pathogenesis and prevention of steroid-induced osteonecrosis. Clin Orthop Relat Res 2000;(370):295–310

90. Pritchett JW. Statin therapy decreases the risk of osteonecrosis in patients receiving steroids. Clin Orthop Relat Res 2001;(386):173–178

91. Glueck CJ, Freiberg RA, Sieve L, Wang P. Enoxaparin prevents progression of stages I and II osteonecrosis of the hip. Clin Orthop Relat Res 2005;(435):164–170

92. Guo P, Gao F, Wang Y, et al. The use of anticoagulants for prevention and treatment of osteonecrosis of the femoral head: a systematic review. Medicine (Baltimore) 2017;96(16):e6646

93. Wang CJ, Huang CC, Yip HK, Yang YJ. Dosage effects of extracorporeal shockwave therapy in early hip necrosis. Int J Surg 2016;35:179–186

94. Lieberman JR, Berry DJ, Mont MA, et al. Osteonecrosis of the hip: management in the 21st century. Instr Course Lect 2003;52:337–355

95. Al Omran A. Multiple drilling compared with standard core decompression for avascular necrosis of the femoral head in sickle cell disease patients. Arch Orthop Trauma Surg 2013;133(5):609–613

96. Lavernia CJ, Sierra RJ, Grieco FR. Osteonecrosis of the femoral head. J Am Acad Orthop Surg 1999;7(4):250–261

97. Koo KH, Kim R, Ko GH, Song HR, Jeong ST, Cho SH. Preventing collapse in early osteonecrosis of the femoral head. A randomised clinical trial of core decompression. J Bone Joint Surg Br 1995;77(6):870–874

98. Stulberg BN, Davis AW, Bauer TW, Levine M, Easley K. Osteonecrosis of the femoral head. A prospective randomized treatment protocol. Clin Orthop Relat Res 1991;(268):140–151

99. Cao L, Guo C, Chen J, Chen Z, Yan Z. Free vascularized fibular grafting improves vascularity compared with core decompression in femoral head osteonecrosis: a randomized clinical trial. Clin Orthop Relat Res 2017;475(9):2230–2240

100. Ligh CA, Nelson JA, Fischer JP, Kovach SJ, Levin LS. The effectiveness of free vascularized fibular flaps in osteonecrosis of the femoral head and neck: a systematic review. J Reconstr Microsurg 2017;33(3):163–172

101. Sabesan VJ, Pedrotty DM, Urbaniak JR, Ghareeb GM, Aldridge JM. Free vascularized fibular grafting preserves athletic activity level in patients with osteonecrosis. J Surg Orthop Adv 2012;21(4):242–245

102. Vail TP, Urbaniak JR. Donor-site morbidity with use of vascularized autogenous fibular grafts. J Bone Joint Surg Am 1996;78(2):204–211

103. Tang CL, Mahoney JL, McKee MD, Richards RR, Waddell JP, Louie B. Donor site morbidity following vascularized fibular grafting. Microsurgery 1998;18(6):383–386

104. Aluisio FV, Urbaniak JR. Proximal femur fractures after free vascularized fibular grafting to the hip. Clin Orthop Relat Res 1998;(356):192–201

105. Seyler TM, Marker DR, Ulrich SD, Fatscher T, Mont MA. Nonvascularized bone grafting defers joint arthroplasty in hip osteonecrosis. Clin Orthop Relat Res 2008;466(5):1125–1132

106. Piuzzi NS, Chahla J, Jiandong H, et al. Analysis of cell therapies used in clinical trials for the treatment of osteonecrosis of the femoral head: a systematic review of the literature. J Arthroplasty 2017;32(8):2612–2618

107. Hernigou P, Poignard A, Zilber S, Rouard H. Cell therapy of hip osteonecrosis with autologous bone marrow grafting. Indian J Orthop 2009;43(1):40–45

108. Gangji V, Hauzeur JP, Matos C, De Maertelaer V, Toungouz M, Lambermont M. Treatment of osteonecrosis of the femoral head with implantation of autologous bone-marrow cells. A pilot study. J Bone Joint Surg Am 2004;86(6):1153–1160

109. Gangji V, De Maertelaer V, Hauzeur JP. Autologous bone marrow cell implantation in the treatment of non-traumatic osteonecrosis of the femoral head: Five year follow-up of a prospective controlled study. Bone 2011;49(5):1005–1009

110. Sen RK, Tripathy SK, Aggarwal S, Marwaha N, Sharma RR, Khandelwal N. Early results of core decompression and autologous bone marrow mononuclear cells instillation in femoral head osteonecrosis: a randomized control study. J Arthroplasty 2012;27(5):679–686

111. Ma Y, Wang T, Liao J, et al. Efficacy of autologous bone marrow buffy coat grafting combined with core decompression in patients with avascular necrosis of femoral head: a prospective, double-blinded, randomized, controlled study. Stem Cell Res Ther 2014;5(5):115

112. Tabatabaee RM, Saberi S, Parvizi J, Mortazavi SM, Farzan M. Combining concentrated autologous bone marrow stem cells injection with core decompression improves outcome for patients with early-stage osteonecrosis of the femoral head: a comparative study. J Arthroplasty 2015;30(9, Suppl)11–15

113. Pepke W, Kasten P, Beckmann NA, Janicki P, Egermann M. Core decompression and autologous bone marrow concentrate for treatment of femoral head osteonecrosis: a randomized prospective study. Orthop Rev (Pavia) 2016;8(1):6162

114. Shannon BD, Trousdale RT. Femoral osteotomies for avascular necrosis of the femoral head. Clin Orthop Relat Res 2004;(418):34–40

115. Lee YK, Park CH, Ha YC, Kim DY, Lyu SH, Koo KH. Comparison of surgical parameters and results between curved varus osteotomy and rotational osteotomy for osteonecrosis of the femoral head. Clin Orthop Surg 2017;9(2):160–168

116. Utsunomiya T, Motomura G, Ikemura S, Hamai S, Fukushi JI, Nakashima Y. The results of total hip arthroplasty after sugioka transtrochanteric anterior rotational osteotomy for osteonecrosis. J Arthroplasty 2017;32(9):2768–2773

117. Pyda M, Koczy B, Widuchowski W, et al. Hip resurfacing arthroplasty in treatment of avascular necrosis of the femoral head. Med Sci Monit 2015;21:304–309

118. Daniel J, Pradhan C, Ziaee H, McMinn D. Survival of birmingham hip resurfacing in patients with femoral head osteonecrosis. J Bone Joint Surg Br 2012;94-B(Suppl IV):7

119. Scheerlinck T, Dezillie M, Monsaert A, Opdecam P. Bipolar versus total hip arthroplasty in the treatment of avascular necrosis of the femoral head in young patients. Hip Int 2002;12(2):142–149
120. Mankar SH, Dwidmuthe SC, Faizan M, Sakhare R. A comparative study of bipolar hemi-arthroplasty and total hip joint replacement for the treatment of grade III osteonecrosis of femoral head. Panacea J Med Sci 2015;5(2):73
121. Cabanela ME. Femoral endoprostheses and total hip replacement for avascular necrosis. Semin Arthroplasty 1998;9:253–260
122. Kim KJ, Rubash HE. Large amounts of polyethylene debris in the interface tissue surrounding bipolar endoprostheses. Comparison to total hip prostheses. J Arthroplasty 1997;12(1):32–39
123. McGrory BJ, York SC, Iorio R, et al. Current practices of AAHKS members in the treatment of adult osteonecrosis of the femoral head. J Bone Joint Surg Am 2007;89(6):1194–1204
124. Chandler HP, Reineck FT, Wixson RL, McCarthy JC. Total hip replacement in patients younger than thirty years old. A five-year follow-up study. J Bone Joint Surg Am 1981;63(9):1426–1434
125. Cornell CN, Salvati EA, Pellicci PM. Long-term follow-up of total hip replacement in patients with osteonecrosis. Orthop Clin North Am 1985;16(4):757–769
126. Stauffer RN. Ten-year follow-up study of total hip replacement. J Bone Joint Surg Am 1982;64(7):983–990
127. Wang TI, Hung SH, Su YP, Feng CQ, Chiu FY, Liu CL. Noncemented total hip arthroplasty for osteonecrosis of the femoral head in elderly patients. Orthopedics 2013;36(3):e271–e275
128. Issa K, Naziri Q, Maheshwari AV, Rasquinha VJ, Delanois RE, Mont MA. Excellent results and minimal complications of total hip arthroplasty in sickle cell hemoglobinopathy at mid-term follow-up using cementless prosthetic components. J Arthroplasty 2013;28(9):1693–1698
129. Kim YH, Kim JS, Park JW, Joo JH. Contemporary total hip arthroplasty with and without cement in patients with osteonecrosis of the femoral head: a concise follow-up, at an average of seventeen years, of a previous report. J Bone Joint Surg Am 2011;93(19):1806–1810
130. Martz P, Maczynski A, Elsair S, Labattut L, Viard B, Baulot E. Total hip arthroplasty with dual mobility cup in osteonecrosis of the femoral head in young patients: over ten years of follow-up. Int Orthop 2017;41(3):605–610
131. Singh JA, Chen J, Inacio MC, Namba RS, Paxton EW. An underlying diagnosis of osteonecrosis of bone is associated with worse outcomes than osteoarthritis after total hip arthroplasty. BMC Musculoskelet Disord 2017;18(1):8
132. Johannson HR, Zywiel MG, Marker DR, Jones LC, McGrath MS, Mont MA. Osteonecrosis is not a predictor of poor outcomes in primary total hip arthroplasty: a systematic literature review. Int Orthop 2011;35(4):465–473
133. Swarup I, Shields M, Mayer EN, Hendow CJ, Burket JC, Figgie MP. Outcomes after total hip arthroplasty in young patients with osteonecrosis of the hip. Hip Int 2017;27(3):286–292

26 Septic Arthritis of the Hip

Robert Axel Sershon, Joshua Alan Bell

Native Hip

I. Background[1-6]: Septic arthritis of the hip is a relatively rare condition in healthy adults and is more common in the pediatric setting. Due to the destructive nature of an infection on native cartilage, septic arthritis is typically treated emergently to prevent future sequelae.

   A. Epidemiology:

   1. Most commonly monoarticular and in large joints:

      a. Hip is the second most common location, involved in 13% of cases.

      b. Knee is most common (~50% of cases).

   2. Low incidence of native septic hip infections in adults:

      a. Two to 10 out of 100,000.

   3. Higher incidence in the pediatric population:

      a. 0.25% of all hospitalizations

      b. Ninety-five percent single joint infections.

   4. Adult risk factors:

      a. Elderly, intravenous drug users, recent sepsis, malnutrition, prior surgery, and immunocompromised (HIV/AIDS, diabetics, rheumatoid, cirrhosis).

   5. Pediatric risk factors:

      a. Fifty percent occur in children younger than 2 years.

      b. Immunocompromised, prematurity, and cesarean section.

   6. Origins of inoculation:

      a. Pneumonia, endocarditis, dermatologic, urinary tract infection, various gastrointestinal infections.

II. Differential diagnosis[1,2,7-9]:

   A. Intra-articular injury.

   B. Osteomyelitis.

   C. Inflammatory arthroplasty (rheumatoid arthritis, gout and pseudogout, reactive arthritis, systemic lupus erythematosus, Lyme arthritis, psoriatic arthritis).

   D. Sickle cell disease.

   E. Transient synovitis of the hip (pediatric).

   F. Pigmented villonodular synovitis.

   G. Hemarthrosis.

   H. Neuropathic arthropathy.

   I. Osteoarthritis.

    J.   Osteonecrosis of the femoral head.

    K. Pediatric hip disorders (slipped capital femoral epiphysis, Legg–Calvé–Perthes, hip dysplasia, etc.).

    L. Soft-tissue infection—septic bursa, psoas abscess, or cellulitis.

III. Pathophysiology[2,9]:

    A. Joint inoculation occurs in one of three ways:

        1. Bacteremia (e.g., pneumonia).

        2. Direct inoculation (e.g., trauma).

        3. Contiguous spread (e.g., nearby osteomyelitis—common with intra-articular metaphysis of the hip).

    B. Seeding pathway:

        1. Bacteria enters through the highly permeable and vascular synovial membrane, depositing on the membrane:

            a. High vascularity and permeability allow for production of synovial fluid, exchange of nutrients, and waste removal.

        2. Lack of robust immunologic barriers and absence of a limiting membrane allows bacteria to seed the synovial fluid and precipitously proliferate in the nutrient-filled environment.

    C. Bacterial proliferation results in release of destructive toxins and enzymes:

        1. Alpha, β, delta toxins in the *Staphylococcus* species break down cell membranes and proteins.

        2. Adhesins allow for bacterial adhesion, facilitating stability and growth.

        3. Cartilage degradation can occur within 8 hours and gross destruction is typically apparent within 1 week following an untreated infection.

    D. Bacterial cell wall and intracellular proteins initiate the inflammatory cascade:

        1. B-cells, T-cells, and macrophages release inflammatory cytokines:

            a. B-cell: interleukin-1 (IL-1) and IL-10.

            b. T-cell: IL-4 and IL-10.

            c. Macrophage: IL-1, IL-10, and tumor necrosis factor-α (TNF-α).

    E. Inflammatory response from host further contributes to cartilaginous breakdown via matrix metalloproteinases:

        1. Bacterial presence alters normal synovial fluid production and filtration:

            a. Gradual increase of toxic enzymes and inflammatory concentrations.

            b. Abnormal filtration results in increased intra-articular pressure, which further contributes to joint destruction and increases the risk of femoral head osteonecrosis.

    F. Histological findings from acute to chronic inflammation show an increase from neutrophils to mononuclear leukocytes and lymphocytes:

        1. Lymphocytes are predominate cells by 3 weeks.

    G. Blood supply:

        1. Robust pediatric blood supply of the hip renders infants and children more susceptible to hematogenous seeding:

    a. Medial femoral circumflex artery:

      i. Dominant blood supply to the femoral head after 4 years of age.

    b. Lateral femoral circumflex artery:

      i. Smaller contribution to femoral head as the child ages.

    c. Artery of the ligamentum teres:

      i. Begins to regress at 4 years of age.

    d. Metaphyseal vessels:

      i. Abundant supply to metaphysis.

IV. Microbiology[2,9,10]:

  A. Common organisms[9,11]:

    1. *Staphylococcus aureus* (40–75%; **Fig. 26.1**):

      a. Most common pathogen, except for:

        i. Young, healthy, sexually active adults (*Neisseria gonorrhoeae*—75%).

        ii. *Haemophilus influenza* in unvaccinated infants and toddlers.

      b. Methicillin-sensitive *S. aureus* (MSSA).

        i. Beta-lactamase confers penicillin resistance; however, it remains susceptible to methicillin.

        ii. Antibiotic: methicillin (or similar penicillin derivative).

      c. Methicillin-resistant *S. aureus* (MRSA):

        i. Bacteria carrying the mecA gene produce penicillin-binding protein 2A, which results in poor bacterial binding to penicillin. These bacteria are resistant to penicillin and methicillin (MRSA).

        ii. Commonly hospital or health care acquired, although becoming more common in the public domain:

          (1) Obtained from hospitals, surgery, catheters, advanced-care facilities.

          (2) More commonly multiple drug-resistant forms.

        iii. Community acquired; becoming a more common source:

          (1) Typically less virulent with less drug resistance.

          (2) At risk: intravenous (IV) drug users, athletes, military.

        iv. Antibiotics: vancomycin, daptomycin, or linezolid.

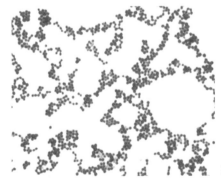

Fig. 26.1 *Staphylococcus aureus.*

2. Other staphylococcal species:

    a. Uncommon in the setting of primary infection.

3. *Streptococcus* species (20%):

    a. Group A most common form isolated.

    b. Group B: often found susceptible populations: infants, diabetics, and elderly.

4. Gram negative (<5% of cases):

    a. *Escherichia coli, Salmonella, Pseudomonas, Klebsiella*, and *Enterobacter* species.

    b. IV drug users, neonates, and elderly are at highest risk.

5. *N. gonorrhoeae* (10%; **Fig. 26.2**):

    a. Most common source in young, healthy, sexually active adults (75%):

        i. Incidence of 3 to 5% of all patients infected with *N. gonorrhoeae*.

    b. Polyarticular and migratory with associated rash.

    c. Diagnosis typically made by polymerase chain reaction (PCR), as joint cultures are often negative:

        i. Cultures from urethra or pharynx may be positive.

    d. Less morbid and destructive than most other pathogens.

    e. Responds quickly and well to antibiotics, and formal incision and drainage is often unnecessary.

6. Special cases:

    a. *Salmonella*—more common with sickle cell disease.

    b. *Bartonella henselae*—common in HIV patients.

    c. *Pseudomonas aeruginosa*—often found in IV drug users.

    d. *Pasteurella multocida*—typically associated with a dog or cat bite.

    e. *Eikenella corrodens*—seen after a human bite injury.

B. Fungal:

1. Unlike bacteria, fungal infections undergo granulomatous reactions, resulting in thickened synovium, effusions, and fibrin "rice bodies."

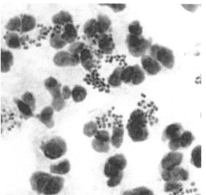

Fig. 26.2 *Neisseria gonorrhoeae.*

    2. Cartilage progressively destroyed via infiltration of granulation tissue.

    3. Risk factors: Found with substance abusers, immunocompromised, organ transplant patients, those on broad-spectrum antibiotics, and presence of an indwelling catheter (ref—Bariteau, JAAOS 2014).

V. Clinical presentation[2,9,12]:

A. Acute onset of pain, swelling, stiffness, and inability or unwillingness to bear weight through the affected extremity.

B. Pain is typically located in the groin:

    1. Be aware of referred pain to thigh and knee, especially in the pediatric population.

    2. Often will not allow the hip to be taken through any range of motion.

C. Fever, chills, malaise, erythema are variable in presence and severity.

D. Concurrent infection or sepsis.

E. Kocher's criteria for pediatrics:

    1. White blood cell (WBC) greater than 12,000 cells/µL.

    2. Inability to bear weight in the affected extremity.

    3. Fever greater than 38.5°C (101.3°F).

    4. Erythrocyte sedimentation rate (ESR) greater than 40 mm/h.

    5. Sensitivity as high as 99.6% when all four criteria are met.

VI. Examination[2,9,12]:

A. Unable to bear weight or severe antalgic gait.

B. Hip held in flexion, abduction, external rotation: affords greatest capsular volume.

C. Significant pain with short arcs of motion.

D. Systemic physical examination for primary infectious source.

VII. Diagnosis[2,6,7,9,10,12–14]:

A. Combination of clinical history, examination, and diagnostic studies:

    1. Important criteria include fever → elevated inflammatory markers → refusal to walk/bear weight.

B. Serum laboratory:

    1. Serum WBC greater than 12,000/L.

    2. ESR greater than 30 mm/h.

    3. C-reactive protein (CRP) greater than 10.5 mg/L is predictive of infection.

C. Synovial fluid aspiration:

    1. Gold standard.

    2. Cell count and differential:

        a. WBC greater than 50,000 cells/µL:

            i. High sensitivity, low specificity.

            ii. Leukocyte counts greater than 28,000/µL or less in immunocompromised.

        b. Margaretten et al[9] report counts of less than 25,000/mm³, more than 25,000/mm³, more than 50 000/mm³, and more than 100 000/mm³ gave a septic arthritis likelihood ratio of 0.32, 2.9, 7.7, and 28.0, respectively.

  c. Polymorphonuclear (PMN) neutrophils greater than 90% indicates infection (historically >75% considered positive).

  d. Glucose and protein have low sensitivity and specificity.

3. Gram stain:

  a. Not a recommended tool for guidance of treatment due to variable sensitivity and specificity.

  b. Nonpyogenic arthritis often presents with false negatives.

4. Synovial culture:

  a. Can be negative in up to 75% of cases.

  b. Obtained prior to administration of IV antibiotics.

  c. Blood cultures obtained in the cases of systemic sepsis.

5. Crystal analysis:

  a. Presence of crystals does not necessarily rule out infection.

  b. Urate crystals are negatively birefringent and highly suggestive of gout.

  c. Calcium pyrophosphate dehydrate crystals are positively birefringent and are highly suggestive of pseudogout.

  d. Presence of crystals in the setting of concomitant septic arthritis is 1.5% of cases.

D. Aspiration technique:

1. Sterile prep.

2. Fluoroscopic guidance (**Fig. 26.3**).

3. An 18-gauge needle or larger, preferably 6 inches in length.

4. Approaches: anterior, anterolateral, and lateral.

5. Air arthrogram upon entering joint capsule.

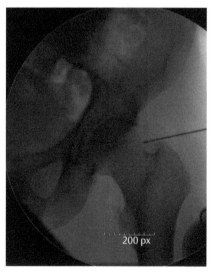

200 px

Fig. 26.3 Hip aspiration.

VIII. Imaging[2,7,9,12]:

A. Limited role in diagnosis.

B. Plain radiographs:

1. Anteroposterior of the hip and pelvis.

2. Lateral hip.

3. May be used to monitor the response to treatment:

a. Joint destruction or degeneration, osteomyelitis, bone loss, etc.

C. Ultrasound:

1. Can determine location and extent of effusion.

2. Echo-free effusion has low false-positive rate.

3. Can also assist in aspiration.

D. Advanced imaging:

1. Computed tomography (CT):

a. Detects soft-tissue swelling, joint effusion, and abscess formation.

b. Often utilized to guide joint aspiration in small or difficult-to-access areas.

c. More readily obtained and less costly than MRI.

2. Magnetic resonance imaging (MRI):

a. Superior soft-tissue detail compared with CT and bone scans.

b. Useful in differentiating between osteomyelitis, soft-tissue abscesses, and joint effusion.

c. Costly and difficult to obtain in a timely fashion.

3. Radionucleotide bone scan:

a. Detect localized areas of inflammation.

b. Areas with increased technetium-99m uptake are correlated with increased osteoblasts activity and vascularity:

i. Poor sensitivity and specificity when used alone.

c. Gallium citrate indium-111 chloride are taken up rapidly of inflammation:

i. Overall poor sensitivity for septic arthritis when used alone (60%) with high incidence of false positives.

d. Rarely indicated in the setting of acute septic arthritis.

4. All advanced imaging modalities have the potential to delay appropriate treatment and are best reserved for instances of diagnostic uncertainty.

IX. Treatment[2,8,10,15–18]:

A. Emergent condition that is indicated for prompt fluid evacuation, irrigation and debridement, and empiric antibiotic therapy.

B. Hip arthroscopy:

1. Native hip arthroscopy with irrigation and debridement has been shown to be as effective as open arthrotomy.

2. Less morbid procedure with more rapid discharge and return to function.

C. Open arthrotomy with irrigation and debridement:
   1. Current gold standard.
   2. Approach based upon surgeon preference and planned future interventions:
      a. Anterior-based approaches (direct anterior, Smith-Petersen, or antero-lateral, Watson-Jones) allow easy access to the hip joint while better preserving the blood supply to the femoral head.
   3. Increased risk of instability regardless of approach utilized.
D. Resection arthroplasty:
   1. Necessary in the cases where the femoral head is extensively involved.
   2. May be definitive in the elderly, nonambulatory, and severely immuno-compromised patients.
   3. Antibiotic spacer placement used when considering future arthroplasty:
      a. May also be used as definitive treatment in select individuals.
E. Two-stage arthroplasty:
   1. Conversion from resection arthroplasty with or without insertion of an antibiotic spacer.
   2. Second stage once:
      a. Laboratory results have normalized.
      b. Patient is off antibiotics for several weeks without reoccurrence.
      c. Repeat aspiration is negative for infection.
   3. Increased reinfection rate (7–14%) compared healthy patients without prior infection (<1%), but overall excellent outcomes.
F. Antibiotics:
   1. Empiric antibiotics begin immediately following aspiration and culture and are based on the clinical condition and/or the local antibiogram:
      a. Choice of coverage dictated by final culture.
      b. Broad spectrum with MRSA coverage preferable.
   2. Consultation with infectious disease for final recommendations.
   3. Length of treatment typically ranges from 4 to 6 weeks.

X. Outcomes[2,15,16,19]:
A. Time to diagnosis remains most crucial element of treatment, as an exponential rise in joint pressure and destruction continues until treatment.
B. Delay or missed diagnosis carries serious consequences, both locally and systemically.
C. Recent literature has shown majority of patients (>95%) go on to have excellent functional outcomes when treated early with either open or arthroscopy techniques.
D. Negative consequences include:
   1. Joint contractures.
   2. Growth abnormalities—pediatrics.

3. Osteonecrosis.

4. Gait abnormalities.

5. Postseptic arthritis degenerative joint disease.

Periprosthetic Infection of the Hip

I.   Background[2,20–22]:

A. Epidemiology:

1. Third most common indication for revision THA.

2. Estimated to be 0.5 to 2.2% of all THAs.

3. Estimated to approach cost of $600 million per year by 2020.

B. Risk factors[22–24]:

1. Superficial wound infection.

2. Morbid obesity (>40 kg/m^2).

3. Transfusion of allogenic blood.

4. Urinary tract infection.

5. American Society of Anesthesiologists (ASA) score greater than 2.

6. Extended operative time (>2 hours) and excessive room traffic during surgery.

7. Recent bacteremia (<1 year).

8. IV drug use.

9. Metachronous prosthetic joint infection (PJI).

10. Skin disorders (e.g., psoriasis, chronic cellulitis, lymphedema, chronic venous stasis, skin ulcers).

11. Active infection at other site.

12. MRSA infection within 3 years or colonization.

II. Differential diagnosis[2]:

A. Aseptic loosening.

B. Osteolysis.

C. Metallosis and aseptic lymphocyte–dominant vasculitis-associated lesion (ALVAL) reaction.

D. Hemarthrosis.

E. Periprosthetic fracture.

F. Superficial infection.

III. Pathophysiology[2,25]:

A. Mechanisms of infection:

1. Exogenous (e.g., aspiration).

2. Contiguous (e.g., superficial surgical site infection, osteomyelitis).

3. Hematogenous (e.g., seeding of implant following dental procedure or process associated with a bacteremic event).

B. Prosthetic surfaces promote infection:

1. Decrease efficacy of host neutrophils.

2. Decease the number of pathogens needed for infection.

3. Surface for biofilm formation.

C. Biofilms:

1. Rapid adhesion and aggregation of pathogens with surface glycocalyx leads to formation of biofilm.

2. Organisms can exist in sessile state or become free floating.

3. *Antibiotic resistant*:

   a. Limits antibiotic diffusion.

   b. Cell division targets not available to antibiotics while pathogen in quiescent state.

   c. Local chemistry changes prevents antibiotic effectiveness.

IV. Microbiology[22,26–30]:

A. Common organisms in PJI:

1. *S. aureus* (24–36%):

   a. MSSA and MRSA.

   b. Local epidemiology.

2. Coagulase-negative *Staphylococci* (11–51%).

3. *Streptococci* spp. (4–25%).

4. Gram-negative pathogens:

   a. Enteric gram-negative rods (0–15%).

   b. *Pseudomonas* (0–11%).

   c. Occur more commonly in older patients with older prostheses.

5. Anaerobic pathogens (0–25%):

   a. Require anaerobic culture medium.

   b. Longer incubation time.

6. Culture negative (7–26%):

   a. Fastidious organisms.

   b. Prior antibiotic usage.

7. Multidrug-resistant organisms (MDRO):

   a. Growing incidence of multidrug resistance worldwide with very limited number of new antimicrobial agents in development.

   b. Definitions:

      i. MDR defined as acquired nonsusceptibility to at least one agent in three or more antimicrobial categories.

      ii. Extremely drug resistant (XDR): nonsusceptibility to at least one agent in all but two or fewer antimicrobial categories.

      iii. Pandrug resistant (PDR): nonsusceptibility to all agents in all antimicrobial categories.

    c. MDRO:

      i. MRSA.

      ii. Methicillin-resistant *S. epidermidis* (MRSE).

      iii. Vancomycin-resistant Enterococci (VRE):

        (1) Increasing problem: hospitalizations with VRE-related infections more than doubled from 2003 to 2006.

        (2) Second most common cause of nosocomial infection in the United States.

        (3) Only account for 3 to 10% of PJIs, but is challenging to treat.

        (4) Currently only linezolid is approved by the U.S. Food and Drug Administration (FDA) for treatment of VRE.

    d. Carbapenemase-producing *Klebsiella pneumonia* (CPKP) and *Acinetobacter* spp.:

      i. Highly resistant gram-negative bacteria.

      ii. Typically susceptible only to older, more toxic agents such as polymyxins.

    e. Extended-spectrum β-lactamase (ESBL) producing *Enterobacteriaceae.*

    f. MDR *P. aeruginosa.*

V. Clinical presentation[2,22,25]:

  A. Pain is typically located in the groin:

    1. Be aware of referred pain to thigh and knee.

  B. Variable presence of fever, chills, malaise, erythema.

  C. Concurrent infection or sepsis.

  D. Acute hematogenous:

    1. Duration of symptoms less than 3 weeks following an inciting event.

    2. Acute onset of joint pain.

    3. Typically preceded by systemic infection (e.g., pneumonia, urinary tract infection [UTI], sepsis).

  E. Acute postoperative:

    1. Occurring within 6 weeks of index procedure.

    2. Acute onset of joint pain, fever, malaise, possible wound drainage/effusion.

  F. Early postinterventional:

    1. Infection within 4 to 6 weeks after invasive procedure.

    2. Increase or return of pain.

    3. Protracted drainage.

    4. Signs of local inflammation.

  G. Chronic:

    1. Infection with presence of symptoms for greater than 3 weeks or occurring after the early postinterventional period (4–6 weeks).

    2. Pain.

    3. Chronic joint effusion.

    4. Implant loosening on imaging.

VI. Examination[2,25]:

  A. Antalgic or altered gait mechanics.

  B. Incision site with signs of acute inflammation or drainage.

  C. Pain with short-arc range of motion less reliable than the same in native hip.

  D. Close examination for systemic infection.

VII. Diagnosis[22,31,32]:

  A. Musculoskeletal Infection Society Criteria for Periprosthetic Joint Infection:

    1. Greater than or equal to 1 major or ≥3 minor criteria.

    2. Major criteria:

      a. Two positive cultures with identical organisms.

      b. Sinus tract communicating with joint.

    3. Minor criteria:

      a. ESR greater than 30 mm/hour.

      b. CRP greater than 10 mg/L.

      c. Elevated synovial WBC or ++ change on leukocyte esterase test strip.

      d. Elevated synovial PMN%.

      e. Positive histological analysis of periprosthetic tissue.

      f. A single positive culture.

  B. Combination of pretest probability based on risk factors, serum laboratory markers, and synovial fluid analysis.

  C. Serum laboratory:

    1. CRP, ESR:

      a. Screening tests: inexpensive, ubiquitous, easily obtained.

      b. Sensitivity: 95% (ESR) and 94% (CRP).

    2. Threshold for aspiration:

      a. Acute (<6 weeks): CRP > 93 mg/L.

      b. Chronic (>4–6 weeks): CRP elevation above laboratory normal value.

  D. Synovial analysis:

    1. Cell count with differential:

      a. Acute (<6 weeks): WBC > 12,800, PMN > 89%.

      b. Chronic (>6 weeks): WBC > 3,000, PMN > 80%.

    2. Alpha defensin:

      a. Recent data showing high sensitivity and specificity (100%, 96%).

      b. Expensive and not readily available at this time.

    3. Gram stain:

      a. Not recommended to diagnosis PJI.

      b. High false-positive rate (1–8%).

      c. Low sensitivity (14–23%).

    4. Culture:

       a. Sensitivity: 50 to 92.8%; specificity 91 to 94%.

       b. Utility: confirm infection and antibiotic sensitivity.

    5. Leukocyte esterase:

       a. Moderate sensitivity and high specificity (81%; 97%).

       b. Controversial screening due to moderate sensitivity.

       c. Cheap and readily available across the world.

VIII. Imaging[2,22,31,33–35]:

  A. Plain radiographs:

    1. Low accuracy for diagnosing PJI.

    2. Used to assess for other cause of failure.

    3. Radiographic loosening within first few years or osteolysis within first postoperative decade should cause suspicion for PJI.

  B. Nuclear medicine:

    1. Expensive, requires specialized equipment and expert consultation.

    2. Utility in patients with high probability of infection, but aspiration results are inconclusive.

    3. Technetium-99:

       a. Unable to differentiate septic from aseptic failure.

    4. Indium-111 WBC scan:

       a. High negative predictive value (utility in ruling out infection).

       b. Use in combination with sulfur colloid bone marrow scan to account for marrow packing artifact.

  C. MRI and CT:

    1. Insufficient evidence of utility, role unclear.

    2. MRI is highly sensitive for detecting osteomyelitis and soft-tissue infection but limited to diagnosis PJI due to metallic artifact.

    3. CT identification of bone abnormalities not useful to diagnose PJI.

IX. Treatment[2,22,36–39]:

  A. Hold antibiotics until synovial cultures have been obtained:

    1. Prophylactic preoperative antibiotics should not be withheld for patients at low probability of infection.

  B. Irrigation and debridement with head and liner exchange:

    1. Controversial.

    2. Typically indicated for early postoperative infections that occur within 4 weeks of the index procedure or in the cases of acute hematogenous infection:

       a. Strep species and nonresistant gram negatives have best response.

    3. Lower success rate than one-stage or two-stage exchange.

  C. One-stage exchange:

    1. Explant of colonized implants, aggressive debridement of bone and soft tissues, and new implant placement with antibiotic cement.

2. Benefits over two-stage exchange:

   a. Shorter hospital stay.

   b. Improved post-op mobility and pain.

   c. Lower cost.

   d. No second-stage surgery.

D. Two-stage exchange:

   1. Most common in the United States.

   2. Consistently highest success rates in the literature (80–90%).

   3. Recommended for patients if:

      a. Chronic symptoms.

      b. Draining sinus tract.

      c. Virulent organisms.

   4. Complete explant of implants, thorough debridement, placement of antibiotic eluting spacer, and minimum treatment of 6 weeks of IV antibiotics directed by an infectious disease specialist.

E. Chronic antibiotic suppression:

   1. Criteria:

      a. Medical contraindications.

      b. Susceptibility to oral antibiotic.

      c. Patient can tolerate long-term therapy.

      d. Stable prosthesis.

F. Resection arthroplasty:

   1. Good results in eradicating infection.

   2. Poor functional outcomes:

      a. Ambulation in patients with excellent upper body strength.

      b. Fifty-nine percent of patients satisfied with functional outcome.

   3. Indications:

      a. Recurrent infection with severe bone loss.

      b. Medical comorbidities preclude complex reconstructive surgery.

X. Outcomes[2,22,37–42]:

A. Irrigation and debridement with retention of components.

   1. Variable success rates (~40–50%) in acute PJI.

   2. Higher failure with:

      a. *S. aureus.*

      b. Sinus tract.

      c. Duration of symptom ≥2 weeks prior to debridement.

B. One-stage exchange:

   1. Approximately 80 to 90% success rate.

   2. More successful with:

     a. Monomicrobial infections.

     b. Low-virulence organisms.

     c. Susceptible to common antibiotics.

     d. Prolonged antimicrobial therapy.

     e. Thorough debridement of tissues.

     f. Use of cemented implants with high dose, organism-specific antibiotics added.

   C. Two-stage exchange.

1. Success rates of 75 to 90%:

     a. Four times higher failure rate with MRSA.

     b. Higher failure rate with prior irrigation and debridement.

2. Associated with substantial:

     a. One series: 90-day mortality rate of 4%.

     b. Medical comorbidities may preclude two-stage implantation.

References

1. Goldenberg DL. Septic arthritis. Lancet 1998;351(9097):197–202
2. Callaghan JJ. The Adult Hip. Philadelphia, PA: Lippincott Williams & Wilkins; 2016:582–588
3. Saraux A, Taelman H, Blanche P, et al. HIV infection as a risk factor for septic arthritis. Br J Rheumatol 1997;36(3):333–337
4. Kaandorp CJ, Van Schaardenburg D, Krijnen P, Habbema JD, van de Laar MA. Risk factors for septic arthritis in patients with joint disease. A prospective study. Arthritis Rheum 1995;38(12):1819–1825
5. Gupta MN, Sturrock RD, Field M. Prospective comparative study of patients with culture proven and high suspicion of adult onset septic arthritis. Ann Rheum Dis 2003;62(4):327–331
6. Herring JA. Tachdjian's Pediatric Orthopedics. 5th ed. Philadelphia, PA: Elsevier; 2014:582–588
7. Sack K. Monarthritis: differential diagnosis. Am J Med 1997;102(1A, 1a):30S–34S
8. Chen CE, Wang JW, Juhn RJ. Total hip arthroplasty for primary septic arthritis of the hip in adults. Int Orthop 2008;32(5):573–580
9. Margaretten ME, Kohlwes J, Moore D, Bent S. Does this adult patient have septic arthritis? JAMA 2007;297(13):1478–1488
10. Canale STB. J.H. Campbell's Operative Orthopaedics. 12th ed. Philadelphia, PA: Mosby; 2012:582–588
11. Dubost JJ, Soubrier M, De Champs C, Ristori JM, Bussiére JL, Sauvezie B. No changes in the distribution of organisms responsible for septic arthritis over a 20 year period. Ann Rheum Dis 2002;61(3):267–269
12. Dubost JJ, Soubrier M, Sauvezie B. Pyogenic arthritis in adults. Joint Bone Spine 2000;67(1):11–21
13. Mathews CJ, Coakley G. Septic arthritis: current diagnostic and therapeutic algorithm. Curr Opin Rheumatol 2008;20(4):457–462
14. Shah K, Spear J, Nathanson LA, McCauley J, Edlow JA. Does the presence of crystal arthritis rule out septic arthritis? J Emerg Med 2007;32(1):23–26
15. de SA D, Cargnelli S, Catapano M, et al. Efficacy of hip arthroscopy for the management of septic arthritis: a systematic review. Arthroscopy 2015;31(7):1358–1370
16. Nusem I, Jabur MK, Playford EG. Arthroscopic treatment of septic arthritis of the hip. Arthroscopy 2006;22(8):902.e1–902.e3

17. Fleck EE, Spangehl MJ, Rapuri VR, Beauchamp CP. An articulating antibiotic spacer controls infection and improves pain and function in a degenerative septic hip. Clin Orthop Relat Res 2011;469(11):3055–3064

18. Klein N, Moore T, Capen D, Green S. Sepsis of the hip in paraplegic patients. J Bone Joint Surg Am 1988;70(6):839–843

19. Matthews PC, Dean BJ, Medagoda K, et al. Native hip joint septic arthritis in 20 adults: delayed presentation beyond three weeks predicts need for excision arthroplasty. J Infect 2008;57(3):185–190

20. Pulido L, Ghanem E, Joshi A, Purtill JJ, Parvizi J. Periprosthetic joint infection: the incidence, timing, and predisposing factors. Clin Orthop Relat Res 2008;466(7):1710–1715

21. Kurtz SM, Lau E, Watson H, Schmier JK, Parvizi J. Economic burden of periprosthetic joint infection in the United States. J Arthroplasty 2012;27(8, Suppl):61–5.e1

22. Parvizi J, Gehrke T, Chen AF. Proceedings of the International Consensus on Periprosthetic Joint Infection. Bone Joint J 2013;95-B(11):1450–1452

23. Ridgeway S, Wilson J, Charlet A, Kafatos G, Pearson A, Coello R. Infection of the surgical site after arthroplasty of the hip. J Bone Joint Surg Br 2005;87(6):844–850

24. Småbrekke A, Espehaug B, Havelin LI, Furnes O. Operating time and survival of primary total hip replacements: an analysis of 31,745 primary cemented and uncemented total hip replacements from local hospitals reported to the Norwegian Arthroplasty Register 1987-2001. Acta Orthop Scand 2004;75(5):524–532

25. Zimmerli W. Clinical presentation and treatment of orthopaedic implant-associated infection. J Intern Med 2014;276(2):111–119

26. Hsieh PH, Lee MS, Hsu KY, Chang YH, Shih HN, Ueng SW. Gram-negative prosthetic joint infections: risk factors and outcome of treatment. Clin Infect Dis 2009;49(7):1036–1043

27. Brook I. Microbiology and management of joint and bone infections due to anaerobic bacteria. J Orthop Sci 2008;13(2):160–169

28. Magiorakos AP, Srinivasan A, Carey RB, et al. Multidrug-resistant, extensively drug-resistant and pandrug-resistant bacteria: an international expert proposal for interim standard definitions for acquired resistance. Clin Microbiol Infect 2012;18(3):268–281

29. Ip D, Yam SK, Chen CK. Implications of the changing pattern of bacterial infections following total joint replacements. J Orthop Surg (Hong Kong) 2005;13(2):125–130

30. Si S, Durkin MJ, Mercier MM, Yarbrough ML, Liang SY. Successful treatment of prosthetic joint infection due to vancomycin-resistant Enterococci with Tedizolid. Infect Dis Clin Pract (Baltim Md) 2017;25(2):105–107 (Baltim Md)

31. Della Valle C, Parvizi J, Bauer TW, et al; American Academy of Orthopaedic Surgeons. Diagnosis of periprosthetic joint infections of the hip and knee. J Am Acad Orthop Surg 2010;18(12):760–770

32. Wyatt MC, Beswick AD, Kunutsor SK, Wilson MJ, Whitehouse MR, Blom AW. The alpha-defensin immunoassay and leukocyte esterase colorimetric strip test for the diagnosis of periprosthetic infection: a systematic review and meta-analysis. J Bone Joint Surg Am 2016;98(12):992–1000

33. Tigges S, Stiles RG, Roberson JR. Appearance of septic hip prostheses on plain radiographs. AJR Am J Roentgenol 1994;163(2):377–380

34. Prandini N, Lazzeri E, Rossi B, Erba P, Parisella MG, Signore A. Nuclear medicine imaging of bone infections. Nucl Med Commun 2006;27(8):633–644

35. Cyteval C, Hamm V, Sarrabère MP, Lopez FM, Maury P, Taourel P. Painful infection at the site of hip prosthesis: CT imaging. Radiology 2002;224(2):477–483

36. Esenwein SA, Robert K, Kollig E, Ambacher T, Kutscha-Lissberg F, Muhr G. Long-term results after resection arthroplasty according to Girdlestone for treatment of persisting infections of the hip joint. Chirurg 2001;72(11):1336–1343

37. Leonard HA, Liddle AD, Burke O, Murray DW, Pandit H. Single- or two-stage revision for infected total hip arthroplasty? A systematic review of the literature. Clin Orthop Relat Res 2014;472(3):1036–1042

38. Kuzyk PR, Dhotar HS, Sternheim A, Gross AE, Safir O, Backstein D. Two-stage revision arthroplasty for management of chronic periprosthetic hip and knee infection: techniques, controversies, and outcomes. J Am Acad Orthop Surg 2014;22(3):153–164

39. Koyonos L, Zmistowski B, Della Valle CJ, Parvizi J. Infection control rate of irrigation and débridement for periprosthetic joint infection. Clin Orthop Relat Res 2011;469(11):3043–3048

40. Haddad FS, Muirhead-Allwood SK, Manktelow AR, Bacarese-Hamilton I. Two-stage uncemented revision hip arthroplasty for infection. J Bone Joint Surg Br 2000;82(5):689–694

41. Berend KR, Lombardi AV Jr, Morris MJ, Bergeson AG, Adams JB, Sneller MA. Two-stage treatment of hip periprosthetic joint infection is associated with a high rate of infection control but high mortality. Clin Orthop Relat Res 2013;471(2):510–518

42. Sherrell JC, Fehring TK, Odum S, et al; Periprosthetic Infection Consortium. The Chitranjan Ranawat Award: fate of two-stage reimplantation after failed irrigation and débridement for periprosthetic knee infection. Clin Orthop Relat Res 2011;469(1):18–25

Index